Lung Cancer: From Diagnosis to Treatment

Lung Cancer: From Diagnosis to Treatment

Editor: Jute Cassie

AMERICAN
MEDICAL PUBLISHERS
www.americanmedicalpublishers.com

AMERICAN
MEDICAL PUBLISHERS
www.americanmedicalpublishers.com

Cataloging-in-Publication Data

Lung cancer : from diagnosis to treatment / edited by Jute Cassie.
p. cm.
Includes bibliographical references and index.
ISBN 978-1-63927-712-4
1. Lungs--Cancer. 2. Lungs--Cancer--Diagnosis. 3. Lungs--Cancer--Treatment.
4. Lungs--Diseases. I. Cassie, Jute.
RC280.L8 L86 2023
616.994 24--dc23

American Medical Publishers,
41 Flatbush Avenue,
1st Floor, New York,
NY 11217, USA

ISBN 978-1-63927-712-4 (Hardback)

Contents

Preface

Lung cancer is a malignant lung tumor that causes uncontrolled cell growth in lung tissues. There are two most common types of lung cancer, namely, small cell lung cancer and non-small cell lung cancer. Majority of the lung cancer cases are caused by long-term tobacco smoking. The symptoms and signs of lung cancer include chest pain, headache, a new cough that won't go away, shortness of breath, bone pain, and hoarseness. Computed tomography (CT) scans and chest radiographs are commonly used to view lung cancer. The diagnosis of lung cancer is done through a biopsy, which is commonly performed using CT guidance or bronchoscopy. The primary method for preventing lung cancer is to minimize risk factors, such as air pollution and smoking. The treatments and long-term outcomes of lung cancer rely on the stage and the type of cancer, as well as the person's overall health condition. Some of the common treatments are radiotherapy, surgery and chemotherapy. This book unravels the recent studies on lung cancer. It contains a detailed explanation of the various diagnostic and therapeutic techniques associated with this disease. The extensive content of this book provides the readers with a thorough understanding of the subject.

Various studies have approached the subject by analyzing it with a single perspective, but the present book provides diverse methodologies and techniques to address this field. This book contains theories and applications needed for understanding the subject from different perspectives. The aim is to keep the readers informed about the progresses in the field; therefore, the contributions were carefully examined to compile novel researches by specialists from across the globe.

Indeed, the job of the editor is the most crucial and challenging in compiling all chapters into a single book. In the end, I would extend my sincere thanks to the chapter authors for their profound work. I am also thankful for the support provided by my family and colleagues during the compilation of this book.

Editor

1

The Desire to Better Understand Older Adults with Solid Tumors to Improve Management: Assessment and Guided Interventions—The French PACA EST Cohort Experience

Rabia Boulahssass [1,2,3,*], Sebastien Gonfrier [1], Noémie Champigny [1], Sandra Lassalle [2,3,4,5], Eric François [6], Paul Hofman [2,3,4,5] and Olivier Guerin [1,2,3]

1 Geriatric Coordination Unit for Geriatric Oncology (UCOG) PACA Est CHU de Nice, 06000 Nice, France; gonfrier.s@chu-nice.fr (S.G.); champigny.n@chu-nice.fr (N.C.); guerin.o@chu-nice.fr (O.G.)
2 FHU OncoAge, 06000 Nice, France; lassalle.s@chu-nice.fr (S.L.); hofman.p@chu-nice.fr (P.H.)
3 University Côte d'Azur, 06000 Nice, France
4 Laboratory of Clinical and Experimental Pathology, Pasteur Hospital, 06000 Nice, France
5 Hospital-related Biobank (BB-0033-00025), 06000 Nice, France
6 Department of Medical Oncology, Lacassagne Center, 06000 Nice, France; eric.francois@nice.unicancer.fr
* Correspondence: boulahssass.r@chu-nice.fr

Abstract: Todays challenge in geriatric oncology is to screen patients who need geriatric follow-up. The main goal of this study was to analyze factors that identify patients, in a large cohort of patients with solid tumors, who need more geriatric interventions and therefore specific follow-up. Between April 2012 and May 2018, 3530 consecutive patients were enrolled in the PACA EST cohort (France). A total of 3140 patients were finally enrolled in the study. A Comprehensive Geriatric Assessment (CGA) was performed at baseline. We analyzed the associations between factors at baseline (geriatric and oncologic factors) and the need to perform more than three geriatric interventions. The mean age of the population was 82 years old with 59% of patients aged older than 80 years old. A total of 8819 geriatric interventions were implemented for the 3140 patients. The percentage of patients with three or more geriatric interventions represented 31.8% (n = 999) of the population. In multivariate analyses, a Mini Nutritional assessment (MNA) <17, an MNA $\leq$23·5 and $\geq$17, a performans status (PS) >2, a dependence on Instrumental Activities of Daily Living (IADL), a Geriatric Depression Scale (GDS) $\geq$5, a Mini Mental State Examination (MMSE) <24, and a Screening tool G8 $\leq$14 were independent risk factors associated with more geriatric interventions. Factors associated with more geriatric interventions could assist practitioners in selecting patients for specific geriatric follow-up.

Keywords: cancer; older adults; geriatric assessment; geriatric interventions

---

1. Introduction

Cancer is significantly associated with aging, and life expectancy is increasing in France and worldwide [1]. Thus, the proportion of older adults with cancer is rising [2]. Despite this "demographic tsunami," elderly patients are under-represented in clinical studies [3]. The population of the French Riviera is one the oldest populations in France; a quarter of the population is over 60 years old, and the proportion of the population over 80 years old has increased by nearly 40% within the past decade [4]. In this context, this region is a "living laboratory" for elderly patients. In 2011, we set up the geriatric coordination unit for geriatric oncology (UCOG PACA EST) with the support of the French National Cancer Institute (INCA). It aims to upgrade care, research, and teaching in geriatric oncology field in

Southeast France. To study this population, we decided to create a database called the "PACA EST Cohort" by developing a strong partnership between the Lacassagne Cancer Center (Nice, France) and the geriatric department of the University Hospital of Nice. In 2016, to participate in further collaborative research, the UCOG PACA EST team joined the Hospital Federation for research, OncoAge, a consortium of skills of a high level from several fields in health care, research, and education dedicated to cancer in the elderly.

In a clinical routine, the International Society of Geriatric Oncology (SIOG) and the American Society of Clinical Oncology (ASCO) recommend performing a comprehensive geriatric assessment (CGA) due to the substantial heterogeneity among elderly patients [5,6]. A CGA as defined by Rubenstein is a "multidimensional interdisciplinary diagnostic process focused on determining a frail elderly person's medical, psychological, and functional capability in order to develop coordinated and integrated plan for treatment" [7]. The CGA is time-consuming, but specific tools for frailty screening are available to detect patients who really need to perform a complete CGA [8–10]. During the past decade, the partnership between geriatricians and oncologists has improved patient care by profiling the level of patient frailty with this process. Therefore, the CGA has been shown to predict outcomes (chemotherapy toxicity, life expectancy) to help make therapeutic decisions but also provide the best interventions [11,12]. Previous studies have described adherence of geriatric assessment recommendations [13,14] as well as guidelines for practical assessment and management of older patients receiving chemotherapy [6]. Now, the challenge in geriatric oncology is to screen patients who require geriatric follow-up with specific guided interventions. The main purpose is to determine which patients need to have repeated geriatric assessment in the follow-up. Therefore, the goal of this study was to analyze a large cohort of patients with solid tumors, for factors that provide a profile of the phenotype of patients who need more geriatric interventions and therefore specific follow-up.

2. Results

2.1. Patient Characteristics

The mean age of the population was 81.9 years old (range 70–102) with 59% of patients aged older than 80 years old. Fifty-five percent were women and 33% had a metastatic status. The most common cancers observed in the cohort were breast cancers (n = 548/17.5%), colorectal cancer (n = 527/16.7%), and lung cancers (n = 356/11.3%) (Table 1).

Table 1. Demographic and tumor characteristics.

Demographic and Tumor Characteristics	n = 3140	%
Age, years		
Median 81.9 Range (70–102)		
<80	1286	41
80–85	978	31.1
>85	876	27.9
Gender		
Male	1395	44.4
Cancer Site		
Breast	548	17.5
Colorectal	525	16.7
Lung	356	11.3
Cholangiocarcinoma/pancreatic	281	8.9
Gynecological	226	7.2
Dermatologic	246	7.8
Bladder	219	7
Upper digestive	198	6.3
Head and neck	176	5.6
Prostatic	157	5
Kidney	94	3
Hepatocarcinoma	73	2.3
Other	41	1.4
Stage IV	1028	32.9
ECOG-PS		
0	260	8.3
1	966	30.8

Table 1. *Cont.*

Demographic and Tumor Characteristics	n = 3140	%
2	855	27.2
3	807	25.7
4	226	7.2
>2	1033	32.9
Missing	26	0.8

PS: performance status.

2.2. Geriatric Assessment Model

Only 13.5% of patients had a G8 >14, which allows practitioners to not perform a full CGA in clinical routines.

In the whole cohort, 16% felt homebound, 48.6% had dependence on ADL, and 16% were malnourished according to the MNA. Table 2 shows a description of the domains that were explored in the standardized CGA at baseline.

Table 2. Comprehensive geriatric assessment (CGA) at baseline.

Comprehensive Geriatric Assessment Heading Title	n = 3140	%
Activity of Daily Living (ADL)		
≥5.5	1528	48.6
Missing	7	0.2
Instrumental Activity of Daily Living (IADL)		
>0	1885	60
Missing	8	0.3
Speed Gait		
<0.8 m/s	1482	47.2
Missing	5	0.2
One leg stand		
<5 s	2232	71.2
Missing	8	0.3
Isolation	242	7.7
Missing	6	0.2
Home confinement	896	28,6
Missing	4	0.1
Balducci Score		
1	146	4.6
2	1568	49.9
3	1426	45,4
Missing	0	
MNA		
>23.5	1030	32.8
17–23.5	1500	47.8
<17	502	16
Missing	108	3.4
MMSE		
≤24	1230	39.2
Missing	104	3.3
GDS		
<5	1912	69.9
Missing	249	7.9
G8 > 14	424	13.5
Missing	68	2.2
Lee Score		
0–5	52	1.7
0–9	763	24.3
0–13	1083	34.5
>14	1210	38
Missing	32	1
Ponderated Charlson		
<5	277	8.9
Missing	26	0.8
NCASS		
0–6	1592	50.7
7 to 9	762	24.2
8 to 9	490	15.6
11	138	4.5
Missing	158	5

ADL: Activity Daily Living; IADL: Instrumental Activity Daily Living; MNA: Mini Nutritional Assessment; GDS: Geriatric Depression Scale; MMSE: Mini Mental State Evaluation; NCCAS: Nice Cancer Aging Survival Score.

2.3. *Treatments Proposed and Influence of the CGA*

Patients were referred to a geriatrician; 47.7% were referred for treatment with chemotherapy or a combined treatment, 28% for surgery, 10.2% for radiotherapy, 8.3% for best supportive care, and 6% for other treatments. In 22% of patients, the CGA modified the therapeutic decision.

2.4. *Geriatric Interventions*

2.4.1. Description

A total of 8819 geriatric interventions were implemented for the 3140 patients. On average, fit patients benefited from 1.5 geriatric interventions, patients classified as "Balducci 2" from 2.4 interventions, and frail patients from 3.3 interventions. In the whole cohort, the medium number of interventions per patient was 2.8. Vulnerable and frail patients had significantly more geriatric interventions ($p < 0.0001$). The guided geriatric interventions are listed in Table 3.

Table 3. Geriatric guided interventions.

Geriatric Interventions	n = 8819	%
Nutritional care	2231	71.1
Physiotherapist intervention	1462	46.6
Delirium prevention	599	19.1
Social worker interventions	733	23.3
Psychological/Psychiatric care	510	16.2
Treatment modification for optimization	667	21.2
Adjustment medication for iatrogenic disorders	351	11.2
Comorbidity management	970	30.9
Nursing interventions	580	18.5
Specialized pain management	96	3.1
Caregiver care	355	11.3
Care pathway modification	265	8.4

2.4.2. Factors Associated with an Increased Need of Geriatric Interventions

Patients with three or more geriatric interventions represented 31.8% (n = 999) of the population. Univariate significant factors associated with an increased need of geriatric interventions are listed in Table 4. In multivariate analyses, an MNA <17, an MNA ≤23.5 and ≥17, a PS >2, a dependence on IADL, a GDS ≥5, an MMSE ≤24, and a G8 ≤14 are independent risk factors associated with this requirement (Table 5).

Table 4. Univariate significant factors of an increased need of geriatric interventions.

Geriatric Interventions (GI)	3 GI n = 999	%	<3 GI n = 2137	%	*p* value
Dependence on ADL	598	59.9	935	43.8	$p < 0.0001$
Dependence on IADL	743	74.4	1147	53.7	$p < 0.0001$
Speed gait					
<0.8m/s	572	57.4	908	42.5	$p < 0.0001$
Isolation	103	10.3	140	6.6	$p < 0.0001$
Delirium	79	7.9	97	4.5	$p < 0.0001$
Home Confinement	436	43.6	461	21.6	$p < 0.0001$
MNA score					
17–23.5	531	55.3	968	46.8	$p < 0.0001$
<17	256	27.0	242	11.7	$p < 0.0001$
MMSE					
≤24	508	52.6	721	34.9	$p < 0.0001$
GDS					
≥5	427	46.9	550	27.8	$p < 0.0001$
G8 score					
>14	928	94.6	1716	82.2	$p < 0.0001$
Charlson score					
≥6	931	93.8	1904	89.9	$p < 0.0001$
Stage IV					
	361	36.4	666	31.3	$p = 0.005$
Performance status					
>2	472	47.4	562	26.6	$p < 0.0001$

ADL: Activity Daily Living; IADL: Instrumental Activity Daily Living; MNA: Mini Nutritional Assessment, GDS: Geriatric Depression Scale; MMSE: Mini Mental State Evaluation.

Table 5. Independent factors associated with an increased need of geriatric interventions.

Factors	p	OR	95%CI
G8 $\leq$ 14	0.023	1.5	(1.1–2.1)
Dependence on IADL	0.013	1.3	(1.1–1.6)
MNA score			
>23.5			Reference
17–23.5	<0.0001	1.9	(1.5–2.4)
<17	<0.0001	3.1	(2.2–4.3)
GDS $\geq$ 5	<0.0001	1.5	(1.2–1.8)
MMS $\leq$ 24	0.009	1.3	(1.1–1.5)
PS > 2	p = 0.003	1.4	(1.1–1.8)

MNA: Mini Nutritional Assessment; PS: Performance Status; MMS: Mini Mental State; GDS: Geriatric Depression Scale. Adjusted to metastatic status, age, comorbidity index, and ADL.

3. Discussion

3.1. The Challenge in Geriatric Oncology Is to Screen Patients for Follow-Up

The first step in geriatric oncology is to screen patients who need a complete geriatric assessment. A number of tools are available and recommended for screening [8–10]. Thus, practitioners can propose a comprehensive assessment and elaborate recommendations according to the deficits observed [6]. In 2013, Kenis et al. [15] demonstrated that screening and CGA are feasible in clinical practice and detected unknown geriatric problems in 51% of cases. This study also showed that oncologists were aware of the geriatric assessment results only in 2/3 of the patients, and recommendations were planned in only 25%. This cohort study highlights the difficulty of implementing geriatric interventions and of the necessity of follow-up. Recent studies have listed the types of interventions and their implementation, but they did not analyze the factors that can lead to more interventions [13,14]. Baitar et al. [16] in 2015 described an adherence of 35.5% to geriatric interventions, and Kenis et al. [14] in 2018 adherence of over 40% in the most important domains. These three studies were conducted by the same team and suggest that the increased rate of implementation is obviously due to the learning curve. To our knowledge, there are no studies exploring the phenotype of patients who need more geriatric interventions. Screening patients who may need follow-up to check for intervention is new.

3.2. Influence of the CGA on Treatment Changes

This study confirms the influence of the CGA on 22% of therapeutic decisions. This rate is very similar to that found in other studies. Kenis et al. [12] found 25%, Caillet et al. [17], 20%. Feasibility of treatment and guided geriatric interventions seem to have different mechanisms, but they are probably two sides of the same coin. Changes in treatment plan according to the CGA certainly influence the level and type of guided interventions. Furthermore, geriatricians implement different types of interventions depending on the type of treatment (chemotherapy, surgery, palliative care, etc.), and this process could probably lead to support deficits in areas of geriatric assessment and help in the treatment feasibility. These considerations need to be confirmed in further prospective studies in the PACA EST cohort.

3.3. Factors Associated with an Increase in the Need for Intervention

In multivariate analyses, to be malnourished or at risk of being malnourished regarding the MNA, a PS >2, a dependence on IADL, a positive screening for depression regarding the GDS, cognitive disorders regarding an MMSE <24, and a positive screening regarding a G8 $\leq$14 are independent risk factors associated with an increased requirement of geriatric interventions.

These are well-known factors for a worse outcome in geriatric oncology. Regarding the PS, there are several studies showing a prediction of an increased risk of death in this population [18–20]. In addition, there is abundant literature showing that the nutritional status and the MNA predict outcomes such as early death, early discontinuation of chemotherapy, poor tolerance of chemotherapy, and an increased risk of morbidities [21–24]. Mood disorders and cognitive impairment have also been explored in other studies showing early functional decline on chemotherapy and decreased survival [25–27]. Moreover, dependence on IADL was associated with increased mortality, morbidity, hospitalization, and functional decline [6]. These data invite us to take into account these factors to optimize the management and the follow up of elderly patients. However, we do not yet have robust data (randomized studies) in geriatric oncology supporting the fact that interventions improve the outcome, but some studies are underway to analyze the impact of a multimodal approach [6]. For example, the PREPARE study in France plans an interventional multimodal approach using "case management." We hope that this study by Soubeyran et al. will supply abundant information and evidence in favor of guided interventions. (PREPARE, ClinicalTrials.gov Identifier: NCT02704832) [28].

3.4. A Call for Co-Management

This study shows that elderly patients require different interventions with various health partners. Creating individualized "care" and "take care" plans require a strong partnership between a network including geriatricians, oncologists, specialized doctors, but also nurses, psychologists, dieticians, social workers, physiotherapists, and many other actors. The task of the UCOG teams in France is to coordinate and streamline patient care, offering easy lines of communication and shortening referral times. In the domain of co-management, perspectives in geriatric oncology from innovative professions coordinating the development of specific e-health tools are plentiful [29].

3.5. How This Model Could Add Value in Clinical Practice?

The utility of the multivariable model lies in the determination of independent factors strongly associated with the establishment of more geriatric interventions. This model underlines some domains of the GA that can be assessed by other health partners, such as dieticians, nutritionists, psychologists, or psychiatrists, even if there is no geriatrician on the team. A nurse could coordinate and educate patients who present these factors and link them to general practitioners that can provide them with simple interventions such as nutritional support, advice, physiotherapy, and so on.

3.6. Improving Together Prediction and Outcome

Clinicians and researchers are working together to elaborate scoring systems or factors aimed at improving the outcome and patient care of older adults with cancer. The PACA EST cohort is a prospective and multicentric cohort (n > 3800) created to better understand elderly cancer patients. Prospective and systematic follow-up improve substantially the quality of care and connect general practitioners and heath partners. The UCOG PACA EST team joined the Hospital Federation University in research into OncoAge so that research and care become a continuum in the future. Subsequent studies will focus on adherence and on the impact of geriatric interventions in this cohort, but also on the barriers and difficulties of implementation. An OncoAge work package aims to improve and analyze a lifestyle plan. Educating patients and caregivers about the options of care, including guided geriatric interventions, is crucial.

3.7. Strengths and Limitations

The strengths of this study lie in the large cohort studied, which enrolled a "true life population" with a mean age of 82 years old. A complete and standardize CGA was performed at baseline. Interventions were guided by the deficits observed in the CGA. However, this study did not analyze the level of intervention and adherence at follow-up. A pilot study conducted in the PACA EST cohort (n = 50) had shown that, after one month, the adherence to interventions ranged from 73 to 89 % depending on the domains. This is probably because geriatricians in the PACA EST cohort implemented the interventions at baseline and did not propose recommendations only.

4. Materials and Methods

4.1. Patient Population

Between April 2012 and May 2018, 3530 consecutive patients were enrolled in the PACA EST cohort. The UCOG PACA EST cohort is an observational, multicentric cohort (five centers in Southeast France: a teaching hospital, a specialized cancer center, and three cancer clinics). Three thousand one hundred and forty patients with various types of solid cancers at any stage and aged older than 70 years old (no upper limit) were enrolled in this study at the time of diagnosis and before the final therapeutic decision. Patients could be outpatients or hospitalized. Patients were referred by more than 60 practitioners (oncologists, surgeons, and radiotherapists) to the UCOG PACA EST team (Geriatric Oncology Coordination Unit) for a CGA before a final therapeutic decision.

4.2. Ethics

At the first visit of inclusion, patients gave informed consent and were registered at baseline in compliance with the French database and privacy law (CNIL, Commission Nationale de l'Informatique et Liberté, registration number CILS: 188). This study was approved by an ethics committee (Espace Ethique Gériatrique Report 04-2012).

4.3. Study Methods

4.3.1. CGA and Data Collected at Baseline

Four geriatricians received the same training at baseline and performed a standardized comprehensive geriatric baseline assessment as described in Table 1. The CGA included cognitive function screening using the Mini-Mental Test (MMSE) [30], an autonomy assessment using Activity in Daily Living (ADL) [31] and Instrumental Activity of Daily Living (IADL) [32,33], a nutritional status assessment using the Mini Nutritional Assessment [34], a gait assessment using gait speed [35], and the one leg balance test, screening for depression using the Geriatric Depression Scale 15 for patients with an MMSE score higher than 15 (GDS) [36], and acomorbidities assessment using the Charlson Index [37]. Prediction of early death was assessed with the Nice Cancer Aging Survival Score (NCASS) [21], and mortality at 4 years was assessed with the Lee score [38]. Demographic data and the perception of isolation and being homebound were also determined (homebound was defined in the study as going out of home with or without assistance only for important activities, e.g., a medical visit). Finally, the Balducci score was assessed [39]. The validated cut-offs for scales are specified in Table 2. In addition, data on guided geriatric interventions, on oncologic treatments proposed by oncologists, and on tumor type and tumor stage were collected during follow-up. Geriatric interventions were defined by interventions implemented by a geriatrician at baseline in 12 domains (nutrition, psychological care, specialized pain management, prevention of delirium, comorbidities management, nursing interventions, social worker interventions, treatment modification for optimization, adjustment medication for iatrogenic disorders, physiotherapy, caregiver care, and care pathway modification). Geriatric interventions are standardized (based on guidelines when available) and individualized (focused on specific deficits). Some interventions as caregiver care or social interventions are based on experience (no guidelines available). Geriatric interventions are described in Table 6. Within a month, geriatricians who included patients in the cohort received a specific training on the CGA and on guided interventions. They received a prescription book with standardized recommendations.

Table 6. Guided geriatric intervention description.

Interventions	Description
Nutritional Care	Nutritional Advice Nutritional supplements Artificial nutrition **Based on guidelines [40,41], standardized prescription**
Physiotherapist Interventions	Balance Strength Pain management Recommendations of walking aids Coordination Promotion of physical activity **Based on patient deficits, standardized prescription (list)**
Delirium Prevention	Checklist for patient, caregiver and medical team: advice, recommendations for prescription for surgical team. **Based on guidelines [42], standardized check list**
Social Worker Interventions	Prevention, In home health services, housing, social inclusion, financial accommodations, legal action, end of life services, institutional placement, nutrition accommodations. **Based on social worker and geriatrician experiences.**
Psychological/Psychiatric Care	Consultation with psychologist or psychiatrist **Duration and methods based on patient needs and practitioners experience**
Treatment Modification for Optimization	Medical treatment assessment, optimization of treatment **Based on geriatrician experience**
Adjustment Medication for Iatrogenic Disorders	Inappropriate medication assessment. **Based on geriatrician experience**
Comorbidity Management	Advice, treatment modification, referral to others clinicians or paramedical, medical checkup **Based on geriatrician experience**
Nursing Interventions	
Specialized Pain Management	Drug or non-drug therapy, referral to specific pain management **Based on guidelines [43]**
Caregiver Care	Counselling, training courses, social supports, medical supports, psychological care, assistance bureaucracies, advocacy, crisis interventions **Based on geriatrician and social worker experiences**
Care Pathway Modification	Identification of appropriate resources, coordination of the care process, coordination of admission in acute care unit rehabilitation unit (rehabilitation/prehabilitation), long stay hospitalization, referral to a one-day hospital, integration on specific organization (palliative care, home care hospitalization) **Based on geriatrician and social worker experiences**

4.3.2. Statistics

The primary aim of the study was to analyze the association between geriatric and oncologic factors and the need to implement more than three geriatric interventions (the median number of guided interventions in the whole cohort) using a logistic regression model in a univariate analysis. A multivariable analysis was performed with all geriatric and oncologic items that reached a significant level of $p < 0.05$. Regarding frailty levels and interventions, we compared the medium number of geriatric interventions in the three groups according to the Balducci classification by using an ANOVA test and the Bonferroni adjusted p-value.

5. Conclusions

Nutritional status, a PS >2, a dependence on IADL, a positive screening for depression, cognitive impairment, and a G8 $\leq$14 were independent risk factors associated with more geriatric interventions. Factors associated with more geriatric interventions could assist practitioners in selecting patients for specific geriatric follow-up. Further studies on the PACA EST cohort will focus on the level of intervention and adherence at follow-up. Research needs to not only focus on interventions but also on the quality of the implementation according to the guidelines. Standardization of the interventions is an important task, and research is underway in a number of studies being performed in the world [11].

Author Contributions: Conceptualization: R.B., S.G., N.C., S.L., E.F., P.H. and O.G.; methodology: S.G. and R.B.; software, S.G.; validation: R.B., S.G., N.C., S.L., E.F., P.H. and O.G.; formal analysis: S.G.; investigation: all authors; writing—original draft preparation: R.B., S.G., N.C., S.L., E.F., P.H. and O.G.; writing—review and editing: R.B., S.G., N.C., S.L., E.F., P.H. and O.G.; visualization: R.B.; supervision: R.B., O.G. and E.F.; project administration: R.B.

Acknowledgments: The authors would like to thank the patients, their caregivers, and all the health partners at the Nice Teaching Hospital, the Lacassagne Cancer Center, the Tzanck Clinic, the St Jean Clinic, and the Mougins Cancer Center.

References

1. Yancik, R. Population aging and cancer: A cross-national concern. *Cancer J.* **2005**, *11*, 437–441. [CrossRef] [PubMed]
2. Michel, A.; Mugno, E.; Krogh, V.; Quinn, M.J.; Coleman, M.; Hakulinen, T.; Gatta, G.; Berrino, F.; Capocaccia, R.; EUROPREVAL Working Group. Cancer prevalence in European registry areas. *Ann. Oncol.* **2002**, *13*, 840–865. [CrossRef]
3. Talarico, L.; Chen, G.; Pazdur, R. Enrollment of elderly patients in clinical trials for cancer drug registration: a 7-year experience by the US Food and Drug Administration. *J. Clin. Oncol.* **2004**, *22*, 4626–4631. [CrossRef] [PubMed]
4. INSEE (Institut national de la statistique et des études économiques). Available online: https://www.insee.fr (accessed on 27 October 2010).
5. Wildiers, H.; Heeren, P.; Puts, M.; Topinkova, E.; Janssen-Heijnen, M.L.; Extermann, M.; Falandry, C.; Artz, A.; Brain, E.; Colloca, G.; et al. International Society of Geriatric Oncology consensus on geriatric assessment in older patients with cancer. *J. Clin. Oncol.* **2014**, *32*, 2595–2603. [CrossRef] [PubMed]
6. Mohile, S.G.; Dale, W.; Somerfield, M.R.; Hurria, A. Practical Assessment and Management of Vulnerabilities in Older Patients Receiving Chemotherapy: ASCO Guideline for Geriatric Oncology Summary. *J. Oncol. Pract.* **2018**, *14*, 442–446. [CrossRef] [PubMed]
7. Rubenstein, L.Z.; Stuck, A.E.; Siu, A.L.; Wieland, D. Impact of geriatric evaluation and management programs on defined outcomes: overview of the evidence. *J. Am. Geriatr. Soc.* **1991**, *39*, 8–16. [CrossRef]
8. Hamaker, M.E.; Jonker, J.M.; de Rooij, S.E.; Vos, A.G.; Smorenburg, C.H.; van Munster, B.C. Frailty screening methods for predicting outcome of a comprehensive geriatric assessment in elderly patients with cancer: A systematic review. *Lancet Oncol.* **2012**, *13*, 437–444. [CrossRef]
9. Soubeyran, P.; Bellera, C.; Goyard, J.; Heitz, D.; Curé, H.; Rousselot, H.; Albrand, G.; Servent, V.; Jean, O.S.; van Praagh, I.; et al. Screening for vulnerability in older cancer patients: The ONCODAGE Prospective Multicenter Cohort Study. *PLoS ONE* **2014**, *9*, e115060. [CrossRef]
10. Saliba, D.; Elliott, M.; Rubenstein, L.Z.; Solomon, D.H.; Young, R.T.; Kamberg, C.J.; Roth, C.; MacLean, C.H.; Shekelle, P.G.; Sloss, E.M.; et al. The Vulnerable Elders Survey: A tool for identifying vulnerable older people in the community. *J. Am. Geriatr. Soc.* **2001**, *49*, 1691–1699. [CrossRef]
11. Hurria, A.; Togawa, K.; Mohile, S.G.; Owusu, C.; Klepin, H.D.; Gross, C.P.; Lichtman, S.M.; Gajra, A.; Bhatia, S.; Katheria, V.; et al. Predicting chemotherapy toxicity in older adults with cancer: A prospective multicenter study. *J. Clin. Oncol.* **2011**, *29*, 3457–3465. [CrossRef]
12. Extermann, M.; Boler, I.; Reich, R.R.; Lyman, G.H.; Brown, R.H.; DeFelice, J.; Levine, R.M.; Lubiner, E.T.; Reyes, P.; Schreiber, F.J., 3rd; et al. Predicting the risk of chemotherapy toxicity in older patients: The Chemotherapy Risk Assessment Scalefor High-Age Patients (CRASH) score. *Cancer* **2012**, *118*, 3377–3386. [CrossRef] [PubMed]
13. Magnuson, A.; Allore, H.; Cohen, H.J.; Mohile, S.G.; Williams, G.R.; Chapman, A.; Extermann, M.; Olin, R.L.; Targia, V.; Mackenzie, A.; et al. Geriatric assessment with management in cancer care: Current evidence and potential mechanisms for future research. *J. Geriatr. Oncol.* **2016**, *7*, 242–248. [CrossRef] [PubMed]

14. Kenis, C.; Decoster, L.; Flamaing, J.; Debruyne, P.R.; De Groof, I.; Focan, C.; Cornélis, F.; Verschaeve, V.; Bachmann, C.; Bron, D.; et al. Adherence to geriatric assessment-based recommendations in older patients with cancer: A multicenter prospective cohort study in Belgium. *Ann. Oncol.* **2018**, *29*, 1987–1994. [CrossRef] [PubMed]
15. Kenis, C.; Bron, D.; Libert, Y.; Decoster, L.; van Puyvelde, K.; Scalliet, P.; Cornette, P.; Pepersack, T.; Luce, S.; Langenaeken, C.; et al. Relevance of a systematic geriatric screening and assessment in older patients with cancer: results of aprospective multicentric study. *Ann. Oncol.* **2013**, *24*, 1306–1312. [CrossRef] [PubMed]
16. Baitar, A.; Kenis, C.; Moor, R.; Decoster, L.; Luce, S.; Bron, D.; van Rijswijk, R.; Rasschaert, M.; Langenaeken, C.; Jerusalem, G.; et al. Implementation of geriatric assessment-based recommendations in older patients with cancer: A multicentre prospective study. *J. Geriatr. Oncol.* **2015**, *6*, 401–410. [CrossRef]
17. Caillet, P.; Canoui-Poitrine, F.; Vouriot, J.; Berle, M.; Reinald, N.; Krypciak, S.; Bastuji-Garin, S.; Culine, S.; Paillaud, E. Comprehensive geriatric assessment in the decision-making process in elderly patients with cancer: ELCAPA study. *J. Clin. Oncol.* **2011**, *29*, 3636–3642. [CrossRef] [PubMed]
18. Kanesvaran, R.; Li, H.; Koo, K.N.; Poon, D. Analysis of prognostic factors of comprehensive geriatric assessment and development of a clinical scoring system in elderly Asian patients with cancer. *J. Clin. Oncol.* **2011**, *29*, 3620–3627. [CrossRef] [PubMed]
19. Bamias, A.; Lainakis, G.; Kastritis, E.; Antoniou, N.; Alivizatos, G.; Koureas, A.; Chrisofos, M.; Skolarikos, A.; Karayiotis, E.; Dimopoulos, M.A. Biweekly carboplatin/gemcitabine in patients with advanced urothelial cancer who are unfit for cisplatin-based chemotherapy: Report of efficacy, quality of life and geriatric assessment. *Oncology* **2007**, *73*, 290–297. [CrossRef]
20. Kristjansson, S.R.; Nesbakken, A.; Jordhøy, M.S.; Skovlund, E.; Audisio, R.A.; Johannessen, H.O.; Bakka, A.; Wyller, T.B. Comprehensive geriatric assessment can predict complications in elderly patients after elective surgery for colorectal cancer: A prospective observational cohort study. *Crit. Rev. Oncol. Hematol.* **2010**, *76*, 208–217. [CrossRef]
21. Boulahssass, R.; Gonfrier, S.; Ferrero, J.M.; Sanchez, M.; Mari, V.; Moranne, O.; Rambaud, C.; Auben, F.; Hannoun Levi, J.M.; Bereder, J.M.; et al. Predicting early death in older adults with cancer. *Eur. J. Cancer* **2018**, *100*, 65–74. [CrossRef]
22. Bourdel-Marchasson, I.; Diallo, A.; Bellera, C.; Blanc-Bisson, C.; Durrieu, J.; Germain, C.; Mathoulin-Pélissier, S.; Soubeyran, P.; Rainfray, M.; Fonck, M.; et al. One-Year Mortality in Older Patients with Cancer: Development and External Validation of an MNA-Based Prognostic Score. *PLoS ONE* **2016**, *11*, e0148523. [CrossRef]
23. Ferrat, E.; Paillaud, E.; Laurent, M.; Le Thuaut, A.; Caillet, P.; Tournigand, C.; Lagrange, J.L.; Canouï-Poitrine, F.; Bastuji-Garin, S.; ELPACA Study Group. Predictors of 1-Year Mortality in a Prospective Cohort of Elderly Patients with Cancer. *J. Gerontol. A Biol. Sci. Med. Sci.* **2015**, *70*, 1148–1155. [CrossRef] [PubMed]
24. Caillet, P.; Liuu, E.; Raynaud Simon, A.; Bonnefoy, M.; Guerin, O.; Berrut, G.; Lesourd, B.; Jeandel, C.; Ferry, M.; Rolland, Y.; et al. Association between cachexia, chemotherapy and outcomes in older cancer patients: A systematic review. *Clin. Nutr.* **2017**, *36*, 1473–1482. [CrossRef] [PubMed]
25. Freyer, G.; Geay, J.F.; Touzet, S.; Provencal, J.; Weber, B.; Jacquin, J.P.; Ganem, G.; Tubiana-Mathieu, N.; Gisserot, O.; Pujade-Lauraine, E. Comprehensive geriatric assessment predicts tolerance to chemotherapy and survival in elderly patientswith advanced ovarian carcinoma: a GINECO study. *Ann. Oncol.* **2005**, *16*, 1795–1800. [CrossRef]
26. Biesma, B.; Wymenga, A.N.; Vincent, A.; Dalesio, O.; Smit, H.J.; Stigt, J.A.; Smit, E.F.; van Felius, C.L.; van Putten, J.W.; Slaets, J.P.; et al. Quality of life, geriatric assessment and survival in elderly patients with non-small-cell lung cancer treated with carboplatin-gemcitabine or carboplatin-paclitaxel: NVALT-3 a phase III study. *Ann. Oncol.* **2011**, *22*, 1520–1527. [CrossRef]
27. Magnuson, A.; Mohile, S.; Janelsins, M. Cognition and Cognitive Impairment in Older Adults with Cancer. *Curr. Geriatr. Rep.* **2016**, *5*, 213–219. [CrossRef]
28. Soubeyran, P.; Terret, C.; Bellera, C.; Bonnetain, F.; Jean, O.S.; Galvin, A.; Chakiba, C.; Zwolakowski, M.D.; Mathoulin-Pélissier, S.; Rainfray, M. Role of geriatric intervention in the treatment of older patients with cancer: rationale and design of a phase III multicenter trial. *BMC Cancer* **2016**, *16*, 932. [CrossRef]

29. Loh, K.P.; Ramsdale, E.; Culakova, E.; Mendler, J.H.; Liesveld, J.L.; O'Dwyer, K.M.; McHugh, C.; Gilles, M.; Lloyd, T.; Goodman, M.; et al. Novel mHealth App to Deliver Geriatric Assessment-Driven Interventions for Older Adults with Cancer: Pilot Feasibility and Usability Study. *JMIR Cancer* **2018**, *4*, e10296. [CrossRef] [PubMed]
30. Folstein, M.F.; Folstein, S.E.; McHugh, P.R. Mini-mental state. A practical method for grading the cognitive state of patients for the clinician. *J. Psychiatr. Res.* **1975**, *12*, 189–198. [CrossRef]
31. Katz, S.; Downs, T.D.; Cash, H.; Grotz, R.C. Progress in development of the index of ADL. *Gerontologist* **1970**, *10*, 20–30. [CrossRef]
32. Lawton, M.P.; Brody, E.M. Assessment of older people: self-maintaining and instrumental activities of daily living. *Gerontologist* **1969**, *9*, 179–186. [CrossRef] [PubMed]
33. Barberger-Gateau, P.; Dartigues, J.F.; Letenneur, L. Four Instrumental Activities of Daily Living Score as a predictor of one-year incident dementia. *Age Ageing* **1993**, *22*, 457–463. [CrossRef] [PubMed]
34. Vellas, B.; Guigoz, Y.; Garry, P.J.; Nourhashemi, F.; Bennahum, D.; Lauque, S.; Albarede, J.L. The Mini Nutritional Assessment (MNA) and its use in grading the nutritional state of elderly patients. *Nutrition* **1999**, *15*, 116–122. [CrossRef]
35. Pamoukdjian, F.; Paillaud, E.; Zelek, L.; Laurent, M.; Lévy, V.; Landre, T.; Sebbane, G. Measurement of gait speed in older adults to identify complications associated with frailty: A systematic review. *J. Geriatr. Oncol.* **2015**, *6*, 484–496. [CrossRef] [PubMed]
36. Yesavage, J.A.; Brink, T.L.; Rose, T.L.; Lum, O.; Huang, V.; Adey, M.; Leirer, V.O. Development and validation of a geriatric depression screening scale: a preliminary report. *J. Psychiatr. Res.* **1982**, *17*, 37–49. [CrossRef]
37. Charlson, M.E.; Pompei, P.; Ales, K.L.; MacKenzie, C.R. A new method of classifying prognostic comorbidity in longitudinal studies: development and validation. *J. Chronic Dis.* **1987**, *40*, 373–383. [CrossRef]
38. Lee, S.; Lindquist, K.; Segal, M.R.; Covinsky, K.E. Development and validation of a prognostic index for 4-year mortality in older adults. *JAMA* **2006**, *295*, 801–808. [CrossRef]
39. Balducci, L.; Yates, J. General guidelines for the management of older patients with cancer. *Oncology* **2000**, *14*, 221–227.
40. Haute Autorité de Santé. Nutritional Support Strategy for Protein-Energy. Malnutrition in the Elderly. 2007. Available online: http://www.hassante.fr (accessed on 29 January 2014).
41. French Speaking Society of Clinical Nutrition and Metabolism (SFNEP). Clinical nutrition guidelines of the French Speaking Society of Clinical Nutrition and Metabolism (SFNEP): Summary of recommendations for adults undergoing non-surgical anticancer treatment. *Dig. Liver Dis.* **2014**, *46*, 667–674. [CrossRef]
42. Bush, S.H.; Lawlor, P.G.; Ryan, K.; Centeno, C.; Lucchesi, M.; Kanji, S.; Siddiqi, N.; Morandi, A.; Davis, D.H.J.; Laurent, M.; et al. ESMO Guidelines Committee. Delirium in adult cancer patients: ESMO Clinical Practice Guidelines. *Ann. Oncol.* **2018**, *29*, iv143–iv165. [CrossRef]
43. Evaluation et Suivi de la Douleur Chronique Chez L'adulte en Médecine Ambulatoire, ANAES. Available online: http://www.has-sante.fr/portail/jcms/c_540915/evaluation-et-suivi-de-la-douleur-chronique-chez-l-adulte-en-medecine-ambulatoire (accessed on 1 December 2009).

2

Macrophage Origin, Metabolic Reprogramming and IL-1β Signaling: Promises and Pitfalls in Lung Cancer

Emma Guilbaud [1], Emmanuel L. Gautier [2] and Laurent Yvan-Charvet [1,*]

[1] Institut National de la Santé et de la Recherche Médicale (Inserm) U1065, Université Côte d'Azur, Centre Méditerranéen de Médecine Moléculaire (C3M), Atip-Avenir, Fédération Hospitalo-Universitaire (FHU) Oncoage, 06204 Nice, France; eguilbaud@unice.fr

[2] Institut National de la Santé et de la Recherche Médicale (Inserm) UMR_S 1166, Sorbonnes Universités, Hôpital de la Pitié Salpêtrière, 75013 Paris, France; emmanuel-laurent.gautier@inserm.fr

* Correspondence: yvancharvet@unice.fr

Abstract: Macrophages are tissue-resident cells that act as immune sentinels to maintain tissue integrity, preserve self-tolerance and protect against invading pathogens. Lung macrophages within the distal airways face around 8000–9000 L of air every day and for that reason are continuously exposed to a variety of inhaled particles, allergens or airborne microbes. Chronic exposure to irritant particles can prime macrophages to mediate a smoldering inflammatory response creating a mutagenic environment and favoring cancer initiation. Tumor-associated macrophages (TAMs) represent the majority of the tumor stroma and maintain intricate interactions with malignant cells within the tumor microenvironment (TME) largely influencing the outcome of cancer growth and metastasis. A number of macrophage-centered approaches have been investigated as potential cancer therapy and include strategies to limit their infiltration or exploit their antitumor effector functions. Recently, strategies aimed at targeting IL-1β signaling pathway using a blocking antibody have unexpectedly shown great promise on incident lung cancer. Here, we review the current understanding of the bridge between TAM metabolism, IL-1β signaling, and effector functions in lung adenocarcinoma and address the challenges to successfully incorporating these pathways into current anticancer regimens.

Keywords: lung adenocarcinoma; macrophage; immunotherapy; interleukin-1β and immunometabolism

---

1. Introduction

Lung cancer is the leading cause of cancer-related death and the second most common malignancy with non-small cell lung cancer (NSCLC) referring for lung adeno and squamous carcinomas and accounting for up to 80% of all newly diagnosed lung cancer cases [1,2]. The overall five-year survival rate among newly diagnosed lung cancer patients remains in the low range of 15% [3]. This is in part because (1) the majority of lung cancer cases are diagnosed relatively late in the course of the disease despite advances in lung cancer screening and diagnosis and (2) lung adenocarcinomas are extremely diverse in terms of histopathology, radiology, and molecular spectrum impeding treatments despite multimodality therapeutics [4]. Since the 80's, macrophage density from biopsies of dozen types of cancer, including lung adenocarcinoma, has been linked to tumor growth and poor outcomes for cancer patients [5–8]. However, distinct subsets of tumor-associated macrophages (TAMs) exist within tumors and these cells can adopt a wide array of phenotypes depending on their environment. We are just starting to better appreciate the ontogeny and effector functions of these TAMs and how they can influence the initiation and growth of the tumor depending on a dynamic equilibrium influenced by the tumor microenvironment (TME) [5,6,9–11].

The plasticity of macrophages has now been largely accepted [12] and is reflected by their ability to sense, respond, and rapidly adapt to their local environment [13–17] to maintain tissue integrity and preserve self-tolerance [18–20]. However, when the host is chronically challenged, upon chronic exposure to irritant particles or infection, for example, macrophages may play a detrimental role contributing to a low-grade inflammatory state that leads to disease progression or even cancer initiation [21,22]. This is illustrated by the increased lung cancer risk in smokers and patients with chronic obstructive pulmonary disease (COPD).

The origin of TAMs within lung adenocarcinoma and their selective functions are currently a topic for debate but a mixed ontogeny and immunosuppressive functions are emerging depending of the stage and location of the tumors [23–26]. For instance, tumors can early on secrete the colony-stimulating factor 1 (CSF-1 or M-CSF) that expands the pool of macrophages towards the cancer supporting TAM phenotype and later on the chemokine (C-C motif) ligand 2 (CCL2) that attracts monocytes [5,6,9–11]. Once infiltrated within the tumor, TAMs maintain intricate interactions with malignant cells within the TME and this is most likely the key culprit of their antitumoral response largely influencing the outcome of tumor growth and metastasis.

In this review, we describe recent advances made on the ontogeny of lung resident macrophages and their expansion and metabolic rewiring towards the lung cancer supporting TAM phenotype, which depend on a specialized TME. We discuss therapeutic promises of general therapies to block macrophage recruitment to tumors or more selective therapies to reeducate their tumoricidal functions, both having reached clinical trials. We further outline the contribution of the IL-1β signaling pathway, and how its metabolic-dependent modulation in TAMs could explain part of the anti-tumorigenic potential of IL-1β inhibition.

2. Environment-Dependent Maintenance of Lung Macrophages during Homeostasis

2.1. *Lung Macrophage Ontogeny and Maintenance*

Macrophages are tissue-resident cells that act as immune sentinels to maintain tissue integrity, preserve self-tolerance, and protect against invading pathogens [18–20]. In the lung, early preclinical studies have suggested that monocytes poorly contribute to tissue-resident macrophages at steady state and their maintenance mainly relies on homeostatic self-renewal [27–29]. Modern tools using fate mapping and tracing methods in mice have confirmed that a specific population of lung alveolar macrophages (AMs) originates from fetal liver progenitors and relies in large part on their ability to self-renew at steady state [30–36]. Alveolar macrophages remain the main macrophage population investigated in the lung and reside in the airspace lumen where they are specialized in recycling surfactant molecules and clearing inhaled particles and debris [37–41]. Alveolar macrophages are long-lived, with a turnover rate of only approximately 40% in a year [41]. By contrast to most of tissue-resident macrophages, the maintenance of AMs is not supported by CSF-1 as illustrated in op/op mice that harbor a mutation in this gene [18–20]. Indeed, mouse AMs are highly dependent on the granulocyte-macrophage colony-stimulating factor (GM-CSF) and the transforming growth factor beta (TGF-β) for their genesis and survival [42,43]. Three additional subpopulations of mouse interstitial macrophages (IMs) have been identified in the pulmonary interstitium, comprising up to 4% of lung macrophages and presumably existing between the blood compartment and the airways [44,45]. These macrophage populations are defined by their location and site of origin, and distinguished by specific cell surface markers (Figure 1, left panel) [46]. As for AMs, two populations of mouse IMs may self-maintain independently of adult hematopoiesis [44,45]. Emphasizing the complexity of IMs, the third population of IMs could be maintained by circulating monocytes to exert their tissue remodeling and immunoregulatory activities [47–49]. Consistently, there is a strong interest to develop new tools to specifically target these different macrophage populations in vivo and address their transcriptional signature and immune function during lung homeostasis and diseases [50].

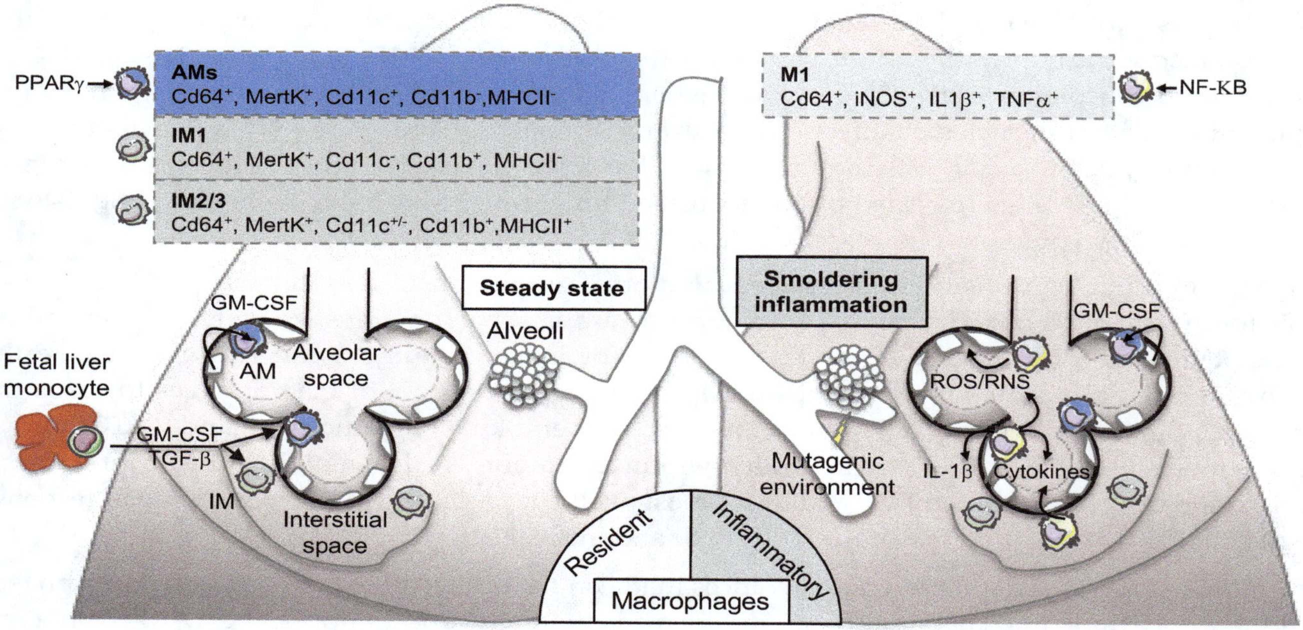

Figure 1. Lung macrophage origin and contribution to "smoldering inflammation". Left panel: lung-resident macrophages are derived from fetal liver monocytes originating during embryogenesis. The genesis and self-maintenance of macrophages depend on granulocyte-macrophage colony-stimulating factor (GM-CSF) and transforming growth factor β (TGF-β). Four populations of macrophages are present in the lung and are defined by their locations and expression of specific cell surface markers (please refer to boxes): alveolar macrophages (AMs) reside in the airspaces of lung where they self-renew thanks to GM-CSF-expressing alveolar cells. AMs express peroxisome proliferator-activated receptor γ (PPARγ) to maintain lipid homeostasis most likely required for surfactant lipid recycling. Three interstitial macrophage (IMs) populations are located in the lung interstitium and have potential immunoregulatory properties. Right panel: upon exposure to irritant particles or chronic inflammation, macrophages can be primed into an inflammatory M1 phenotype participating to a "smorldering inflammation". This inflammation is illustrated by the secretion inflammatory cytokines such as interleukin-1β (IL-1β) or tumor necrosis factor α (TNFα) that are under the control of the transcriptional factor NF-kB and the production of reactive oxygen or nitrogen species (ROS/RNS) that favor the induction of somatic mutations in surrounding epithelial cells.

2.2. *Environment-Dependent Lung Macrophage Identity during Homeostasis*

The plasticity of macrophages has now been largely accepted [12] and is reflected by their ability to sense, respond and rapidly adapt to their local environment, including inflammatory signals [13], ectopic nutrient deposition [14,15] or apoptotic debris [16,17]. Consistently, gene expression patterns of mouse macrophages are diverse among various peripheral tissues reflecting their propensity to sense environmental cues and the wide array of phenotypes they can adopt [51–53]. For instance, macrophages within the distal airways face around 8000–9000 L of air every day and for that reason are continuously exposed to a variety of inhaled particles, allergens or airborne microbes [37–40]. A handy and consequently persistent shorthand for understanding macrophage function divides these cells into two extreme phenotypes of a large spectrum in vitro by polarizing them into a pro-inflammatory M1 phenotype induced by LPS (alone or in combination with INFγ) or an alternative M2 phenotype induced after IL-4 stimulation [54–56]. Although oversimplified, this in vitro classification has provided a useful guide for investigating the mechanisms that dictate macrophage switch during lung inflammation or repair [57,58]. For instance, while the inflammatory properties of M1 macrophages contribute to early host defense or injury responses, the repair functions of M2 macrophages play a crucial role during wound healing. This adaptation to the environment could explain why macrophage effector functions is intimately linked to intracellular metabolic reprograming to rapidly respond to the adequate energy demand [59–62]. However, this classification limits our ability to clearly define a boundary and categorize cells during homeostasis as macrophages respond to a vast number of steady state single or combined environmental cues, thus complicating our understanding of the precise mechanisms and metabolic flows that maintain macrophage basic cellular functions in vivo. At least, compared to other tissue resident macrophages, AMs are better equipped with genes involved in gas exchange such as the carbonic anhydrase Car4 due to their proximity to the airways or genes regulating lipid metabolism in order to catabolize the surfactant, which are in large part controlled by the transcription factor peroxisome proliferator-activated receptor γ (PPARγ) [51,53]. Consistently, PPARγ expression is important to maintain lung macrophage transcriptome, functionality, and surfactant catabolism as well as response to infection in mice [63–66]. This tissue specific transcriptional signature is in part the consequence of a chromatin landscape reshaping induced by the local microenvironment [53] that could largely be influenced by acute and chronic inflammation [57,67] and epigenetic-dependent reprogramming [67,68]. In contrast, little is known about the regulation of IM populations. Besides sensing microbial products [47], IMs may be impacted by low oxygen tension (i.e., hypoxia) to exert their immunoregulatory activities in mouse pulmonary hypertension or allergenic contexts [69,70]. Thus, given their different phenotypes and ontogenies, it is now clear that AMs and IMs perform different functions in the lung that are so far been linked to tissue maintenance (i.e., surfactant catabolism and luminal infection) and innate immunoregulatory mechanisms (i.e., hypoxia and allergen sensing and tissular infection).

3. Lung Macrophage Origin and Diversity in Lung Adenocarcinoma

3.1. Smoldering Inflammation

Environmental and genetic factors influence lung cancer pathogenesis with cigarette smoke being the major environmental risk factor, followed by chronic infection and dietary factors. Chronic inflammatory diseases are linked to the initiation of tumorigenesis in part by creating a mutagenic environment in sub-epithelial stroma [21,22]. This type of inflammation with increased cancer risk is often referred to "smoldering inflammation". Immune cells, especially macrophages, participate to the mutagenic environment by producing various cytokines (including IL-1β) and generating reactive nitrogen and oxygen species that promote genetic instability and induce somatic mutations in epithelial cells (Figure 1, right panel). Even if detailed mechanisms underlying tobacco-induced cancerogenesis are not completely elucidated [71], there is strong evidence that cigarette smoke contributes to this smoldering inflammation by inducing secretion of inflammatory cytokines and macrophage apoptosis [72,73] along with the formation of lung nodules [74]. The two most frequent oncogenic mutations in lung adenocarcinoma, which are generally mutually exclusive, include the activating mutations in a small GTPase transductor protein KRAS (V-KI-ras2 Kirsten rat sarcoma viral oncogene homolog) and the epidermal growth factor receptor (EGFR) [4]. In preclinical and clinical studies, chronic obstructive pulmonary disease (COPD) leads to increased lung cancer risk [75,76]. This disease is predicted to rank in the top five of overall burden of disease by 2020 according to the World Heathy Organization (WHO) [77] because of increased tobacco use and its relationship to the metabolic syndrome [78,79]. There are also evidences that COPD could be driven by chronic exposure to irritant particles such as asbestos or silica through NOD-like receptor family, pyrin domain containing 3 (NLRP3) inflammasome-dependent IL-1β secretion [80,81]. Thus, chronic inflammatory diseases, dominated by macrophage inflammation, is a culprit of cancer initiation.

3.2. Resident Tumor-Associated Macrophages (rTAMs)

On the site where a tumor develops, malignant cells are surrounded by non-malignant stroma cells that are part of the TME. Non-malignant populations include connective tissue cells and leucocytes, with TAMs representing the majority of the leukocyte population [82,83]. The specific maintenance of tissue-resident macrophages through in situ proliferation and the diversity of TAMs within tumors have challenged our understanding of their role in tumors. Indeed, in mouse models of brain tumors and pancreatic cancer, TAMs can originate from both circulating monocytes and tissue-resident macrophages where they could facilitate tumor growth by contributing to tissue remodeling [25,84]. After inoculation of TC-1 lung carcinoma cells in mice, the group of Boissonnas identified a specific population of mouse rTAMs that originated from tissue-resident IMs already present in healthy lungs that could support lung tumor development (Figure 2, left panel) [85]. In comparison to other macrophage subsets, profiling of rTAMs revealed a transcriptional signature associated to tissue remodeling including transcripts related to extracellular matrix (ECM) and vasculature interactions that supported tumor cell growth [85]. Using single-cell and mass cytometry by time of-flight (CyTOF) analyses in early human lung adenocarcinomas, the group of Merad also identified a unique tumor-specific macrophage population that dissociated from tissue-resident macrophages (Figure 2, left panel) [86]. These rTAMs exhibited an upregulation of transcripts involved in macrophage effector functions such as triggering receptor expressed on myeloid cells-2 (TREM2), tetraspanin CD81 or macrophage receptor with collagenous structure (MARCO) that were associated with a significant survival disadvantage [86]. As reviewed elsewhere, it was previously reported that both TREM2 and MARCO are critical in mouse airway macrophages to limit pro-inflammatory or Toll-like receptor responses [41]. Intriguingly, these human rTAMs also expressed higher levels of the transcription factor PPARγ involved in tissue-resident AM immunomodulatory functions and surfactant catabolism [86]. These findings suggest that rTAMs signature may be associated with a tumor-specific metabolic rewiring opening therapeutic perspectives for lung cancer diagnosis and treatment [87]. For instance, pro-surfactant protein B (SFTPB), known to be transcriptionally controlled by PPARγ, is used as a serum biomarker of lung adenocarcinoma both in preclinical and clinical studies [88–90]. Additionally, higher density of anti-tumoral TAMs were observed in human lung tumor nests and stroma [21] and stroma TAMs were associated with systemic blood inflammation (i.e., elevated plasma CRP levels), adverse prognostic factors (i.e., lymph node metastasis) or poor overall survival [91,92].

3.3. Monocyte-Derived TAMs (MoTAMs)

While the role of rTAMs in promoting cancers spread (i.e., metastasis) is well documented, the role of MoTAMs remains much less understood beyond their potential roles in continuously replenishing tumors [6,93]. The TAMs were originally hypothesized to originate from circulating monocytes that were recruited in response to chemotactic signals released from tumor cells with a subset of these cells being called myeloid-derived-suppressor cells [94,95]. Targeting chemokine interactions and subsequent recruitment of macrophages within tumors, including the CCL2/CCR2 or CXCL12/CXCR4/7 chemokine-chemokine receptor axes, have shown great potential for cancer therapies in various mouse models of cancer metastasis [96–98]. In the clinic, antibodies that selectively target CCL2 (CNTO888) have produced mixed results as antitumor activity [99–101]. By contrast, CCR2 inhibitors (i.e., PF04136309 or CCX872) are currently tested in metastatic pancreatic cancer (Figure 3) [102,103]. Using, a mouse model of lung cancer metastasis driven by p53 deficiency and the oncogenic mutation $Kras^{G12D}$ the group of Pittet showed that circulating classical inflammatory monocytes employ the chemokine receptor CCR2 to promote a potent macrophage amplification program that generated TAMs within the lung (Figure 2, right panel) [23,94]. A role for the CXCL12/CXCR4/7 chemokine–chemokine receptor axes has also been proposed in mouse lung cancer metastasis-induced by lung carcinoma cell transplantation [104,105] most likely by shaping infiltrated immune cell population and promoting angiogenesis [106]. By contrast to classical monocytes, the group of Hedrick recently identified that nonclassical "patrolling" monocytes, enriched in the microvasculature of multiple mouse metastatic tumor models, prevented tumor invasion and reduced lung metastasis by scavenging tumor material from the lung vasculature (Figure 2, right panel) [107]. Further investigations will be required to pinpoint at with stage the imbalance between classical and non-classical MoTAMs occurs in lung cancer. Still, some evidences in humans indicate that the lymphocyte–monocyte ratio (LMR) could not only be an independent prognostic factor in patient with

NSCLC (Figure 3) [108] but also a predictor of survival and clinical outcome before complete resection for primary lung cancer or after treatment with anti-angiogenic therapy plus chemotherapy [109–112]. However, whether this ratio predicts a chemokine gradient, a switch between MoTAMs and/or the pathologic role for infiltrated MoTAMs remain to be fully elucidated.

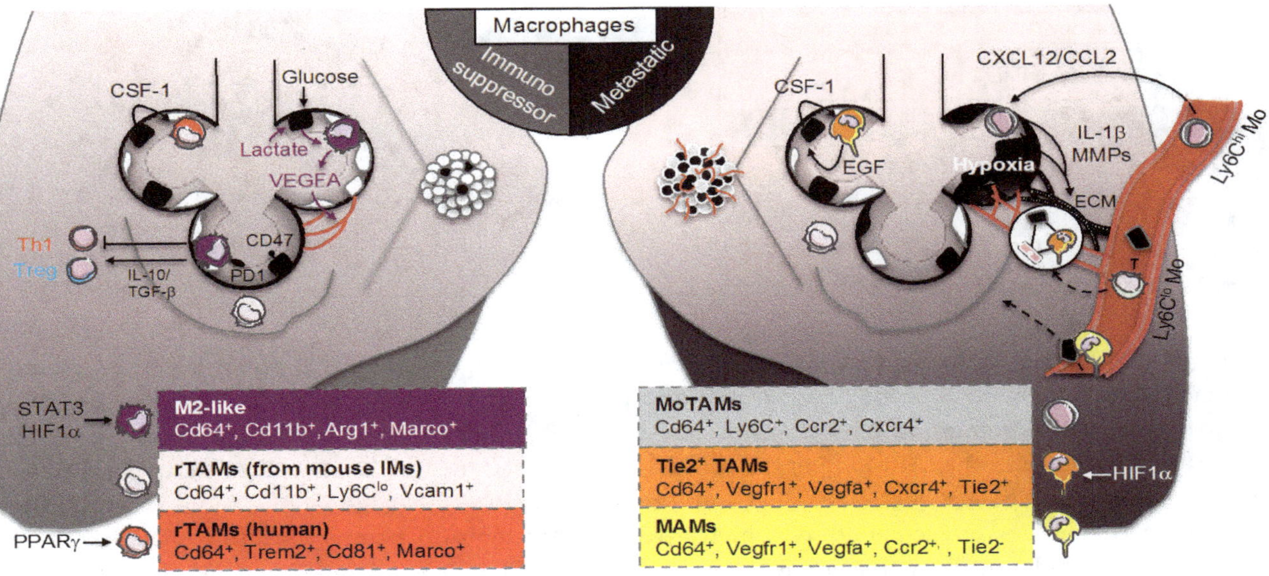

Figure 2. Macrophage effector functions as part of the 7th hallmark of cancer. Right panel: In established tumors, tumor-associated macrophages (TAMs) are the major part of the immune infiltrate that constitutes the tumor microenvironment (TME). Malignant cells produce the colony stimulating factor 1 (CSF-1), which participates to the conversion of tissue-resident macrophages into resident-TAMs (rTAMs). Their origin and cell surface makers may differ between mice and humans, with PPARγ being highly expressed in human rTAMs. Tumor cells also produce lactate through anaerobic glycolysis referred as the "Warburg effect" that can feed cancer cells in a cell-autonomous fashion for proliferation or act in a paracrine fashion to stabilize the hypoxia-inducible factor 1α (HIF1α) and promote a non-classical "M2-like" macrophage polarization. The signal transducer and activator of transcription 3 (STAT3) is another key transcription factor of M2 polarization. These M2-like macrophages participate to the tumor growth through at least 4 mechanisms: (1) secretion of the angiogenic vascular endothelial growth factor A (VEGFA), (2) expression of the immune checkpoint programmed death-1 (PD-1), (3) defect in recognizing and phagocytosing CD47-expressing tumor cells and (4) immunosuppression through inhibition of Th1 helper cells (Th1) and recruitment of regulatory T cells (Treg). Left panel: TAMs are also involved in more chaotic metastatic tumors. A feed-forward loop between CSF-1-expressing tumor cells and EGF-expressing TAMs contributes to intensive proliferation and oxygen consumption leading to a hypoxic environment. Tumor cells also secrete chemokine ligands such as CXCL12 and CCL2, involved in the recruitment into the tumor site of newly monocyte-derived TAMs (MoTAMs) from circulating Ly6C^{hi} monocytes contributing to the expansion of the tumor and the hypoxic niche. Hypoxia within tumor nest alters tumor cells and surrounding MoTAMs promoting extracellular matrix (ECM) remodeling through secretion of IL-1β and metalloproteases (MMPs). This remodeling favors the "angiogenic switch". A population of Tie2$^+$ TAMs, which most likely derives from a subpopulation of circulating Ly6C^{lo} monocytes, is located within the tumor vasculature interacting with mammalian-enabled (MENA)-expressing tumor cells and endothelial cells to further promote angiogenesis and create a metastatic environment. Circulating Ly6C^{lo} monocytes also scavenge tumor materials to prevent tumor invasion whereas metastasis-associated macrophages (MAMs) allow the extravasation of tumor cells into the lung.

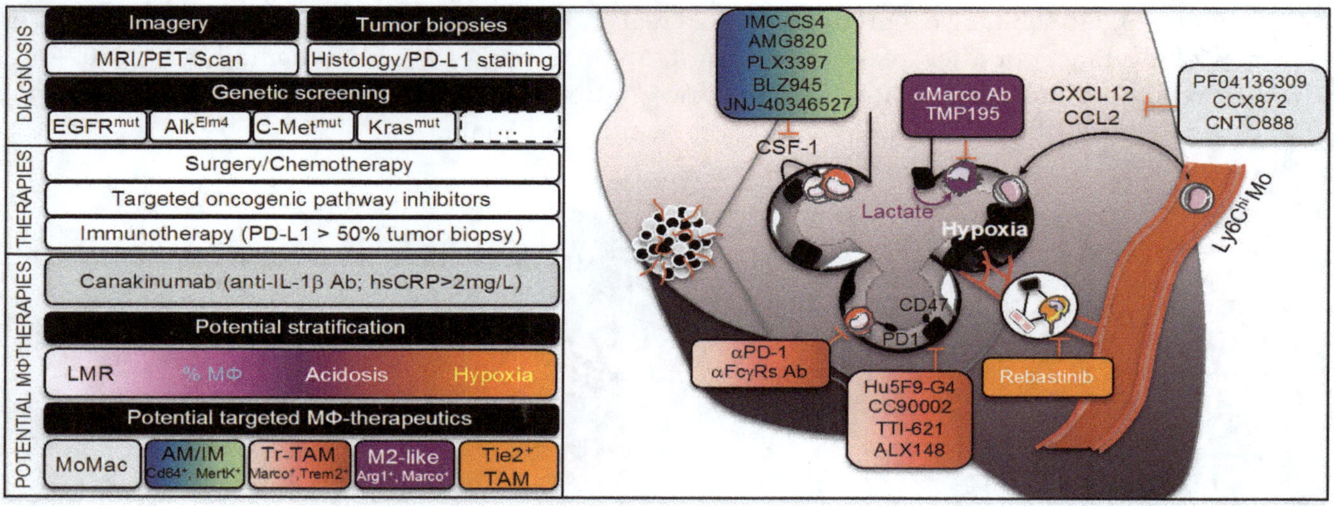

Figure 3. Lung adenocarcinoma treatment and emerging therapeutic potential of targeting macrophages. Diagnosis of lung adenocarcinoma patient requires at first magnetic resonance imaging (MRI) or positron-emission tomography scan (PET-scan). Tumor biopsies were also performed to further characterize the histology of the tumor and to determine the cancer cell's origin, the disease progression, and the expression of PD-L1 among other features. Oncogenic mutations driving lung adenocarcinomas were screened, of which V-KI-ras2 Kirsten rat sarcoma viral oncogene homolog (KRAS) and epidermal growth factor receptor (EGFR) mutations were the most frequent. These different diagnoses allow personalized treatment options with targeted oncogenic pathway inhibitors and/or chemotherapy. Immunotherapy is highly patient-dependent since the treatment with a checkpoint inhibitor that targets the PD-1/PD-L1 pathway requires tumors expressing levels of PD-L1 higher than 50%. These therapies are generally not exclusive and different strategies are employed for a better healing without remission. Novel potential therapies are aimed at targeting tumor-associated macrophages (TAMs). Whether or not IL-1β inhibitory antibody (Canakinumab) targets macrophages, its use on patients with C-reactive protein (CRP) levels higher than 2 mg/L reduced the rate of lung cancer. Composition of the tumor microenvironment (TME) may allow patient stratification. For instance, lymphocyte-monocyte ratio (LMR), a prognostic factor and a predictor survival, could be modified with CCR2 inhibitors (PF04136309 or CCX872) or with CCL2 inhibitors (CNTO888), preventing the recruitment of circulating Ly6C^{hi} monocytes into tumors. To limit the conversion of tissue-resident macrophages (i.e., alveolar macrophages AMs and interstitial macrophages IMs) into TAMs, blocking antibodies anti-CSF-1R (IMC-CS4 or AMG820) and tyrosine kinase inhibitors (PLX3397, BLZ945 or JNJ-40346527) are used. Cancer cells express CD47 on their surface, known to be a "don't eat me" signal and recognized by SIRP1α expressed on macrophages, which triggers a cascade of events that inhibit phagocytosis: anti-CD47 (Hu5F9-G4 or CC90002) or competitive recombinant SIRP1αFC (TTI-621 or ALX148) are developed as a way to reeducate TAMs for eliminating cancer cells. As for T-cells, TAMs also express the immune checkpoint receptor PD-1, inducing immune tolerance and TAMs PD-1 expression reduced the phagocytic potency against tumor cells. Immunotherapy with the use of αPD-1 not only targets PD-1/PD-L1 pathway on T-cells but is efficient to reactivate phagocytic potency of macrophages. However, TAMs could limit anti-PD-1 therapeutic benefits by stealing and capturing αPD-1 antibody from the CD8+ T-cells via FcγRIIb/III receptors unless if αFcγRs antibodies are administrated before. Another way to reeducate TAMs is to convert M2-like macrophages to an antitumor phenotype in targeting MARCO (αMarco Ab) or in inhibiting histone deacetylase (TMP195) to reprogram macrophage-dependent T-cell immune responses. Rebastinib reduced cancer cell metastasis by inhibiting a specific Tie2^{+} TAMs population implicated in the angiogenic switch.

4. Lung Macrophage Immunometabolism and Function in Lung Adenocarcinoma

4.1. TAM Immunomodulation

Understanding the distinct functions of different TAM populations within tumors remains an intense area of research. Nevertheless, in the vast majority of cancers, macrophages exhibit an overall immunosuppressive phenotype characterized by low levels of inflammatory molecules and an increased expression of transcripts expressed by alternatively activated M2 macrophages (Figure 2, left panel) [6]. Their in vitro and in vivo responses are associated with TGF-β and other growth factor such as vascular endothelial growth factor (VEGFA), interleukin or metalloprotease production that could impact their proliferation and differentiation in an autocrine manner and their surrounding environment in a paracrine manner [113,114]. This macrophage switch was recently highlighted in a transcriptional single cell analysis of human lung adenocarcinomas [115]. This antitumor response is thought to be mediated by the local environment created by the tumor to educate and take advantage of them. Although the M1/M2 distinction is oversimplified, therapies aimed at reprogramming TAMs towards a pro-inflammatory phenotype have emerged as a way to promote tumoricidal functions of TAMs. In animal models, drugs that inhibit key signaling molecules involved in M2 polarization (i.e., IL-4, STAT3 or PI3-kinase) successfully limited the immunosuppressive functions of TAMs and shrank tumors [116–120]. Macrophage-specific deletion of c-MYC also reduced tumor growth by preventing alternative TAM polarization [121]. Similarly, targeting the macrophage receptor with collagenous structure (MARCO), which is a key M2 marker, reprogrammed macrophage-dependent T-cell immune responses restricting tumor development and metastasis in mice (Figure 3) [122]. These findings add on the original Weissman's work on how cancer cells escape TAM's cancer-killing potential. Indeed, almost every type of cancer cell expresses CD47 at their cell surface, which is a molecule known for its role on normal, healthy cells as a "don't eat me" signal to phagocytosing macrophages (Figure 2, left panel) [123]. By expressing CD47, cancer cells will block "eat me" signals (such as the molecule calreticulin, which marks the cells for phagocytosis) by engaging the signal regulatory protein alpha (SIRP1α) on the surface of macrophages and limiting their cellular rearrangement for efficient engulfment. These findings led to novel therapeutic approaches targeting CD47 or SIRP1α (i.e., anti-CD47 antibodies such as Hu5F9-G4 or CC90002 and competitive recombinant SIRP1αFC such as TTI-621 and ALX148) as a way to reeducate TAMs for eliminating cancer cells in humans (Figure 3) [124,125]. Another example to reeducate the tumoricidal activity of TAMs is the use of CD40 agonists [126] that have also found their ways to the clinic [11]. Despite major efforts in precision medicine in the era of personalized medicine [127], identifying the type of cancer and patient population who will benefit the most from these emerging "macro-immunotherapies" is still a matter of intense investigations. At least in mouse models of lung cancer metastasis-induced by lung carcinoma cell transplantation or xenograft, therapeutic targeting of intracellular signaling pathways that regulate the switch between macrophage polarization states or the efferocytic function of TAMs was efficient to promote tumor regression and synergized with checkpoint inhibitor therapy [116,117,124,128–131].

4.2. Adaptation of TAM to the "Warburg Effect"

Although the immunosuppression of TAMs is anticipated to be highly complex and context-dependent, recent evidence suggest that metabolic changes in tumor cells could create a metabolic imbalance within the TME that can significantly impact TAM effector functions [132,133]. This environment is generally characterized by hypoxia and acidosis. The latter arises from the propensity for cancer cells to convert glucose to lactate despite the presence of oxygen, a mechanism originally described by Otto Warburg and referred as the "Warburg effect" [134]. Consistently, positron emission tomography (PET) scans using 18F-labeled 2-deoxyglucose as a non-metabolizable glucose analog light up primary and metastatic mouse and human lung cancers (Figure 3). Additionally, an inverse association between the tumor expression of the hypoxia-inducible factor (HIF)-1α, glucose transporter GLUT1 or the lactate dehydrogenase LDHA and the prognostic of patients was observed in lung adenocarcinoma [135–138]. Recent works from the group of DeBerardinis elegantly showed that human NSCLC heterogeneously oxidize glucose in the tricarboxylic acid (TCA) cycle [139] and even use a larger amount of lactate in a cell-autonomous fashion [140]. Some preclinical evidence in a lung cancer murine xenograft model suggest that targeting GLUT1 inhibits cancer cell growth [141,142]. In a murine model of $Kras^{G12D}$-driven lung cancer, pharmaceutical LDHA inhibition also inhibited both tumor progression and regression [143]. Thus, optimization of GLUT1 (BAY and DRB-18) or LDHA inhibitors may offer novel therapeutic strategies for treating lung cancer [144–146]. The importance of this metabolic pathway for TAM effector functions has been revealed by Colegio et al. who demonstrated in a murine model of Lewis lung carcinoma that lactic acid produced by tumors stabilizes HIF1α in TAMs, leading to an "M2-like" phenotype that was independent of IL-4R signaling (Figure 2, left panel) [147]. In other mouse model of cancer, the immunosuppression of TAMs was rather attributed to a role of HIF2α in accelerating tumor burden [148]. These discrepancies may reflect the specific metabolic rewiring of tumors depending on the oncogenic driver mutation, the local TME organization or the tissue where they develop and how TAMs form an alliance with cancer cells for metabolic symbiosis or compete for precious nutrients [132,149,150]. Recently, Carmona-Fontaine et al. showed that the modular organization of hypoxia and acidosis within the mouse TME may not only dictate the metabolic rewiring of TAMs but may also be sufficient to recapitulate their spatial diversity in vitro [151,152]. Although oxidative phosphorylation (OXPHOS) is a hallmark of anti-inflammatory M2 macrophages by contrast to glycolytic M1 macrophages in vitro [59,60] and the high glucose requirement of the tumor competes with the surrounding cells present in the mouse TME [153], reports on the glucose utilization and OXPHOS by TAMs in lung adenocarcinoma remain scarce [133].

4.3. TAM Immunometabolism beyond Glycolytic Activity

Besides glucose metabolism, modulation of lipid and amino acid metabolism by tumors could also impact the metabolic flexibility and mitochondrial OXPHOS in TAMs [133,149,150]. Although current knowledge on whether modulation of peripheral lipid flux affects cancer pathogenesis is still elusive and controversial [154], an original study from the group of Hoefler revealed that inhibition of peripheral lipolysis was not sufficient to locally affect tumor burden [155]. Moreover, the importance of the pathophysiological tissue context for cancer growth has recently been highlighted by the metabolic phenotyping of a murine model of $Kras^{G12D}$-driven lung tumor revealing that glutamine utilization was minimal in contrast to in vitro culture or other types of cancer [156]. Thus, the origin of alteration of lipid and amino acid metabolism in lung adenocarcinoma remains to be fully understood. On one hand, it could be linked to local acidosis that reprogram mitochondrial metabolism and promote histone deacetylation [157–159]. In line with these observations, checkpoint blockade therapy to restore immune cell nutrition restriction, nutritional intervention or treatment with a histone deacetylase inhibitor (TMP195) converted immune cells to an antitumor phenotype in mouse models of cancer metastasis (Figure 3) [153,160–162] including a shift from an M2 phenotype to a more efferocytic function of TAMs against cancer cells [160]. Alternatively, there is emerging evidence of local communication between cancer cells and TAMs through energy metabolism-derived (i.e., lipid and amino acid) mediators, referred to nowadays as "oncometabolites" or "metabokines" [163–165], even though their identification in lung adenocarcinoma has been limited [156,163–165]. At least, alteration of lipid metabolism within different populations of macrophages, especially AMs, in an immunocompetent syngeneic murine model injected with Lewis lung carcinoma cell correlated with selective expression of eicosanoids from both tumor cells and TAMs [166,167]. Although a new fatty acid-synthesis inhibitor (ND-646) was shown to blunt lung tumor growth in xenograft and genetically engineered mouse models of NSCLC [168], it is unknown if this compound may restore the functional polarization of TAMs as it has been shown by metformin in other cancer models [169,170]. Apart from glutamine, other amino acids such as arginine derived from the urea cycle may also be involved in the communication between cancer cells and TAMs. Indeed, knockdown of arginase 1 (ARG1) in macrophages prevented lung tumor growth by limiting the hydrolysis of arginine to ornithine [147]. Most of these metabolic pathways converge to increase localized ROS in cancer cells, which activate signaling pathways and transcription factors such as the transcription factor nuclear factor (erythroid-derived 2)–related factor-2 (NRF2) to promote tumorigenesis [160]. For instance, NRF2 regulates serine biosynthesis in NSCLC to generate NADPH and recycle oxidized glutathione, which is critical for the redox balance of cancer cells. Thus, emerging mechanistic insights linking tumor cells to the metabolic reprogramming of TAMs in lung adenocarcinoma hold promise for novel cancer therapy.

4.4. Tie2+ TAMs and Metastasis-Associated Macrophages (MAMs)

From original works by the group of Pollard and others [5,6], it has been well appreciated that, by supporting tumor angiogenesis, TAMs not only supply oxygen, nutrients and growth factors for tumor's development but also lay out a path for metastatic cells to reach new sites in the body, a process known as the "angiogenic switch" [171]. In the mid-1990s, evidence arose from CSF-1 deficient mice that the maturation and survival of macrophages had to do with cancer's spread (i.e., metastasis), rather than cancer tumor growth [5,6,9–11]. This led to the development of several anti-CSF-1R therapies (including CSF-1R blocking antibodies IMC-CS4 or AMG820 or tyrosine kinase inhibitors such as PLX3397, BLZ945 or JNJ-40346527) for patients with advanced solid tumors refractory to standard therapy (Figure 3) [11]. A specific Tie2-positive TAM population has been identified to mediate tumor angiogenesis and support tumor cell intravasation [172,173]. These TAMs could originate from Tie2-positive monocytes that are a subpopulation of nonclassical "patrolling" monocytes playing a role during mouse tumor neovascularization [174–177]. Mechanistically, these TAMs secrete VEGFA and proteases that degrade basement membranes of the ECM and participate in the formation of a TME of metastasis that comprises a pyramid-type structure on the vessel wall with mammalian-enabled (MENA)-expressing tumor cells that allow interactions with Tie2+ TAMs and blood vessel endothelial cells (Figure 2, right panel) [172,173]. These interactions suggest cell–cell contact for short-range transmission of growth and survival signals as recently illustrated for macrophage-fibroblast circuit [178] and resembles the paracrine EGF–CSF-1 interactions previously observed between TAMs and tumor cells [5,6]. Hypoxia is a major determinant of angiogenesis and HIF1α in TAMs acts as a major regulator of the "angiogenic switch" by inducing a switch from aerobic to anaerobic metabolism and increasing expression of diverse range of factors including VEGFA [174]. Despite mitigated cancer patient outcomes with VEGFR tyrosine kinase inhibitors or VEGFR2 antibodies [4,179], these findings have set up the stage for therapeutic approaches aimed at reducing cancer cell metastasis using a selective Tie2 inhibitor Rebastinib (Figure 3). In mice, the cooperation of the two oncogenes *Kras* and *Myc* has been recently shown to be required for the "angiogenic switch" and the transition to invasive adenocarcinoma [180]. It will remain to be carefully investigated in lung adenocarcinoma whether these Tie2+ TAMs also impact the epithelial–mesenchymal transition (EMT) that has been linked to invasive potential of various cancer cells [113,114,181,182]. Additionally, another population of TAMs seeding at distant sites and being recruited by CCL2 were dubbed metastasis-associated macrophages (MAMs) (Figure 2, right panel). These MAMs allow the extravasation of mouse tumor cells by secreting the chemokine ligand CCL3 and CSF-1 that facilitates metastatic seeding of breast cancer cells in the lung [183,184] and potentially VCAM-1 that transmits survival signals to these tumor cells [185]. The relevance of these MAMs in helping cancer cells to leave blood vessels and promote lung adenocarcinoma metastasis in mice was previously illustrated through their recruitment to extravasating pulmonary metastatic cells regardless of species of origin [186].

4.5. Bone Marrow Macrophages and Bone Metastasis

Osteolytic bone metastasis is a frequent event in late stage of lung cancer and is associated with high mortality of lung adenocarcinoma [187–189]. Once metastatic tumor cells reach the bone marrow (BM) after adhesion to the mineralized matrix through their invadopodia [190], they promote resorption and bone destruction by interfering with the osteoblastic bone-forming cells and osteoclastic bone-resorbing cells [191]. Osteoclasts are large multinucleated cells that differentiate from macrophage lineage precursors by increasing tartrate-resistant acid phosphatase (TRAP) expression following coregulation by CSF-1 and the receptor activator of nuclear factor κB ligand (RANKL) among other growth factors [192,193]. These growth factors can all be secreted by metastatic lung tumor cells [194–196]. Two different populations of macrophage have been described in the BM namely $CD11b^{hi}$ osteomacs [197] and $CD11b^{int}CD169^{+}$ macrophages [198] that are localized in different hypoxic area of the BM [199]. Targeting of these macrophage populations influences tumor-induced bone modelling in mouse models of prostate or Lewis lung cancer-induced bone metastasis [200,201]. The underlying mechanisms are not fully understood but could be linked to perturbation of osteoclast differentiation and disruption of the endosteal "osteoblastic niche" through bone resorption (i.e., mineral dissolution, followed by a degradation of the organic phase) and demineralization (i.e., acidification of the extracellular microenvironment and exposure to proteases) [138]. Future studies will be required to investigate whether tumor cells could also locally impact bone tissue, which is a specialized connective tissue consisting of cells and mineralized extracellular matrix (i.e., hydroxyapatite, a type of calcium phosphate) that could be responsible for the production of the calcified matrix in lung nodules [202–204].

5. IL-1β Signaling and Immunometabolism: A New Role in Lung Adenocarcinoma?

5.1. CANTOS Trial and Lung Adenocarcinoma

A recent retrospective analysis by Ridker et al. [205] reveal an unexpected dramatic reduction in the number of incident cases of lung cancer in the large, randomized CANTOS trial (Canakinumab Anti-inflammatory Thrombosis Outcomes Study) originally designed to test the hypothesis that canakinumab, an interleukin 1β (IL-1β) inhibitory antibody, could reduce a secondary cardiovascular event in very high-risk patients with prior myocardial infarction and inflamed setting (i.e., C-reactive protein (CRP) levels > 2 mg/L) (Figure 3). Of note, the incidence rate for all non-lung cancers was not statistically significant and one has to be cautious with hypothesis-based retrospective analysis [206,207]. Nevertheless, these findings led to a follow-up phase I study aimed at testing the combination of canakinumab and PD-1 inhibitor in NSCLC patients. As discussed above the relationship between inflammation and cancer is complicated, probably driven by an immunosuppression within TME. However, the concept of immunotherapy came from Coley's observation that cancer regression can be achieved by active bacterial infection [208,209]. Thus, the higher incidence of bacterial infection in the CANTOS trial [210] may suggest that by dampening chronic low-grade inflammation, canakinumab has unlocked an unspecific bacterial lung antitumoral activity. However, there are several evidences that blocking IL-1β signaling or upstream NLRP3 inflammasome regulation may have direct anticancer activity [211–215]. First, anti-IL-1β antibody dampens low-grade inflammation [211,216], which could prevent "smoldering inflammation" and reduce the mutagenic environment created by inflammatory immune cells [21,22]. Consistently, expression of specific inflammasome gene modules stratifies older individuals into two extreme clinical and immunological states that was associated with all-cause mortality [217]. Since IL-1β has been linked to airway inflammation [218,219], it will be of interest to know if the high CRP levels in the CANTOS trial at baseline were associated with an incidence of COPD, known to increase lung cancer risk [75,76]. Reduced COPD incidence could partially explain how canakinumab at the 300 mg dose induced a marked separation of the incidence curves for lung cancer within few months. Additionally, deficiency or inhibition of IL-1β signaling in TME has been shown to inhibit tumor angiogenesis and metastasis in mouse models of lung metastases-induced by various metastatic cells regardless of species of origin [220–225]. These findings may suggest an additional direct effect of canakinumab on established lung tumors. The CANTOS trial has opened the door to the human relevance of the relationship between IL-1β signaling and lung cancer and provides promising avenue with which to explore new anti-cancer therapies.

5.2. *IL-1β Signaling and Lung Adenocarcinoma*

The cell origin of IL-1β secretion and the implication of NLRP3 or other inflammasomes in lung TME remain to be identified and could have crucial therapeutic implications. Indeed, this pathway could promote on one hand leukocyte priming and trafficking or on the other hand, tumor growth. The tumor growth potential could be attributed to (1) an imbalance between cancer cell proliferation and pyroptosis, (2) an increased epithelial–mesenchymal transition (EMT) through secretion of metalloproteases and other ECM remodeling proteins or (3) an effect on lymphangiogenesis and angiogenesis [211–215]. While macrophages are the main source of IL-1β secretion in the immune response to pathogen [226–228], the TME of established tumors is characterized by an immunosuppression dominated by a M2 alternatively activated TAM phenotype that inhibits NLRP3-dependent IL-1β secretion [229]. Consistently, reduced NLRP3-dependent IL-1β secretion is observed in AMs isolated from the bronchoalveolar lavage of lung cancer patients despite a systemic higher NLRP3 inflammasome activation and IL-1β secretion in peripheral blood leukocytes from these patients [230,231]. Thus, the elevated IL-1β concentration in TME [232] could either derive directly from oncogenic lung cancer cells [233] or eventually from another TAM population (i.e., infiltrated MoTAMs) [230]. In the first scenario, combination of canakinumab with anti-PD-1 therapy, as initiated in phase I trial, may be beneficial by dual targeting of cancer and immune cells. However, in the second scenario, outcomes may be mitigated depending on the stage of tumor development and how suppression of an inflammatory response by canakinumab affect the antitumoral anti-PD-1 therapy response [211–215].

5.3. *Immunometabolism: The Missing Link?*

As discussed above, the origin of the tumor immunosuppression could be in part mediated by the hypoxia and acidosis within the TME [147,148], the metabolic restriction imposed by the high energy demand of the tumor [153] or an epigenetic reprogramming of immune cells [160], all these mechanisms being intimately linked to IL-1β secretion [226,234]. However, whether, where and how IL-1β secretion and potentially the activation of the NLRP3 or other inflammasomes could occur in tumor tissues remain elusive. At least, IL-1β secretion in macrophages must be primed by HIF1α and nuclear factor-kappa B (NF-κB)-dependent transcriptional regulation prior cleavage of pro-IL-1β into active IL-1β by caspase 1 [234,235]. Although historically, hypoxia was seen as a main driver of the activation of HIF1α and the expression of glycolytic enzymes to support an anaerobic glycolysis, it has become apparent that other metabolic stimuli can cause HIF1α-dependent metabolic reprogramming, especially in macrophages [59,62]. Are there such metabolic stimuli driving macrophage IL-1β priming in the heterogeneous lung TME [139,156]? As discussed above HIF1α can be stabilized under acidic conditions in TAMs [147]. So, could we envision that IL-1β secretion is dictated by acidosis in TAMs [236]? What we have learned from in vitro studies is that a broken TCA cycle with a concomitant reduction in mitochondrial respiration allows for funneling citrate and succinate out of the mitochondria where succinate acts as an activator of HIF1α turning on the transcriptional expression of pro-IL-1β [237]. Itaconate, one of the most highly induced metabolites in response to pathogens, could be responsible for the upstream regulation of succinate at least in activated macrophages [238]. Thus, it may not be surprising that succinate and itaconate also mediates crosstalk between macrophage metabolism and tumor growth [239,240]. In parallel, perturbed mitochondria metabolism could provide the second signal for proper activation of the inflammasome and subsequent cleavage of pro-IL-1β into active IL-1β by caspase 1 including mitochondrial DNA (mtDNA), calcium and ROS (mROS) among other stimuli [241]. Thus, future studies are warranted to delineate the metabolic communication between cancer cells and macrophages and how it specifically shapes the tumor immune microenvironment response.

6. Lung Adenocarcinoma Treatment and Macrophage Interaction

6.1. Lung Cancer Therapy Options

In recent years, treatments for all the different hallmarks of cancer have been investigated including anti-proliferative therapies (i.e., tyrosine kinase receptor, cyclin-dependent kinase or growth factor receptor inhibitors), pro-apoptotic therapies (i.e., mitochondrial cell death activation, blockade of DNA repair or telomere destabilization) or anti-angiogenic therapies to limit tumor growth and metastasis [82]. In the context of NSCLC, targeted therapies have been embraced thanks to genetic testing [242]. Targeted therapies prior cytotoxic chemotherapies include EGFR antagonists (i.e., tyrosine kinase inhibitors such as erlotinib, gefitinib, afatinib, necitumumab or osimertinib) for patients harboring an EGFR mutation [243–248], ALK inhibitors (i.e., ceretinib, alectinib or crizotinib) for ALK-rearranged NSCLC patients [249] or c-Met inhibitors (i.e., c-Met tyrosine kinase receptor inhibitors) for ALK/c-Met positive NSCLC (Figure 3) [250]. Details on these current therapies are deeply reviewed elsewhere [249–251]. However, the majority of lung tumors do not contain identified oncogenic mutations, thereby limiting the use of targeted oncogenic pathway inhibitors to a small fraction of patients (Figure 3). Moreover, no highly effective therapies have been developed for cancers harboring mutant KRAS. For instance, lung cancer patients who are positive for KRAS mutation have a low response rate to EGF tyrosine kinase receptor in part because KRAS and EGFR mutations are generally mutually exclusive and when they co-exist, KRAS mutations may confer resistance to EGFR mutations [4]. Thus, there continues to be a great need for new therapeutic strategies for patients with lung adenocarcinoma. Although several groups have demonstrated that concomitant use of MEK and phosphoinositide 3-kinase (PI3K) inhibitors (MEKi/PI3Ki) can induce dramatic tumor regressions in mouse models of KRAS-mutant non-small cell lung cancer (NSCLC), clinical trials investigating this strategy have been underwhelming [252,253] most likely because of heterogeneity in induction of cancer cell apoptosis [254]. By determining anti-apoptotic addiction, novel BH3-mimetic compounds have been developed to overwhelm anti-apoptotic defense mechanisms in response to oncogenic stress or anti-cancer therapy and a recent study revealed that this treatment could synergize with chemotherapy to induce tumor regression in $Kras^{G12D}$ mutant lung cancer mouse model [255]. Clinical trials evaluating safety and efficacy of this approach are currently ongoing [252]. Although clinical trials using telomerase inhibitors in NSCLC patients found that overall survival was not improved and this treatment may even causes some adverse decrease in platelet counts [256], they might still be effective in some tumor types (i.e., subgroup of patients with shortened telomers) [257,258] as it was recently observed in preclinical mouse models bearing the $Kras^{G12D}$ oncogenic mutation [259]. Some drug resistant NSCLC cells could also be sensitized by epigenetic drugs to other cytotoxic drugs [260]. As novel molecular mechanisms of cell death emerge [261], pro-apoptotic therapies may find its path to fight NSCLC, especially KRAS-bearing mutations. Nevertheless, these therapies will have to face drug resistance and find their way within immune checkpoint inhibitors that are increasingly being incorporated into lung cancer treatment protocols.

6.2. Emerging Immunotherapy

New paradigms such as targeting tumor immune microenvironments have been tested [262] and from this research, immune checkpoint inhibitors have emerged in the last decade has a new means to treat human cancer. In the context of NSCLC, immunotherapy (i.e., anti-programmed death-1 (PD-1) antibodies such as pembrolizumab or nivolumab and anti-programmed death ligand-1 (PD-L1) antibodies including atezolizumab, durvalumab and avelumab) was used for PD-L1 expression in at least 50% of tumor biopsies (Figure 3) [263–266]. In preclinical and clinical studies, combined anti-PD-L1 and anti-cytotoxic T-lymphocyte antigen-4 (CTLA-4) monoclonal antibodies may result in higher and more durable responses [267,268]. Even though immune checkpoint inhibitors (anti-CTLA-4 and PD-1/PD-L1 antibodies) have signaled a new direction for lung cancer care, the proportion of patients that respond to these agents remains low and the duration of response is often short [4].

Apart from loss of mismatch-repair function of cancer cells [269], driver mutations could also dampen immune checkpoint blockage by shaping TME. For instance, heterogeneity of intratumor neoantigen or EMT could predict sensitivity to immune checkpoint blockage [270,271] and inactivation of the tumor suppressor liver kinase B1 (LKB1), occurring in one-third of KRAS-mutated lung adenocarcinoma promotes the accumulation of immunosuppressive neutrophils and loss of PD-L1 expression, which is associated with fewer cytotoxic lymphocytes responsible for killing the tumor [272]. Therefore, novel methodologies to enhance the efficacy of immunotherapy in lung cancer are highly desirable.

6.3. TAMs and Lung Cancer Therapy Responses

The mechanisms by which TAMs could inhibit antitumor T cell responses involve more than one mechanism. First, TAMs have "tissue-reparative" activity, particularly M2-like macrophages that support tissue remodeling but at the same time suppress type 1 immune response [273]. Indeed, TAMs could inhibit antitumor T cell responses by secreting various factors including interleukin-10, which prevent dendritic cells from activating antitumor T-cell responses [274] or migration inhibitory factor (MIF), TGF-β and amino-acid degrading enzymes such as ARG1 and indoleamine 2,3-dioxygenase 1(IDO1), which promote survival of a subset of anti-inflammatory regulatory T-cells (Figure 2, left panel) [147,274–277]. The influx of new TAMs to tumors after first chemotherapy could also suppress the cytotoxic activity of antimitotic agents and stimulate tumor relapse [278,279], although they can in some cases be required for optimal therapy [280]. The group of Pittet identified an anti-PD-1 steal mechanism by TAMs which depends on FcγRIIb/III receptors and limits binding and activation to tumor-killing T-cells (Figure 3) [281]. Interestingly, PD-L1 and PD-1 expression by TAMs also inhibits phagocytosis and tumor immunity revealing that immune checkpoint therapy functions through a direct effect on macrophage effector functions (Figure 2, left panel) [282,283]. Recently, the specific enrichment of M2-like $CD163^{+}CD33^{+}PDL\text{-}1^{+}$ TAMs was associated with paradoxical boost in tumor growth in patients treated with immunotherapy, a phenomenon referred as "hyperprogression" [284]. Thus, TAMs may limit anti-PD-1 and other therapies by different means both in mice and humans. Altogether, these findings open substantial perspectives for improving immunotherapy efficacy including the combinations with strategies aimed at reeducating TAMs to limit their immunosuppressive functions or drug clearance capacity and help them eat cancer cells.

7. Conclusions

We have entered an exciting era of precision medicine with novel genetic and imaging modalities that should help to better stratify patient populations for which a battery of novel checkpoint blockade therapies will become available. Characterization of TME, especially its immune component, has provided an undoubtful value to our understanding of cancer development. Emerging evidences suggest that targeting macrophages and their metabolic reprogramming may have great therapeutic potential. Although, many large questions remain, there is no doubt that human clinical studies and the recent success of the CANTOS trial using an IL-1β inhibitory antibody will pave the way to the investigation of novel approaches to targeting not only traditional checkpoint blockade therapies but also immune checkpoint therapies to fight the residual burden of unmet need of NSCLC patients.

References

1. Travis, W.D.; Brambilla, E.; Nicholson, A.G.; Yatabe, Y.; Austin, J.H.M.; Beasley, M.B.; Chirieac, L.R.; Dacic, S.; Duhig, E.; Flieder, D.B.; et al. The 2015 World Health Organization Classification of Lung Tumors. *J. Thorac. Oncol.* **2015**, *10*, 1243–1260. [CrossRef] [PubMed]

2. Siegel, R.L.; Miller, K.D.; Jemal, A. Cancer statistics, 2018. *CA Cancer J. Clin.* **2018**, *68*, 7–30. [CrossRef] [PubMed]
3. Siegel, R.; Naishadham, D.; Jemal, A. Cancer statistics, 2012. *CA Cancer J. Clin.* **2012**, *62*, 10–29. [CrossRef] [PubMed]
4. Herbst, R.S.; Morgensztern, D.; Boshoff, C. The biology and management of non-small cell lung cancer. *Nature* **2018**, *553*, 446–454. [CrossRef] [PubMed]
5. Lewis, C.E.; Harney, A.S.; Pollard, J.W. The Multifaceted Role of Perivascular Macrophages in Tumors. *Cancer Cell* **2016**, *30*, 18–25. [CrossRef] [PubMed]
6. Yang, M.; McKay, D.; Pollard, J.W.; Lewis, C.E. Diverse Functions of Macrophages in Different Tumor Microenvironments. *Cancer Res.* **2018**, *78*, 5492–5503. [CrossRef] [PubMed]
7. Fridman, W.H.; Pagès, F.; Sautès-Fridman, C.; Galon, J. The immune contexture in human tumours: Impact on clinical outcome. *Nat. Rev. Cancer* **2012**, *12*, 298–306. [CrossRef] [PubMed]
8. Remark, R.; Becker, C.; Gomez, J.E.; Damotte, D.; Dieu-Nosjean, M.-C.; Sautès-Fridman, C.; Fridman, W.-H.; Powell, C.A.; Altorki, N.K.; Merad, M.; et al. The Non–Small Cell Lung Cancer Immune Contexture. A Major Determinant of Tumor Characteristics and Patient Outcome. *Am. J. Respir. Crit. Care Med.* **2015**, *191*, 377–390. [CrossRef] [PubMed]
9. Schupp, J.; Krebs, F.K.; Zimmer, N.; Trzeciak, E.; Schuppan, D.; Tuettenberg, A. Targeting myeloid cells in the tumor sustaining microenvironment. *Cell Immunol.* **2017**. [CrossRef] [PubMed]
10. Binnewies, M.; Roberts, E.W.; Kersten, K.; Chan, V.; Fearon, D.F.; Merad, M.; Coussens, L.M.; Gabrilovich, D.I.; Ostrand-Rosenberg, S.; Hedrick, C.C.; et al. Understanding the tumor immune microenvironment (TIME) for effective therapy. *Nat. Med.* **2018**, *24*, 541–550. [CrossRef] [PubMed]
11. Poh, A.R.; Ernst, M. Targeting Macrophages in Cancer: From Bench to Bedside. *Front. Oncol.* **2018**, *8*. [CrossRef] [PubMed]
12. Gordon, S.; Taylor, P.R. Monocyte and macrophage heterogeneity. *Nat. Rev. Immunol.* **2005**, *5*, 953–964. [CrossRef] [PubMed]
13. Glass, C.K.; Natoli, G. Molecular control of activation and priming in macrophages. *Nat. Immunol.* **2016**, *17*, 26–33. [CrossRef] [PubMed]
14. Tall, A.R.; Yvan-Charvet, L. Cholesterol, inflammation and innate immunity. *Nat. Rev. Immunol.* **2015**, *15*, 104–116. [CrossRef] [PubMed]
15. Koelwyn, G.J.; Corr, E.M.; Erbay, E.; Moore, K.J. Regulation of macrophage immunometabolism in atherosclerosis. *Nat. Immunol.* **2018**, *19*, 526–537. [CrossRef] [PubMed]
16. Tabas, I. Macrophage death and defective inflammation resolution in atherosclerosis. *Nat. Rev. Immunol.* **2010**, *10*, 36–46. [CrossRef] [PubMed]
17. Han, C.Z.; Ravichandran, K.S. Metabolic connections during apoptotic cell engulfment. *Cell* **2011**, *147*, 1442–1445. [CrossRef] [PubMed]
18. Gautier, E.L.; Yvan-Charvet, L. Understanding macrophage diversity at the ontogenic and transcriptomic levels. *Immunol. Rev.* **2014**, *262*, 85–95. [CrossRef] [PubMed]
19. Ginhoux, F.; Guilliams, M. Tissue-Resident Macrophage Ontogeny and Homeostasis. *Immunity* **2016**, *44*, 439–449. [CrossRef] [PubMed]
20. Wynn, T.A.; Chawla, A.; Pollard, J.W. Macrophage biology in development, homeostasis and disease. *Nature* **2013**, *496*, 445–455. [CrossRef] [PubMed]
21. Conway, E.M.; Pikor, L.A.; Kung, S.H.Y.; Hamilton, M.J.; Lam, S.; Lam, W.L.; Bennewith, K.L. Macrophages, Inflammation, and Lung Cancer. *Am. J. Respir. Crit. Care Med.* **2016**, *193*, 116–130. [CrossRef] [PubMed]
22. Grivennikov, S.I.; Greten, F.R.; Karin, M. Immunity, Inflammation, and Cancer. *Cell* **2010**, *140*, 883–899. [CrossRef] [PubMed]
23. Cortez-Retamozo, V.; Etzrodt, M.; Newton, A.; Ryan, R.; Pucci, F.; Sio, S.W.; Kuswanto, W.; Rauch, P.J.; Chudnovskiy, A.; Iwamoto, Y.; et al. Angiotensin II drives the production of tumor-promoting macrophages. *Immunity* **2013**, *38*, 296–308. [CrossRef] [PubMed]
24. Chen, Z.; Feng, X.; Herting, C.J.; Garcia, V.A.; Nie, K.; Pong, W.W.; Rasmussen, R.; Dwivedi, B.; Seby, S.; Wolf, S.A.; et al. Cellular and Molecular Identity of Tumor-Associated Macrophages in Glioblastoma. *Cancer Res.* **2017**, *77*, 2266–2278. [CrossRef] [PubMed]

25. Zhu, Y.; Herndon, J.M.; Sojka, D.K.; Kim, K.-W.; Knolhoff, B.L.; Zuo, C.; Cullinan, D.R.; Luo, J.; Bearden, A.R.; Lavine, K.J.; et al. Tissue-Resident Macrophages in Pancreatic Ductal Adenocarcinoma Originate from Embryonic Hematopoiesis and Promote Tumor Progression. *Immunity* **2017**, *47*, 323–338.e6. [CrossRef] [PubMed]
26. Qian, B.-Z.; Li, J.; Zhang, H.; Kitamura, T.; Zhang, J.; Campion, L.R.; Kaiser, E.A.; Snyder, L.A.; Pollard, J.W. CCL2 recruits inflammatory monocytes to facilitate breast-tumour metastasis. *Nature* **2011**, *475*, 222–225. [CrossRef] [PubMed]
27. Van Furth, R. The Origin and Kinetics of Mononuclear Phagocytes. *J. Exp. Med.* **1968**, *128*, 415–435. [CrossRef] [PubMed]
28. Coggle, J.E.; Tarling, J.D. The Proliferation Kinetics of Pulmonary Alveolar Macrophages. *J. Leukoc. Biol.* **1984**, *35*, 317–327. [CrossRef] [PubMed]
29. Sawyer, R.T. The Ontogeny of Pulmonary Alveolar Macrophages in Parabiotic Mice. *J. Leukoc. Biol.* **1986**, *40*, 347–354. [CrossRef] [PubMed]
30. Ginhoux, F.; Greter, M.; Leboeuf, M.; Nandi, S.; See, P.; Gokhan, S.; Mehler, M.F.; Conway, S.J.; Ng, L.G.; Stanley, E.R.; et al. Fate Mapping Analysis Reveals That Adult Microglia Derive from Primitive Macrophages. *Science* **2010**, *330*, 841–845. [CrossRef] [PubMed]
31. Schulz, C.; Gomez Perdiguero, E.; Chorro, L.; Szabo-Rogers, H.; Cagnard, N.; Kierdorf, K.; Prinz, M.; Wu, B.; Jacobsen, S.E.W.; Pollard, J.W.; et al. A lineage of myeloid cells independent of Myb and hematopoietic stem cells. *Science* **2012**, *336*, 86–90. [CrossRef] [PubMed]
32. Yona, S.; Kim, K.-W.; Wolf, Y.; Mildner, A.; Varol, D.; Breker, M.; Strauss-Ayali, D.; Viukov, S.; Guilliams, M.; Misharin, A.; et al. Fate Mapping Reveals Origins and Dynamics of Monocytes and Tissue Macrophages under Homeostasis. *Immunity* **2013**, *38*, 79–91. [CrossRef] [PubMed]
33. Hashimoto, D.; Chow, A.; Noizat, C.; Teo, P.; Beasley, M.B.; Leboeuf, M.; Becker, C.D.; See, P.; Price, J.; Lucas, D.; et al. Tissue-Resident Macrophages Self-Maintain Locally throughout Adult Life with Minimal Contribution from Circulating Monocytes. *Immunity* **2013**, *38*, 792–804. [CrossRef] [PubMed]
34. Gomez Perdiguero, E.; Klapproth, K.; Schulz, C.; Busch, K.; Azzoni, E.; Crozet, L.; Garner, H.; Trouillet, C.; de Bruijn, M.F.; Geissmann, F.; et al. Tissue-resident macrophages originate from yolk-sac-derived erythro-myeloid progenitors. *Nature* **2015**, *518*, 547–551. [CrossRef] [PubMed]
35. Geissmann, F.; Manz, M.G.; Jung, S.; Sieweke, M.H.; Merad, M.; Ley, K. Development of Monocytes, Macrophages, and Dendritic Cells. *Science* **2010**, *327*, 656–661. [CrossRef] [PubMed]
36. Sheng, J.; Ruedl, C.; Karjalainen, K. Most Tissue-Resident Macrophages Except Microglia Are Derived from Fetal Hematopoietic Stem Cells. *Immunity* **2015**, *43*, 382–393. [CrossRef] [PubMed]
37. Laskin, D.L.; Sunil, V.R.; Gardner, C.R.; Laskin, J.D. Macrophages and Tissue Injury: Agents of Defense or Destruction? *Annu. Rev. Pharmacol. Toxicol.* **2011**, *51*, 267–288. [CrossRef] [PubMed]
38. Westphalen, K.; Gusarova, G.A.; Islam, M.N.; Subramanian, M.; Cohen, T.S.; Prince, A.S.; Bhattacharya, J. Sessile alveolar macrophages communicate with alveolar epithelium to modulate immunity. *Nature* **2014**, *506*, 503–506. [CrossRef] [PubMed]
39. Guilliams, M.; Lambrecht, B.N.; Hammad, H. Division of labor between lung dendritic cells and macrophages in the defense against pulmonary infections. *Mucosal Immunol.* **2013**, *6*, 464–473. [CrossRef] [PubMed]
40. Kopf, M.; Schneider, C.; Nobs, S.P. The development and function of lung-resident macrophages and dendritic cells. *Nat. Immunol.* **2015**, *16*, 36–44. [CrossRef] [PubMed]
41. Hussell, T.; Bell, T.J. Alveolar macrophages: Plasticity in a tissue-specific context. *Nat. Rev. Immunol.* **2014**, *14*, 81–93. [CrossRef] [PubMed]
42. Guilliams, M.; De Kleer, I.; Henri, S.; Post, S.; Vanhoutte, L.; De Prijck, S.; Deswarte, K.; Malissen, B.; Hammad, H.; Lambrecht, B.N. Alveolar macrophages develop from fetal monocytes that differentiate into long-lived cells in the first week of life via GM-CSF. *J. Exp. Med.* **2013**, *210*, 1977–1992. [CrossRef] [PubMed]
43. Yu, X.; Buttgereit, A.; Lelios, I.; Utz, S.G.; Cansever, D.; Becher, B.; Greter, M. The Cytokine TGF-β Promotes the Development and Homeostasis of Alveolar Macrophages. *Immunity* **2017**, *47*, 903–912.e4. [CrossRef] [PubMed]
44. Tan, S.Y.S.; Krasnow, M.A. Developmental origin of lung macrophage diversity. *Dev. Camb. Engl.* **2016**, *143*, 1318–1327. [CrossRef] [PubMed]

45. Gibbings, S.L.; Thomas, S.M.; Atif, S.M.; McCubbrey, A.L.; Desch, A.N.; Danhorn, T.; Leach, S.M.; Bratton, D.L.; Henson, P.M.; Janssen, W.J.; et al. Three Unique Interstitial Macrophages in the Murine Lung at Steady State. *Am. J. Respir. Cell Mol. Biol.* **2017**, *57*, 66–76. [CrossRef] [PubMed]
46. Liegeois, M.; Legrand, C.; Desmet, C.J.; Marichal, T.; Bureau, F. The interstitial macrophage: A long-neglected piece in the puzzle of lung immunity. *Cell Immunol.* **2018**, *330*, 91–96. [CrossRef] [PubMed]
47. Sabatel, C.; Radermecker, C.; Fievez, L.; Paulissen, G.; Chakarov, S.; Fernandes, C.; Olivier, S.; Toussaint, M.; Pirottin, D.; Xiao, X.; et al. Exposure to Bacterial CpG DNA Protects from Airway Allergic Inflammation by Expanding Regulatory Lung Interstitial Macrophages. *Immunity* **2017**, *46*, 457–473. [CrossRef] [PubMed]
48. Schyns, J.; Bureau, F.; Marichal, T. Lung Interstitial Macrophages: Past, Present, and Future. *J. Immunol. Res.* **2018**, *2018*, 5160794. [CrossRef] [PubMed]
49. Rodero, M.P.; Poupel, L.; Loyher, P.-L.; Hamon, P.; Licata, F.; Pessel, C.; Hume, D.A.; Combadière, C.; Boissonnas, A. Immune surveillance of the lung by migrating tissue monocytes. *eLife* **2015**. [CrossRef] [PubMed]
50. McCubbrey, A.L.; Allison, K.C.; Lee-Sherick, A.B.; Jakubzick, C.V.; Janssen, W.J. Promoter Specificity and Efficacy in Conditional and Inducible Transgenic Targeting of Lung Macrophages. *Front. Immunol.* **2017**, *8*, 1618. [CrossRef] [PubMed]
51. Gautier, E.L.; Shay, T.; Miller, J.; Greter, M.; Jakubzick, C.; Ivanov, S.; Helft, J.; Chow, A.; Elpek, K.G.; Gordonov, S.; et al. Gene-expression profiles and transcriptional regulatory pathways that underlie the identity and diversity of mouse tissue macrophages. *Nat. Immunol.* **2012**, *13*, 1118–1128. [CrossRef] [PubMed]
52. Gosselin, D.; Link, V.M.; Romanoski, C.E.; Fonseca, G.J.; Eichenfield, D.Z.; Spann, N.J.; Stender, J.D.; Chun, H.B.; Garner, H.; Geissmann, F.; et al. Environment Drives Selection and Function of Enhancers Controlling Tissue-Specific Macrophage Identities. *Cell* **2014**, *159*, 1327–1340. [CrossRef] [PubMed]
53. Lavin, Y.; Winter, D.; Blecher-Gonen, R.; David, E.; Keren-Shaul, H.; Merad, M.; Jung, S.; Amit, I. Tissue-Resident Macrophage Enhancer Landscapes Are Shaped by the Local Microenvironment. *Cell* **2014**, *159*, 1312–1326. [CrossRef] [PubMed]
54. Mills, C.D.; Kincaid, K.; Alt, J.M.; Heilman, M.J.; Hill, A.M. M-1/M-2 macrophages and the Th1/Th2 paradigm. *J. Immunol.* **2000**, *164*, 6166–6173. [CrossRef] [PubMed]
55. Mosser, D.M.; Edwards, J.P. Exploring the full spectrum of macrophage activation. *Nat. Rev. Immunol.* **2008**, *8*, 958–969. [CrossRef] [PubMed]
56. Murray, P.J.; Allen, J.E.; Biswas, S.K.; Fisher, E.A.; Gilroy, D.W.; Goerdt, S.; Gordon, S.; Hamilton, J.A.; Ivashkiv, L.B.; Lawrence, T.; et al. Macrophage activation and polarization: Nomenclature and experimental guidelines. *Immunity* **2014**, *41*, 14–20. [CrossRef] [PubMed]
57. Misharin, A.V.; Morales-Nebreda, L.; Reyfman, P.A.; Cuda, C.M.; Walter, J.M.; McQuattie-Pimentel, A.C.; Chen, C.-I.; Anekalla, K.R.; Joshi, N.; Williams, K.J.N.; et al. Monocyte-derived alveolar macrophages drive lung fibrosis and persist in the lung over the life span. *J. Exp. Med.* **2017**, *214*, 2387–2404. [CrossRef] [PubMed]
58. Reyfman, P.A.; Washko, G.R.; Dransfield, M.T.; Spira, A.; Han, M.K.; Kalhan, R. Defining Impaired Respiratory Health. A Paradigm Shift for Pulmonary Medicine. *Am. J. Respir. Crit. Care Med.* **2018**, *198*, 440–446. [CrossRef] [PubMed]
59. Artyomov, M.N.; Sergushichev, A.; Schilling, J.D. Integrating immunometabolism and macrophage diversity. *Semin. Immunol.* **2016**, *28*, 417–424. [CrossRef] [PubMed]
60. O'Neill, L.A.J.; Pearce, E.J. Immunometabolism governs dendritic cell and macrophage function. *J. Exp. Med.* **2016**, *213*, 15–23. [CrossRef] [PubMed]
61. Murphy, M.P.; O'Neill, L.A.J. Krebs Cycle Reimagined: The Emerging Roles of Succinate and Itaconate as Signal Transducers. *Cell* **2018**, *174*, 780–784. [CrossRef] [PubMed]
62. Domínguez-Andrés, J.; Joosten, L.A.; Netea, M.G. Induction of innate immune memory: The role of cellular metabolism. *Curr. Opin. Immunol.* **2018**, *56*, 10–16. [CrossRef] [PubMed]
63. Trapnell, B.C.; Whitsett, J.A. Gm-CSF regulates pulmonary surfactant homeostasis and alveolar macrophage-mediated innate host defense. *Annu. Rev. Physiol.* **2002**, *64*, 775–802. [CrossRef] [PubMed]
64. Baker, A.D.; Malur, A.; Barna, B.P.; Ghosh, S.; Kavuru, M.S.; Malur, A.G.; Thomassen, M.J. Targeted PPAR{gamma} deficiency in alveolar macrophages disrupts surfactant catabolism. *J. Lipid Res.* **2010**, *51*, 1325–1331. [CrossRef] [PubMed]
65. Schneider, C.; Nobs, S.P.; Kurrer, M.; Rehrauer, H.; Thiele, C.; Kopf, M. Induction of the nuclear receptor PPAR-γ by the cytokine GM-CSF is critical for the differentiation of fetal monocytes into alveolar macrophages. *Nat. Immunol.* **2014**, *15*, 1026–1037. [CrossRef] [PubMed]

66. Gautier, E.L.; Chow, A.; Spanbroek, R.; Marcelin, G.; Greter, M.; Jakubzick, C.; Bogunovic, M.; Leboeuf, M.; van Rooijen, N.; Habenicht, A.J.; et al. Systemic analysis of PPARγ in mouse macrophage populations reveals marked diversity in expression with critical roles in resolution of inflammation and airway immunity. *J. Immunol.* **2012**, *189*, 2614–2624. [CrossRef] [PubMed]
67. Yao, Y.; Jeyanathan, M.; Haddadi, S.; Barra, N.G.; Vaseghi-Shanjani, M.; Damjanovic, D.; Lai, R.; Afkhami, S.; Chen, Y.; Dvorkin-Gheva, A.; et al. Induction of Autonomous Memory Alveolar Macrophages Requires T Cell Help and Is Critical to Trained Immunity. *Cell* **2018**, *175*, 1634–1650.e17. [CrossRef] [PubMed]
68. Bekkering, S.; Arts, R.J.W.; Novakovic, B.; Kourtzelis, I.; van der Heijden, C.D.C.C.; Li, Y.; Popa, C.D.; Ter Horst, R.; van Tuijl, J.; Netea-Maier, R.T.; et al. Metabolic Induction of Trained Immunity through the Mevalonate Pathway. *Cell* **2018**, *172*, 135–146.e9. [CrossRef] [PubMed]
69. Toussaint, M.; Fievez, L.; Drion, P.-V.; Cataldo, D.; Bureau, F.; Lekeux, P.; Desmet, C.J. Myeloid hypoxia-inducible factor 1α prevents airway allergy in mice through macrophage-mediated immunoregulation. *Mucosal Immunol.* **2013**, *6*, 485–497. [CrossRef] [PubMed]
70. Pugliese, S.C.; Kumar, S.; Janssen, W.J.; Graham, B.B.; Frid, M.G.; Riddle, S.R.; Kasmi, K.C.E.; Stenmark, K.R. A Time- and Compartment-Specific Activation of Lung Macrophages in Hypoxic Pulmonary Hypertension. *J. Immunol.* **2017**, *198*, 4802–4812. [CrossRef] [PubMed]
71. Maci, E.; Comito, F.; Frezza, A.M.; Tonini, G.; Pezzuto, A. Lung nodule and functional changes in smokers after smoking cessation short-term treatment. *Cancer Investig.* **2014**, *32*, 388–393. [CrossRef] [PubMed]
72. Demirjian, L.; Abboud, R.T.; Li, H.; Duronio, V. Acute effect of cigarette smoke on TNF-alpha release by macrophages mediated through the erk1/2 pathway. *Biochim. Biophys. Acta* **2006**, *1762*, 592–597. [CrossRef] [PubMed]
73. Aoshiba, K.; Tamaoki, J.; Nagai, A. Acute cigarette smoke exposure induces apoptosis of alveolar macrophages. *Am. J. Physiol. Lung Cell. Mol. Physiol.* **2001**, *281*, L1392–L1401. [CrossRef] [PubMed]
74. Tonini, G.; D'Onofrio, L.; Dell'Aquila, E.; Pezzuto, A. New molecular insights in tobacco-induced lung cancer. *Future Oncol.* **2013**, *9*, 649–655. [CrossRef] [PubMed]
75. Shacter, E.; Weitzman, S.A. Chronic inflammation and cancer. *Oncology* **2002**, *16*, 217–226. [PubMed]
76. Moghaddam, S.J.; Li, H.; Cho, S.-N.; Dishop, M.K.; Wistuba, I.I.; Ji, L.; Kurie, J.M.; Dickey, B.F.; DeMayo, F.J. Promotion of Lung Carcinogenesis by Chronic Obstructive Pulmonary Disease–Like Airway Inflammation in a K-ras–Induced Mouse Model. *Am. J. Respir. Cell Mol. Biol.* **2009**, *40*, 443–453. [CrossRef] [PubMed]
77. GBD 2017 SDG Collaborators. Measuring progress from 1990 to 2017 and projecting attainment to 2030 of the health-related Sustainable Development Goals for 195 countries and territories: A systematic analysis for the Global Burden of Disease Study 2017. *Lancet* **2018**, *392*, 2091–2138. [CrossRef]
78. Barnes, P.J.; Burney, P.G.J.; Silverman, E.K.; Celli, B.R.; Vestbo, J.; Wedzicha, J.A.; Wouters, E.F.M. Chronic obstructive pulmonary disease. *Nat. Rev. Dis. Primers* **2015**, *1*, 15076. [CrossRef] [PubMed]
79. Wouters, E.F.M. Obesity and Metabolic Abnormalities in Chronic Obstructive Pulmonary Disease. *Ann. Am. Thorac. Soc.* **2017**, *14*, S389–S394. [CrossRef] [PubMed]
80. Dostert, C.; Pétrilli, V.; Van Bruggen, R.; Steele, C.; Mossman, B.T.; Tschopp, J. Innate immune activation through Nalp3 inflammasome sensing of asbestos and silica. *Science* **2008**, *320*, 674–677. [CrossRef] [PubMed]
81. Cassel, S.L.; Eisenbarth, S.C.; Iyer, S.S.; Sadler, J.J.; Colegio, O.R.; Tephly, L.A.; Carter, A.B.; Rothman, P.B.; Flavell, R.A.; Sutterwala, F.S. The Nalp3 inflammasome is essential for the development of silicosis. *Proc. Natl. Acad. Sci. USA* **2008**, *105*, 9035–9040. [CrossRef] [PubMed]
82. Hanahan, D.; Weinberg, R.A. Hallmarks of Cancer: The Next Generation. *Cell* **2011**, *144*, 646–674. [CrossRef] [PubMed]
83. Balkwill, F.; Mantovani, A. Inflammation and cancer: Back to Virchow? *Lancet* **2001**, *357*, 539–545. [CrossRef]
84. Bowman, R.L.; Klemm, F.; Akkari, L.; Pyonteck, S.M.; Sevenich, L.; Quail, D.F.; Dhara, S.; Simpson, K.; Gardner, E.E.; Iacobuzio-Donahue, C.A.; et al. Macrophage Ontogeny Underlies Differences in Tumor-Specific Education in Brain Malignancies. *Cell Rep.* **2016**, *17*, 2445–2459. [CrossRef] [PubMed]
85. Loyher, P.-L.; Hamon, P.; Laviron, M.; Meghraoui-Kheddar, A.; Goncalves, E.; Deng, Z.; Torstensson, S.; Bercovici, N.; Baudesson de Chanville, C.; Combadière, B.; et al. Macrophages of distinct origins contribute to tumor development in the lung. *J. Exp. Med.* **2018**, *215*, 2536–2553. [CrossRef] [PubMed]
86. Lavin, Y.; Kobayashi, S.; Leader, A.; Amir, E.D.; Elefant, N.; Bigenwald, C.; Remark, R.; Sweeney, R.; Becker, C.D.; Levine, J.H.; et al. Innate Immune Landscape in Early Lung Adenocarcinoma by Paired Single-Cell Analyses. *Cell* **2017**, *169*, 750–765.e17. [CrossRef] [PubMed]

87. Merino Salvador, M.; Gómez de Cedrón, M.; Moreno Rubio, J.; Falagán Martínez, S.; Sánchez Martínez, R.; Casado, E.; Ramírez de Molina, A.; Sereno, M. Lipid metabolism and lung cancer. *Crit. Rev. Oncol. Hematol.* **2017**, *112*, 31–40. [CrossRef] [PubMed]
88. Taguchi, A.; Politi, K.; Pitteri, S.J.; Lockwood, W.W.; Faça, V.M.; Kelly-Spratt, K.; Wong, C.-H.; Zhang, Q.; Chin, A.; Park, K.-S.; et al. Lung Cancer Signatures in Plasma Based on Proteome Profiling of Mouse Tumor Models. *Cancer Cell* **2011**, *20*, 289–299. [CrossRef] [PubMed]
89. Sin, D.D.; Tammemagi, C.M.; Lam, S.; Barnett, M.J.; Duan, X.; Tam, A.; Auman, H.; Feng, Z.; Goodman, G.E.; Hanash, S.; et al. Pro-surfactant protein B as a biomarker for lung cancer prediction. *J. Clin. Oncol.* **2013**, *31*, 4536–4543. [CrossRef] [PubMed]
90. Wikoff, W.R.; Hanash, S.; DeFelice, B.; Miyamoto, S.; Barnett, M.; Zhao, Y.; Goodman, G.; Feng, Z.; Gandara, D.; Fiehn, O.; et al. Diacetylspermine is a Novel Prediagnostic Serum Biomarker for Non-Small-Cell Lung Cancer has Additive Performance with Pro-Surfactant Protein, B. *J. Clin. Oncol.* **2015**, *33*, 3880–3886. [CrossRef] [PubMed]
91. Carus, A.; Ladekarl, M.; Hager, H.; Pilegaard, H.; Nielsen, P.S.; Donskov, F. Tumor-associated neutrophils and macrophages in non-small cell lung cancer: No immediate impact on patient outcome. *Lung Cancer* **2013**, *81*, 130–137. [CrossRef] [PubMed]
92. Wu, P.; Wu, D.; Zhao, L.; Huang, L.; Chen, G.; Shen, G.; Huang, J.; Chai, Y. Inverse role of distinct subsets and distribution of macrophage in lung cancer prognosis: A meta-analysis. *Oncotarget* **2016**, *7*, 40451–40460. [CrossRef] [PubMed]
93. Biswas, S.K.; Mantovani, A. Macrophage plasticity and interaction with lymphocyte subsets: Cancer as a paradigm. *Nat. Immunol.* **2010**, *11*, 889–896. [CrossRef] [PubMed]
94. Cortez-Retamozo, V.; Etzrodt, M.; Newton, A.; Rauch, P.J.; Chudnovskiy, A.; Berger, C.; Ryan, R.J.H.; Iwamoto, Y.; Marinelli, B.; Gorbatov, R.; et al. Origins of tumor-associated macrophages and neutrophils. *Proc. Natl. Acad. Sci. USA* **2012**, *109*, 2491–2496. [CrossRef] [PubMed]
95. Franklin, R.A.; Liao, W.; Sarkar, A.; Kim, M.V.; Bivona, M.R.; Liu, K.; Pamer, E.G.; Li, M.O. The cellular and molecular origin of tumor-associated macrophages. *Science* **2014**, *344*, 921–925. [CrossRef] [PubMed]
96. Nagarsheth, N.; Wicha, M.S.; Zou, W. Chemokines in the cancer microenvironment and their relevance in cancer immunotherapy. *Nat. Rev. Immunol.* **2017**, *17*, 559–572. [CrossRef] [PubMed]
97. D'Agostino, G.; Cecchinato, V.; Uguccioni, M. Chemokine Heterocomplexes and Cancer: A Novel Chapter to Be Written in Tumor Immunity. *Front. Immunol.* **2018**, *9*. [CrossRef] [PubMed]
98. Susek, K.H.; Karvouni, M.; Alici, E.; Lundqvist, A. The Role of CXC Chemokine Receptors 1-4 on Immune Cells in the Tumor Microenvironment. *Front. Immunol.* **2018**, *9*, 2159. [CrossRef] [PubMed]
99. Loberg, R.D.; Ying, C.; Craig, M.; Day, L.L.; Sargent, E.; Neeley, C.; Wojno, K.; Snyder, L.A.; Yan, L.; Pienta, K.J. Targeting CCL2 with systemic delivery of neutralizing antibodies induces prostate cancer tumor regression in vivo. *Cancer Res.* **2007**, *67*, 9417–9424. [CrossRef] [PubMed]
100. Brana, I.; Calles, A.; LoRusso, P.M.; Yee, L.K.; Puchalski, T.A.; Seetharam, S.; Zhong, B.; de Boer, C.J.; Tabernero, J.; Calvo, E. Carlumab, an anti-C-C chemokine ligand 2 monoclonal antibody, in combination with four chemotherapy regimens for the treatment of patients with solid tumors: An open-label, multicenter phase 1b study. *Target. Oncol.* **2015**, *10*, 111–123. [CrossRef] [PubMed]
101. Arakaki, R.; Yamasaki, T.; Kanno, T.; Shibasaki, N.; Sakamoto, H.; Utsunomiya, N.; Sumiyoshi, T.; Shibuya, S.; Tsuruyama, T.; Nakamura, E.; et al. CCL2 as a potential therapeutic target for clear cell renal cell carcinoma. *Cancer Med.* **2016**, *5*, 2920–2933. [CrossRef] [PubMed]
102. Nywening, T.M.; Wang-Gillam, A.; Sanford, D.E.; Belt, B.A.; Panni, R.Z.; Cusworth, B.M.; Toriola, A.T.; Nieman, R.K.; Worley, L.A.; Yano, M.; et al. Targeting tumour-associated macrophages with CCR2 inhibition in combination with FOLFIRINOX in patients with borderline resectable and locally advanced pancreatic cancer: A single-centre, open-label, dose-finding, non-randomised, phase 1b trial. *Lancet Oncol.* **2016**, *17*, 651–662. [CrossRef]
103. Linehan, D.; Noel, M.S.; Hezel, A.F.; Wang-Gillam, A.; Eskens, F.; Sleijfer, S.; Desar, I.M.E.; Erdkamp, F.; Wilmink, J.; Diehl, J.; et al. Overall survival in a trial of orally administered CCR2 inhibitor CCX872 in locally advanced/metastatic pancreatic cancer: Correlation with blood monocyte counts. *J. Clin. Oncol.* **2018**, *36*, 92. [CrossRef]

104. Phillips, R.J.; Burdick, M.D.; Lutz, M.; Belperio, J.A.; Keane, M.P.; Strieter, R.M. The Stromal Derived Factor–1/CXCL12–CXC Chemokine Receptor 4 Biological Axis in Non–Small Cell Lung Cancer Metastases. *Am. J. Respir. Crit. Care Med.* **2003**, *167*, 1676–1686. [CrossRef] [PubMed]
105. Miao, Z.; Luker, K.E.; Summers, B.C.; Berahovich, R.; Bhojani, M.S.; Rehemtulla, A.; Kleer, C.G.; Essner, J.J.; Nasevicius, A.; Luker, G.D.; et al. CXCR7 (RDC1) promotes breast and lung tumor growth in vivo and is expressed on tumor-associated vasculature. *Proc. Natl. Acad. Sci. USA* **2007**, *104*, 15735–15740. [CrossRef] [PubMed]
106. Wald, O. CXCR4 Based Therapeutics for Non-Small Cell Lung Cancer (NSCLC). *J. Clin. Med.* **2018**, *7*, 303. [CrossRef] [PubMed]
107. Hanna, R.N.; Cekic, C.; Sag, D.; Tacke, R.; Thomas, G.D.; Nowyhed, H.; Herrley, E.; Rasquinha, N.; McArdle, S.; Wu, R.; et al. Patrolling monocytes control tumor metastasis to the lung. *Science* **2015**, *350*, 985–990. [CrossRef] [PubMed]
108. Hu, P.; Shen, H.; Wang, G.; Zhang, P.; Liu, Q.; Du, J. Prognostic significance of systemic inflammation-based lymphocyte- monocyte ratio in patients with lung cancer: Based on a large cohort study. *PLoS ONE* **2014**, *9*, e108062. [CrossRef] [PubMed]
109. Sarraf, K.M.; Belcher, E.; Raevsky, E.; Nicholson, A.G.; Goldstraw, P.; Lim, E. Neutrophil/lymphocyte ratio and its association with survival after complete resection in non-small cell lung cancer. *J. Thorac. Cardiovasc. Surg.* **2009**, *137*, 425–428. [CrossRef] [PubMed]
110. Zhang, J.; Huang, S.-H.; Li, H.; Li, Y.; Chen, X.-L.; Zhang, W.-Q.; Chen, H.-G.; Gu, L.-J. Preoperative lymphocyte count is a favorable prognostic factor of disease-free survival in non-small-cell lung cancer. *Med. Oncol.* **2013**, *30*, 352. [CrossRef] [PubMed]
111. Kobayashi, N.; Usui, S.; Kikuchi, S.; Goto, Y.; Sakai, M.; Onizuka, M.; Sato, Y. Preoperative lymphocyte count is an independent prognostic factor in node-negative non-small cell lung cancer. *Lung Cancer* **2012**, *75*, 223–227. [CrossRef] [PubMed]
112. Botta, C.; Barbieri, V.; Ciliberto, D.; Rossi, A.; Rocco, D.; Addeo, R.; Staropoli, N.; Pastina, P.; Marvaso, G.; Martellucci, I.; et al. Systemic inflammatory status at baseline predicts bevacizumab benefit in advanced non-small cell lung cancer patients. *Cancer Biol. Ther.* **2013**, *14*, 469–475. [CrossRef] [PubMed]
113. Zhang, J.; Yao, H.; Song, G.; Liao, X.; Xian, Y.; Li, W. Regulation of epithelial-mesenchymal transition by tumor-associated macrophages in cancer. *Am. J. Transl. Res.* **2015**, *7*, 1699–1711. [PubMed]
114. Song, W.; Mazzieri, R.; Yang, T.; Gobe, G.C. Translational Significance for Tumor Metastasis of Tumor-Associated Macrophages and Epithelial-Mesenchymal Transition. *Front. Immunol.* **2017**, *8*, 1106. [CrossRef] [PubMed]
115. Lambrechts, D.; Wauters, E.; Boeckx, B.; Aibar, S.; Nittner, D.; Burton, O.; Bassez, A.; Decaluwé, H.; Pircher, A.; Van den Eynde, K.; et al. Phenotype molding of stromal cells in the lung tumor microenvironment. *Nat. Med.* **2018**, *24*, 1277–1289. [CrossRef] [PubMed]
116. Sun, L.; Chen, B.; Jiang, R.; Li, J.; Wang, B. Resveratrol inhibits lung cancer growth by suppressing M2-like polarization of tumor associated macrophages. *Cell Immunol.* **2017**, *311*, 86–93. [CrossRef] [PubMed]
117. Kaneda, M.M.; Messer, K.S.; Ralainirina, N.; Li, H.; Leem, C.J.; Gorjestani, S.; Woo, G.; Nguyen, A.V.; Figueiredo, C.C.; Foubert, P.; et al. PI3Kγ is a molecular switch that controls immune suppression. *Nature* **2016**, *539*, 437–442. [CrossRef] [PubMed]
118. Yu, H.; Kortylewski, M.; Pardoll, D. Crosstalk between cancer and immune cells: Role of STAT3 in the tumour microenvironment. *Nat. Rev. Immunol.* **2007**, *7*, 41–51. [CrossRef] [PubMed]
119. DeNardo, D.G.; Barreto, J.B.; Andreu, P.; Vasquez, L.; Tawfik, D.; Kolhatkar, N.; Coussens, L.M. CD4(+) T cells regulate pulmonary metastasis of mammary carcinomas by enhancing protumor properties of macrophages. *Cancer Cell* **2009**, *16*, 91–102. [CrossRef] [PubMed]
120. Gocheva, V.; Wang, H.-W.; Gadea, B.B.; Shree, T.; Hunter, K.E.; Garfall, A.L.; Berman, T.; Joyce, J.A. IL-4 induces cathepsin protease activity in tumor-associated macrophages to promote cancer growth and invasion. *Genes Dev.* **2010**, *24*, 241–255. [CrossRef] [PubMed]
121. Pello, O.M.; Andrés, V. Role of c-MYC in tumor-associated macrophages and cancer progression. *Oncoimmunology* **2013**, *2*, e22984. [CrossRef] [PubMed]
122. Georgoudaki, A.-M.; Prokopec, K.E.; Boura, V.F.; Hellqvist, E.; Sohn, S.; Östling, J.; Dahan, R.; Harris, R.A.; Rantalainen, M.; Klevebring, D.; et al. Reprogramming Tumor-Associated Macrophages by Antibody Targeting Inhibits Cancer Progression and Metastasis. *Cell Rep.* **2016**, *15*, 2000–2011. [CrossRef] [PubMed]
123. Weissman, I. How One Thing Led to Another. *Annu. Rev. Immunol.* **2016**, *34*, 1–30. [CrossRef] [PubMed]

124. Weiskopf, K. Cancer immunotherapy targeting the CD47/SIRPα axis. *Eur. J. Cancer* **2017**, *76*, 100–109. [CrossRef] [PubMed]
125. Ring, N.G.; Herndler-Brandstetter, D.; Weiskopf, K.; Shan, L.; Volkmer, J.-P.; George, B.M.; Lietzenmayer, M.; McKenna, K.M.; Naik, T.J.; McCarty, A.; et al. Anti-SIRPα antibody immunotherapy enhances neutrophil and macrophage antitumor activity. *Proc. Natl. Acad. Sci. USA* **2017**, *114*, E10578–E10585. [CrossRef] [PubMed]
126. Beatty, G.L.; Chiorean, E.G.; Fishman, M.P.; Saboury, B.; Teitelbaum, U.R.; Sun, W.; Huhn, R.D.; Song, W.; Li, D.; Sharp, L.L.; et al. CD40 agonists alter tumor stroma and show efficacy against pancreatic carcinoma in mice and humans. *Science* **2011**, *331*, 1612–1616. [CrossRef] [PubMed]
127. Dugger, S.A.; Platt, A.; Goldstein, D.B. Drug development in the era of precision medicine. *Nat. Rev. Drug Discov.* **2018**, *17*, 183–196. [CrossRef] [PubMed]
128. Sharma, S.K.; Chintala, N.K.; Vadrevu, S.K.; Patel, J.; Karbowniczek, M.; Markiewski, M.M. Pulmonary alveolar macrophages contribute to the premetastatic niche by suppressing antitumor T cell responses in the lungs. *J. Immunol.* **2015**, *194*, 5529–5538. [CrossRef] [PubMed]
129. Zhao, H.; Wang, J.; Kong, X.; Li, E.; Liu, Y.; Du, X.; Kang, Z.; Tang, Y.; Kuang, Y.; Yang, Z.; et al. CD47 Promotes Tumor Invasion and Metastasis in Non-small Cell Lung Cancer. *Sci. Rep.* **2016**, *6*, 29719. [CrossRef] [PubMed]
130. Zhang, X.; Kim, S.; Hundal, J.; Herndon, J.M.; Li, S.; Petti, A.A.; Soysal, S.D.; Li, L.; McLellan, M.D.; Hoog, J.; et al. Breast Cancer Neoantigens Can Induce CD8+ T-Cell Responses and Antitumor Immunity. *Cancer Immunol. Res.* **2017**, *5*, 516–523. [CrossRef] [PubMed]
131. Liu, L.; Zhang, L.; Yang, L.; Li, H.; Li, R.; Yu, J.; Yang, L.; Wei, F.; Yan, C.; Sun, Q.; et al. Anti-CD47 Antibody as a Targeted Therapeutic Agent for Human Lung Cancer and Cancer Stem Cells. *Front. Immunol.* **2017**, *8*, 404. [CrossRef] [PubMed]
132. Dang, C.V.; Kim, J.-W. Convergence of Cancer Metabolism and Immunity: An Overview. *Biomol. Ther.* **2018**, *26*, 4–9. [CrossRef] [PubMed]
133. Netea-Maier, R.T.; Smit, J.W.A.; Netea, M.G. Metabolic changes in tumor cells and tumor-associated macrophages: A mutual relationship. *Cancer Lett.* **2018**, *413*, 102–109. [CrossRef] [PubMed]
134. Vander Heiden, M.G.; Cantley, L.C.; Thompson, C.B. Understanding the Warburg effect: The metabolic requirements of cell proliferation. *Science* **2009**, *324*, 1029–1033. [CrossRef] [PubMed]
135. Maki, Y.; Soh, J.; Ichimura, K.; Shien, K.; Furukawa, M.; Muraoka, T.; Tanaka, N.; Ueno, T.; Yamamoto, H.; Asano, H.; et al. Impact of GLUT1 and Ki-67 expression on early-stage lung adenocarcinoma diagnosed according to a new international multidisciplinary classification. *Oncol. Rep.* **2013**, *29*, 133–140. [CrossRef] [PubMed]
136. Osugi, J.; Yamaura, T.; Muto, S.; Okabe, N.; Matsumura, Y.; Hoshino, M.; Higuchi, M.; Suzuki, H.; Gotoh, M. Prognostic impact of the combination of glucose transporter 1 and ATP citrate lyase in node-negative patients with non-small lung cancer. *Lung Cancer* **2015**, *88*, 310–318. [CrossRef] [PubMed]
137. Miao, P.; Sheng, S.; Sun, X.; Liu, J.; Huang, G. Lactate dehydrogenase A in cancer: A promising target for diagnosis and therapy. *IUBMB Life* **2013**, *65*, 904–910. [CrossRef] [PubMed]
138. Pezzuto, A.; Carico, E. Role of HIF-1 in Cancer Progression: Novel Insights. A Review. *Curr. Mol. Med.* **2018**, *18*, 343–351. [CrossRef] [PubMed]
139. Hensley, C.T.; Faubert, B.; Yuan, Q.; Lev-Cohain, N.; Jin, E.; Kim, J.; Jiang, L.; Ko, B.; Skelton, R.; Loudat, L.; et al. Metabolic Heterogeneity in Human Lung Tumors. *Cell* **2016**, *164*, 681–694. [CrossRef] [PubMed]
140. Faubert, B.; Li, K.Y.; Cai, L.; Hensley, C.T.; Kim, J.; Zacharias, L.G.; Yang, C.; Do, Q.N.; Doucette, S.; Burguete, D.; et al. Lactate Metabolism in Human Lung Tumors. *Cell* **2017**, *171*, 358–371. [CrossRef] [PubMed]
141. Liu, Y.; Cao, Y.; Zhang, W.; Bergmeier, S.; Qian, Y.; Akbar, H.; Colvin, R.; Ding, J.; Tong, L.; Wu, S.; et al. A small-molecule inhibitor of glucose transporter 1 downregulates glycolysis, induces cell-cycle arrest, and inhibits cancer cell growth in vitro and in vivo. *Mol. Cancer Ther.* **2012**, *11*, 1672–1682. [CrossRef] [PubMed]
142. Suzuki, S.; Okada, M.; Takeda, H.; Kuramoto, K.; Sanomachi, T.; Togashi, K.; Seino, S.; Yamamoto, M.; Yoshioka, T.; Kitanaka, C. Involvement of GLUT1-mediated glucose transport and metabolism in gefitinib resistance of non-small-cell lung cancer cells. *Oncotarget* **2018**, *9*, 32667–32679. [CrossRef] [PubMed]
143. Xie, H.; Hanai, J.-I.; Ren, J.-G.; Kats, L.; Burgess, K.; Bhargava, P.; Signoretti, S.; Billiard, J.; Duffy, K.J.; Grant, A.; et al. Targeting lactate dehydrogenase—A inhibits tumorigenesis and tumor progression in mouse models of lung cancer and impacts tumor-initiating cells. *Cell Metab.* **2014**, *19*, 795–809. [CrossRef] [PubMed]

144. Siebeneicher, H.; Cleve, A.; Rehwinkel, H.; Neuhaus, R.; Heisler, I.; Müller, T.; Bauser, M.; Buchmann, B. Identification and Optimization of the First Highly Selective GLUT1 Inhibitor BAY-876. *ChemMedChem* **2016**, *11*, 2261–2271. [CrossRef] [PubMed]
145. Shriwas, P.; Qian, Y.; Wang, X.; Roberts, D.; Bergmeier, S.; Chen, X. Abstract 2799: New-generation glucose transporter inhibitors targeting non-small cell lung cancer and triple-negative breast cancer. *Cancer Res.* **2018**, *78*, 2799. [CrossRef]
146. Rani, R.; Kumar, V. When will small molecule lactate dehydrogenase inhibitors realize their potential in the cancer clinic? *Future Med. Chem.* **2017**, *9*, 1113–1115. [CrossRef] [PubMed]
147. Colegio, O.R.; Chu, N.-Q.; Szabo, A.L.; Chu, T.; Rhebergen, A.M.; Jairam, V.; Cyrus, N.; Brokowski, C.E.; Eisenbarth, S.C.; Phillips, G.M.; et al. Functional polarization of tumour-associated macrophages by tumour-derived lactic acid. *Nature* **2014**, *513*, 559–563. [CrossRef] [PubMed]
148. Imtiyaz, H.Z.; Williams, E.P.; Hickey, M.M.; Patel, S.A.; Durham, A.C.; Yuan, L.-J.; Hammond, R.; Gimotty, P.A.; Keith, B.; Simon, M.C. Hypoxia-inducible factor 2alpha regulates macrophage function in mouse models of acute and tumor inflammation. *J. Clin. Investig.* **2010**, *120*, 2699–2714. [CrossRef] [PubMed]
149. Obre, E.; Rossignol, R. Emerging concepts in bioenergetics and cancer research: Metabolic flexibility, coupling, symbiosis, switch, oxidative tumors, metabolic remodeling, signaling and bioenergetic therapy. *Int. J. Biochem. Cell Biol.* **2015**, *59*, 167–181. [CrossRef] [PubMed]
150. Vander Heiden, M.G.; DeBerardinis, R.J. Understanding the Intersections between Metabolism and Cancer Biology. *Cell* **2017**, *168*, 657–669. [CrossRef] [PubMed]
151. Carmona-Fontaine, C.; Bucci, V.; Akkari, L.; Deforet, M.; Joyce, J.A.; Xavier, J.B. Emergence of spatial structure in the tumor microenvironment due to the Warburg effect. *Proc. Natl. Acad. Sci. USA* **2013**. [CrossRef] [PubMed]
152. Carmona-Fontaine, C.; Deforet, M.; Akkari, L.; Thompson, C.B.; Joyce, J.A.; Xavier, J.B. Metabolic origins of spatial organization in the tumor microenvironment. *Proc. Natl. Acad. Sci. USA* **2017**, *114*, 2934–2939. [CrossRef] [PubMed]
153. Chang, C.-H.; Qiu, J.; O'Sullivan, D.; Buck, M.D.; Noguchi, T.; Curtis, J.D.; Chen, Q.; Gindin, M.; Gubin, M.M.; van der Windt, G.J.W.; et al. Metabolic Competition in the Tumor Microenvironment is a Driver of Cancer Progression. *Cell* **2015**, *162*, 1229–1241. [CrossRef] [PubMed]
154. Schreiber, R.; Xie, H.; Schweiger, M. Of mice and men: The physiological role of adipose triglyceride lipase (ATGL). *Biochim. Biophys. Acta Mol. Cell Biol. Lipids* **2018**. [CrossRef] [PubMed]
155. Das, S.K.; Eder, S.; Schauer, S.; Diwoky, C.; Temmel, H.; Guertl, B.; Gorkiewicz, G.; Tamilarasan, K.P.; Kumari, P.; Trauner, M.; et al. Adipose triglyceride lipase contributes to cancer-associated cachexia. *Science* **2011**, *333*, 233–238. [CrossRef] [PubMed]
156. Davidson, S.M.; Papagiannakopoulos, T.; Olenchock, B.A.; Heyman, J.E.; Keibler, M.A.; Luengo, A.; Bauer, M.R.; Jha, A.K.; O'Brien, J.P.; Pierce, K.A.; et al. Environment Impacts the Metabolic Dependencies of Ras-Driven Non-Small Cell Lung Cancer. *Cell Metab.* **2016**, *23*, 517–528. [CrossRef] [PubMed]
157. Cantor, J.R.; Sabatini, D.M. Cancer cell metabolism: One hallmark, many faces. *Cancer Discov.* **2012**, *2*, 881–898. [CrossRef] [PubMed]
158. Corbet, C.; Feron, O. Tumour acidosis: From the passenger to the driver's seat. *Nat. Rev. Cancer* **2017**, *17*, 577–593. [CrossRef] [PubMed]
159. DeBerardinis, R.J.; Chandel, N.S. Fundamentals of cancer metabolism. *Sci. Adv.* **2016**, *2*, e1600200. [CrossRef] [PubMed]
160. Guerriero, J.L.; Sotayo, A.; Ponichtera, H.E.; Castrillon, J.A.; Pourzia, A.L.; Schad, S.; Johnson, S.F.; Carrasco, R.D.; Lazo, S.; Bronson, R.T.; et al. Class IIa HDAC inhibition reduces breast tumours and metastases through anti-tumour macrophages. *Nature* **2017**, *543*, 428–432. [CrossRef] [PubMed]
161. Rubio-Patiño, C.; Bossowski, J.P.; Donatis, G.M.D.; Mondragón, L.; Villa, E.; Aira, L.E.; Chiche, J.; Mhaidly, R.; Lebeaupin, C.; Marchetti, S.; et al. Low-Protein Diet Induces IRE1α-Dependent Anticancer Immunosurveillance. *Cell Metab.* **2018**, *27*, 828–842.e7. [CrossRef] [PubMed]
162. Orillion, A.; Damayanti, N.P.; Shen, L.; Adelaiye-Ogala, R.; Affronti, H.; Elbanna, M.; Chintala, S.; Ciesielski, M.; Fontana, L.; Kao, C.; et al. Dietary Protein Restriction Reprograms Tumor-Associated Macrophages and Enhances Immunotherapy. *Clin. Cancer Res.* **2018**, *24*. [CrossRef] [PubMed]
163. Wang, D.; Dubois, R.N. Eicosanoids and cancer. *Nat. Rev. Cancer* **2010**, *10*, 181–193. [CrossRef] [PubMed]
164. Beloribi-Djefaflia, S.; Vasseur, S.; Guillaumond, F. Lipid metabolic reprogramming in cancer cells. *Oncogenesis* **2016**, *5*, e189. [CrossRef] [PubMed]

165. Pavlova, N.N.; Thompson, C.B. The Emerging Hallmarks of Cancer Metabolism. *Cell Metab.* **2016**, *23*, 27–47. [CrossRef] [PubMed]
166. Poczobutt, J.M.; Gijon, M.; Amin, J.; Hanson, D.; Li, H.; Walker, D.; Weiser-Evans, M.; Lu, X.; Murphy, R.C.; Nemenoff, R.A. Eicosanoid Profiling in an Orthotopic Model of Lung Cancer Progression by Mass Spectrometry Demonstrates Selective Production of Leukotrienes by Inflammatory Cells of the Microenvironment. *PLoS ONE* **2013**, *8*, e79633. [CrossRef] [PubMed]
167. Poczobutt, J.M.; De, S.; Yadav, V.K.; Nguyen, T.T.; Li, H.; Sippel, T.R.; Weiser-Evans, M.C.M.; Nemenoff, R.A. Expression Profiling of Macrophages Reveals Multiple Populations with Distinct Biological Roles in an Immunocompetent Orthotopic Model of Lung Cancer. *J. Immunol.* **2016**, *196*, 2847–2859. [CrossRef] [PubMed]
168. Svensson, R.U.; Parker, S.J.; Eichner, L.J.; Kolar, M.J.; Wallace, M.; Brun, S.N.; Lombardo, P.S.; Van Nostrand, J.L.; Hutchins, A.; Vera, L.; et al. Inhibition of acetyl-CoA carboxylase suppresses fatty acid synthesis and tumor growth of non-small-cell lung cancer in preclinical models. *Nat. Med.* **2016**, *22*, 1108–1119. [CrossRef] [PubMed]
169. Ding, L.; Liang, G.; Yao, Z.; Zhang, J.; Liu, R.; Chen, H.; Zhou, Y.; Wu, H.; Yang, B.; He, Q. Metformin prevents cancer metastasis by inhibiting M2-like polarization of tumor associated macrophages. *Oncotarget* **2015**, *6*, 36441–36455. [CrossRef] [PubMed]
170. Chiang, C.-F.; Chao, T.-T.; Su, Y.-F.; Hsu, C.-C.; Chien, C.-Y.; Chiu, K.-C.; Shiah, S.-G.; Lee, C.-H.; Liu, S.-Y.; Shieh, Y.-S. Metformin-treated cancer cells modulate macrophage polarization through AMPK-NF-κB signaling. *Oncotarget* **2017**, *8*, 20706–20718. [CrossRef] [PubMed]
171. Hanahan, D.; Folkman, J. Patterns and Emerging Mechanisms of the Angiogenic Switch during Tumorigenesis. *Cell* **1996**, *86*, 353–364. [CrossRef]
172. Wyckoff, J.B.; Wang, Y.; Lin, E.Y.; Li, J.; Goswami, S.; Stanley, E.R.; Segall, J.E.; Pollard, J.W.; Condeelis, J. Direct visualization of macrophage-assisted tumor cell intravasation in mammary tumors. *Cancer Res.* **2007**, *67*, 2649–2656. [CrossRef] [PubMed]
173. Harney, A.S.; Arwert, E.N.; Entenberg, D.; Wang, Y.; Guo, P.; Qian, B.-Z.; Oktay, M.H.; Pollard, J.W.; Jones, J.G.; Condeelis, J.S. Real-Time Imaging Reveals Local, Transient Vascular Permeability, and Tumor Cell Intravasation Stimulated by TIE2hi Macrophage-Derived VEGFA. *Cancer Discov.* **2015**, *5*, 932–943. [CrossRef] [PubMed]
174. Murdoch, C.; Muthana, M.; Coffelt, S.B.; Lewis, C.E. The role of myeloid cells in the promotion of tumour angiogenesis. *Nat. Rev. Cancer* **2008**, *8*, 618–631. [CrossRef] [PubMed]
175. De Palma, M.; Murdoch, C.; Venneri, M.A.; Naldini, L.; Lewis, C.E. Tie2-expressing monocytes: Regulation of tumor angiogenesis and therapeutic implications. *Trends Immunol.* **2007**, *28*, 519–524. [CrossRef] [PubMed]
176. Pucci, F.; Venneri, M.A.; Biziato, D.; Nonis, A.; Moi, D.; Sica, A.; Di Serio, C.; Naldini, L.; De Palma, M. A distinguishing gene signature shared by tumor-infiltrating Tie2-expressing monocytes, blood "resident" monocytes, and embryonic macrophages suggests common functions and developmental relationships. *Blood* **2009**, *114*, 901–914. [CrossRef] [PubMed]
177. Coffelt, S.B.; Tal, A.O.; Scholz, A.; De Palma, M.; Patel, S.; Urbich, C.; Biswas, S.K.; Murdoch, C.; Plate, K.H.; Reiss, Y.; et al. Angiopoietin-2 regulates gene expression in TIE2-expressing monocytes and augments their inherent proangiogenic functions. *Cancer Res.* **2010**, *70*, 5270–5280. [CrossRef] [PubMed]
178. Zhou, X.; Franklin, R.A.; Adler, M.; Jacox, J.B.; Bailis, W.; Shyer, J.A.; Flavell, R.A.; Mayo, A.; Alon, U.; Medzhitov, R. Circuit Design Features of a Stable Two-Cell System. *Cell* **2018**, *172*, 744–757.e17. [CrossRef] [PubMed]
179. Arjaans, M.; Schröder, C.P.; Oosting, S.F.; Dafni, U.; Kleibeuker, J.E.; de Vries, E.G.E. VEGF pathway targeting agents, vessel normalization and tumor drug uptake: From bench to bedside. *Oncotarget* **2016**, *7*, 21247–21258. [CrossRef] [PubMed]
180. Kortlever, R.M.; Sodir, N.M.; Wilson, C.H.; Burkhart, D.L.; Pellegrinet, L.; Brown Swigart, L.; Littlewood, T.D.; Evan, G.I. Myc Cooperates with Ras by Programming Inflammation and Immune Suppression. *Cell* **2017**, *171*, 1301–1315.e14. [CrossRef] [PubMed]
181. Yang, J.; Weinberg, R.A. Epithelial-mesenchymal transition: At the crossroads of development and tumor metastasis. *Dev. Cell* **2008**, *14*, 818–829. [CrossRef] [PubMed]
182. Thiery, J.P.; Acloque, H.; Huang, R.Y.J.; Nieto, M.A. Epithelial-mesenchymal transitions in development and disease. *Cell* **2009**, *139*, 871–890. [CrossRef] [PubMed]

183. Qian, B.-Z.; Zhang, H.; Li, J.; He, T.; Yeo, E.-J.; Soong, D.Y.H.; Carragher, N.O.; Munro, A.; Chang, A.; Bresnick, A.R.; et al. FLT1 signaling in metastasis-associated macrophages activates an inflammatory signature that promotes breast cancer metastasis. *J. Exp. Med.* **2015**, *212*, 1433–1448. [CrossRef] [PubMed]
184. Kitamura, T.; Qian, B.-Z.; Soong, D.; Cassetta, L.; Noy, R.; Sugano, G.; Kato, Y.; Li, J.; Pollard, J.W. CCL2-induced chemokine cascade promotes breast cancer metastasis by enhancing retention of metastasis-associated macrophages. *J. Exp. Med.* **2015**, *212*, 1043–1059. [CrossRef] [PubMed]
185. Chen, Q.; Zhang, X.H.-F.; Massagué, J. Macrophage binding to receptor VCAM-1 transmits survival signals in breast cancer cells that invade the lungs. *Cancer Cell* **2011**, *20*, 538–549. [CrossRef] [PubMed]
186. Qian, B.; Deng, Y.; Im, J.H.; Muschel, R.J.; Zou, Y.; Li, J.; Lang, R.A.; Pollard, J.W. A distinct macrophage population mediates metastatic breast cancer cell extravasation, establishment and growth. *PLoS ONE* **2009**, *4*, e6562. [CrossRef] [PubMed]
187. Weiss, R.J.; Wedin, R. Surgery for skeletal metastases in lung cancer. *Acta Orthop.* **2011**, *82*, 96–101. [CrossRef] [PubMed]
188. Rove, K.O.; Crawford, E.D. Metastatic cancer in solid tumors and clinical outcome: Skeletal-related events. *Oncology* **2009**, *23*, 21–27. [PubMed]
189. Luis-Ravelo, D.; Antón, I.; Zandueta, C.; Valencia, K.; Ormazábal, C.; Martínez-Canarias, S.; Guruceaga, E.; Perurena, N.; Vicent, S.; De Las Rivas, J.; et al. A gene signature of bone metastatic colonization sensitizes for tumor-induced osteolysis and predicts survival in lung cancer. *Oncogene* **2014**, *33*, 5090–5099. [CrossRef] [PubMed]
190. Marx, J. Cell biology. Podosomes and invadopodia help mobile cells step lively. *Science* **2006**, *312*, 1868–1869. [CrossRef] [PubMed]
191. Coughlin, T.R.; Romero-Moreno, R.; Mason, D.E.; Nystrom, L.; Boerckel, J.D.; Niebur, G.; Littlepage, L.E. Bone: A Fertile Soil for Cancer Metastasis. *Curr. Drug Targets* **2017**, *18*, 1281–1295. [CrossRef] [PubMed]
192. Suda, T.; Takahashi, N.; Udagawa, N.; Jimi, E.; Gillespie, M.T.; Martin, T.J. Modulation of osteoclast differentiation and function by the new members of the tumor necrosis factor receptor and ligand families. *Endocr. Rev.* **1999**, *20*, 345–357. [CrossRef] [PubMed]
193. Guerrini, M.M.; Takayanagi, H. The immune system, bone and RANKL. *Arch. Biochem. Biophys.* **2014**, *561*, 118–123. [CrossRef] [PubMed]
194. Shih, L.-Y.; Shih, H.-N.; Chen, T.-H. Bone resorption activity of osteolytic metastatic lung and breast cancers. *J. Orthop. Res.* **2004**, *22*, 1161–1167. [CrossRef] [PubMed]
195. Hernández, I.; Moreno, J.L.; Zandueta, C.; Montuenga, L.; Lecanda, F. Novel alternatively spliced ADAM8 isoforms contribute to the aggressive bone metastatic phenotype of lung cancer. *Oncogene* **2010**, *29*, 3758–3769. [CrossRef] [PubMed]
196. Kuo, P.-L.; Liao, S.-H.; Hung, J.-Y.; Huang, M.-S.; Hsu, Y.-L. MicroRNA-33a functions as a bone metastasis suppressor in lung cancer by targeting parathyroid hormone related protein. *Biochim. Biophys. Acta* **2013**, *1830*, 3756–3766. [CrossRef] [PubMed]
197. Winkler, I.G.; Sims, N.A.; Pettit, A.R.; Barbier, V.; Nowlan, B.; Helwani, F.; Poulton, I.J.; van Rooijen, N.; Alexander, K.A.; Raggatt, L.J.; et al. Bone marrow macrophages maintain hematopoietic stem cell (HSC) niches and their depletion mobilizes HSCs. *Blood* **2010**, *116*, 4815–4828. [CrossRef] [PubMed]
198. Chow, A.; Lucas, D.; Hidalgo, A.; Méndez-Ferrer, S.; Hashimoto, D.; Scheiermann, C.; Battista, M.; Leboeuf, M.; Prophete, C.; van Rooijen, N.; et al. Bone marrow CD169+ macrophages promote the retention of hematopoietic stem and progenitor cells in the mesenchymal stem cell niche. *J. Exp. Med.* **2011**, *208*, 261–271. [CrossRef] [PubMed]
199. Ehninger, A.; Trumpp, A. The bone marrow stem cell niche grows up: Mesenchymal stem cells and macrophages move in. *J. Exp. Med.* **2011**, *208*, 421–428. [CrossRef] [PubMed]
200. Wu, A.C.; He, Y.; Broomfield, A.; Paatan, N.J.; Harrington, B.S.; Tseng, H.-W.; Beaven, E.A.; Kiernan, D.M.; Swindle, P.; Clubb, A.B.; et al. CD169(+) macrophages mediate pathological formation of woven bone in skeletal lesions of prostate cancer. *J. Pathol.* **2016**, *239*, 218–230. [CrossRef] [PubMed]
201. Jing, W.; Zhang, L.; Qin, F.; Li, X.; Guo, X.; Li, Y.; Qiu, C.; Zhao, Y. Targeting macrophages for cancer therapy disrupts bone homeostasis and impairs bone marrow erythropoiesis in mice bearing Lewis lung carcinoma tumors. *Cell Immunol.* **2018**, *331*, 168–177. [CrossRef] [PubMed]
202. Mahoney, M.C.; Shipley, R.T.; Corcoran, H.L.; Dickson, B.A. CT demonstration of calcification in carcinoma of the lung. *AJR Am. J. Roentgenol.* **1990**, *154*, 255–258. [CrossRef] [PubMed]

203. Yoshikawa, J.; Takashima, T.; Miyata, S.; Kitagawa, M. CT demonstration of calcification in an adenoid cystic carcinoma of the lung. *AJR Am. J. Roentgenol.* **1990**, *154*, 419. [CrossRef] [PubMed]
204. Khan, A.N.; Al-Jahdali, H.H.; Allen, C.M.; Irion, K.L.; Al Ghanem, S.; Koteyar, S.S. The calcified lung nodule: What does it mean? *Ann. Thorac. Med.* **2010**, *5*, 67–79. [CrossRef] [PubMed]
205. Ridker, P.M.; MacFadyen, J.G.; Thuren, T.; Everett, B.M.; Libby, P.; Glynn, R.J.; Ridker, P.; Lorenzatti, A.; Krum, H.; Varigos, J.; et al. Effect of interleukin-1β inhibition with canakinumab on incident lung cancer in patients with atherosclerosis: Exploratory results from a randomised, double-blind, placebo-controlled trial. *Lancet* **2017**, *390*, 1833–1842. [CrossRef]
206. Chabner, B.A.; Nabel, C.S. Canakinumab and Lung Cancer: Intriguing, but Is It Real? *Oncologist* **2018**, *23*, 637–638. [CrossRef] [PubMed]
207. Crossman, D.; Rothman, A.M.K. Interleukin-1 β inhibition with canakinumab and reducing lung cancer—Subset analysis of the canakinumab anti-inflammatory thrombosis outcome study trial (CANTOS). *J. Thorac. Dis.* **2018**, *10*, S3084–3087. [CrossRef] [PubMed]
208. Haux, J. Infection and cancer. *Lancet* **2001**, *358*, 155–156. [CrossRef]
209. Vernon, L.F. William Bradley Coley, MD, and the phenomenon of spontaneous regression. *Immunol. Targets Ther.* **2018**, *7*, 29–34. [CrossRef] [PubMed]
210. Ridker, P.M.; Everett, B.M.; Thuren, T.; MacFadyen, J.G.; Chang, W.H.; Ballantyne, C.; Fonseca, F.; Nicolau, J.; Koenig, W.; Anker, S.D.; et al. Antiinflammatory Therapy with Canakinumab for Atherosclerotic Disease. *N. Engl. J. Med.* **2017**, *377*, 1119–1131. [CrossRef] [PubMed]
211. Libby, P. Interleukin-1 β as a Target for Atherosclerosis Therapy: Biological Basis of CANTOS and Beyond. *J. Am. Coll. Cardiol.* **2017**, *70*, 2278–2289. [CrossRef] [PubMed]
212. Apte, R.N.; Dotan, S.; Elkabets, M.; White, M.R.; Reich, E.; Carmi, Y.; Song, X.; Dvozkin, T.; Krelin, Y.; Voronov, E. The involvement of IL-1 in tumorigenesis, tumor invasiveness, metastasis and tumor-host interactions. *Cancer Metastasis Rev.* **2006**, *25*, 387–408. [CrossRef] [PubMed]
213. Dinarello, C.A. Why not treat human cancer with interleukin-1 blockade? *Cancer Metastasis Rev.* **2010**, *29*, 317–329. [CrossRef] [PubMed]
214. Zitvogel, L.; Kepp, O.; Galluzzi, L.; Kroemer, G. Inflammasomes in carcinogenesis and anticancer immune responses. *Nat. Immunol.* **2012**, *13*, 343–351. [CrossRef] [PubMed]
215. Karki, R.; Man, S.M.; Kanneganti, T.-D. Inflammasomes and Cancer. *Cancer Immunol. Res.* **2017**, *5*, 94–99. [CrossRef] [PubMed]
216. Lee, M.K.S.; Yvan-Charvet, L.; Masters, S.L.; Murphy, A.J. The modern interleukin-1 superfamily: Divergent roles in obesity. *Semin. Immunol.* **2016**, *28*, 441–449. [CrossRef] [PubMed]
217. Furman, D.; Chang, J.; Lartigue, L.; Bolen, C.R.; Haddad, F.; Gaudilliere, B.; Ganio, E.A.; Fragiadakis, G.K.; Spitzer, M.H.; Douchet, I.; et al. Expression of specific inflammasome gene modules stratifies older individuals into two extreme clinical and immunological states. *Nat. Med.* **2017**, *23*, 174–184. [CrossRef] [PubMed]
218. Pinkerton, J.W.; Kim, R.Y.; Robertson, A.A.B.; Hirota, J.A.; Wood, L.G.; Knight, D.A.; Cooper, M.A.; O'Neill, L.A.J.; Horvat, J.C.; Hansbro, P.M. Inflammasomes in the lung. *Mol. Immunol.* **2017**, *86*, 44–55. [CrossRef] [PubMed]
219. Howrylak, J.A.; Nakahira, K. Inflammasomes: Key Mediators of Lung Immunity. *Annu. Rev. Physiol.* **2017**, *79*, 471–494. [CrossRef] [PubMed]
220. Chirivi, R.G.; Garofalo, A.; Padura, I.M.; Mantovani, A.; Giavazzi, R. Interleukin 1 receptor antagonist inhibits the augmentation of metastasis induced by interleukin 1 or lipopolysaccharide in a human melanoma/nude mouse system. *Cancer Res.* **1993**, *53*, 5051–5054. [PubMed]
221. Voronov, E.; Shouval, D.S.; Krelin, Y.; Cagnano, E.; Benharroch, D.; Iwakura, Y.; Dinarello, C.A.; Apte, R.N. IL-1 is required for tumor invasiveness and angiogenesis. *Proc. Natl. Acad. Sci. USA* **2003**, *100*, 2645–2650. [CrossRef] [PubMed]
222. Nakao, S.; Kuwano, T.; Tsutsumi-Miyahara, C.; Ueda, S.; Kimura, Y.N.; Hamano, S.; Sonoda, K.; Saijo, Y.; Nukiwa, T.; Strieter, R.M.; et al. Infiltration of COX-2–expressing macrophages is a prerequisite for IL-1β–induced neovascularization and tumor growth. *J. Clin. Investig.* **2005**, *115*, 2979–2991. [CrossRef] [PubMed]

223. Shi, H.; Zhang, J.; Han, X.; Li, H.; Xie, M.; Sun, Y.; Liu, W.; Ba, X.; Zeng, X. Recruited monocytic myeloid-derived suppressor cells promote the arrest of tumor cells in the premetastatic niche through an IL-1β-mediated increase in E-selectin expression. *Int. J. Cancer* **2017**, *140*, 1370–1383. [CrossRef] [PubMed]
224. Guo, B.; Fu, S.; Zhang, J.; Liu, B.; Li, Z. Targeting inflammasome/IL-1 pathways for cancer immunotherapy. *Sci. Rep.* **2016**, *6*, 36107. [CrossRef] [PubMed]
225. Saijo, Y.; Tanaka, M.; Miki, M.; Usui, K.; Suzuki, T.; Maemondo, M.; Hong, X.; Tazawa, R.; Kikuchi, T.; Matsushima, K.; et al. Proinflammatory cytokine IL-1 β promotes tumor growth of Lewis lung carcinoma by induction of angiogenic factors: In vivo analysis of tumor-stromal interaction. *J. Immunol.* **2002**, *169*, 469–475. [CrossRef] [PubMed]
226. Próchnicki, T.; Latz, E. Inflammasomes on the Crossroads of Innate Immune Recognition and Metabolic Control. *Cell Metab.* **2017**, *26*, 71–93. [CrossRef] [PubMed]
227. Ting, J.P.Y.; Duncan, J.A.; Lei, Y. How the noninflammasome NLRs function in the innate immune system. *Science* **2010**, *327*, 286–290. [CrossRef] [PubMed]
228. Lamkanfi, M.; Dixit, V.M. Mechanisms and functions of inflammasomes. *Cell* **2014**, *157*, 1013–1022. [CrossRef] [PubMed]
229. Awad, F.; Assrawi, E.; Jumeau, C.; Georgin-Lavialle, S.; Cobret, L.; Duquesnoy, P.; Piterboth, W.; Thomas, L.; Stankovic-Stojanovic, K.; Louvrier, C.; et al. Impact of human monocyte and macrophage polarization on NLR expression and NLRP3 inflammasome activation. *PLoS ONE* **2017**, *12*, e0175336. [CrossRef] [PubMed]
230. Lasithiotaki, I.; Tsitoura, E.; Samara, K.D.; Trachalaki, A.; Charalambous, I.; Tzanakis, N.; Antoniou, K.M. NLRP3/Caspase-1 inflammasome activation is decreased in alveolar macrophages in patients with lung cancer. *PLoS ONE* **2018**, *13*. [CrossRef] [PubMed]
231. Pouniotis, D.S.; Plebanski, M.; Apostolopoulos, V.; McDonald, C.F. Alveolar macrophage function is altered in patients with lung cancer. *Clin. Exp. Immunol.* **2006**, *143*, 363–372. [CrossRef] [PubMed]
232. Lewis, A.M.; Varghese, S.; Xu, H.; Alexander, H.R. Interleukin-1 and cancer progression: The emerging role of interleukin-1 receptor antagonist as a novel therapeutic agent in cancer treatment. *J. Transl. Med.* **2006**, *4*, 48. [CrossRef] [PubMed]
233. Kong, H.; Wang, Y.; Zeng, X.; Wang, Z.; Wang, H.; Xie, W. Differential expression of inflammasomes in lung cancer cell lines and tissues. *Tumour Biol. J. Int. Soc. Oncodev. Biol. Med.* **2015**, *36*, 7501–7513. [CrossRef] [PubMed]
234. Haneklaus, M.; O'Neill, L.A.J. NLRP3 at the interface of metabolism and inflammation. *Immunol. Rev.* **2015**, *265*, 53–62. [CrossRef] [PubMed]
235. Guo, H.; Callaway, J.B.; Ting, J.P.-Y. Inflammasomes: Mechanism of action, role in disease, and therapeutics. *Nat. Med.* **2015**, *21*, 677–687. [CrossRef] [PubMed]
236. Edye, M.E.; Lopez-Castejon, G.; Allan, S.M.; Brough, D. Acidosis drives DAMP-induced interleukin-1 secretion via a caspase-1-independent pathway. *J. Biol. Chem.* **2013**. [CrossRef] [PubMed]
237. O'Neill, L.A.J. A broken krebs cycle in macrophages. *Immunity* **2015**, *42*, 393–394. [CrossRef] [PubMed]
238. Lampropoulou, V.; Sergushichev, A.; Bambouskova, M.; Nair, S.; Vincent, E.E.; Loginicheva, E.; Cervantes-Barragan, L.; Ma, X.; Huang, S.C.-C.; Griss, T.; et al. Itaconate Links Inhibition of Succinate Dehydrogenase with Macrophage Metabolic Remodeling and Regulation of Inflammation. *Cell Metab.* **2016**, *24*, 158–166. [CrossRef] [PubMed]
239. Jiang, S.; Yan, W. Succinate in the cancer-immune cycle. *Cancer Lett.* **2017**, *390*, 45–47. [CrossRef] [PubMed]
240. Weiss, J.M.; Davies, L.C.; Karwan, M.; Ileva, L.; Ozaki, M.K.; Cheng, R.Y.S.; Ridnour, L.A.; Annunziata, C.M.; Wink, D.A.; McVicar, D.W. Itaconic acid mediates crosstalk between macrophage metabolism and peritoneal tumors. *J. Clin. Investig.* **2018**, *128*. [CrossRef] [PubMed]
241. Weinberg, S.E.; Sena, L.A.; Chandel, N.S. Mitochondria in the regulation of innate and adaptive immunity. *Immunity* **2015**, *42*, 406–417. [CrossRef] [PubMed]
242. Kris, M.G.; Johnson, B.E.; Berry, L.D.; Kwiatkowski, D.J.; Iafrate, A.J.; Wistuba, I.I.; Varella-Garcia, M.; Franklin, W.A.; Aronson, S.L.; Su, P.-F.; et al. Using multiplexed assays of oncogenic drivers in lung cancers to select targeted drugs. *JAMA* **2014**, *311*, 1998–2006. [CrossRef] [PubMed]
243. Mok, T.S.; Wu, Y.-L.; Thongprasert, S.; Yang, C.-H.; Chu, D.-T.; Saijo, N.; Sunpaweravong, P.; Han, B.; Margono, B.; Ichinose, Y.; et al. Gefitinib or Carboplatin–Paclitaxel in Pulmonary Adenocarcinoma. *N. Engl. J. Med.* **2009**, *361*, 947–957. [CrossRef] [PubMed]

244. Zhou, C.; Wu, Y.-L.; Chen, G.; Feng, J.; Liu, X.-Q.; Wang, C.; Zhang, S.; Wang, J.; Zhou, S.; Ren, S.; et al. Erlotinib versus chemotherapy as first-line treatment for patients with advanced EGFR mutation-positive non-small-cell lung cancer (OPTIMAL, CTONG-0802): A multicentre, open-label, randomised, phase 3 study. *Lancet Oncol.* **2011**, *12*, 735–742. [CrossRef]
245. Sequist, L.V.; Yang, J.C.-H.; Yamamoto, N.; O'Byrne, K.; Hirsh, V.; Mok, T.; Geater, S.L.; Orlov, S.; Tsai, C.-M.; Boyer, M.; et al. Phase III study of afatinib or cisplatin plus pemetrexed in patients with metastatic lung adenocarcinoma with EGFR mutations. *J. Clin. Oncol.* **2013**, *31*, 3327–3334. [CrossRef] [PubMed]
246. Douillard, J.-Y.; Ostoros, G.; Cobo, M.; Ciuleanu, T.; McCormack, R.; Webster, A.; Milenkova, T. First-line gefitinib in Caucasian *EGFR* mutation-positive NSCLC patients: A phase-IV, open-label, single-arm study. *Br. J. Cancer* **2014**, *110*, 55–62. [CrossRef] [PubMed]
247. Mok, T.S.; Wu, Y.-L.; Ahn, M.-J.; Garassino, M.C.; Kim, H.R.; Ramalingam, S.S.; Shepherd, F.A.; He, Y.; Akamatsu, H.; Theelen, W.S.M.E.; et al. Osimertinib or Platinum–Pemetrexed in EGFR T790M–Positive Lung Cancer. *N. Engl. J. Med.* **2017**, *376*, 629–640. [CrossRef] [PubMed]
248. Soria, J.-C.; Ohe, Y.; Vansteenkiste, J.; Reungwetwattana, T.; Chewaskulyong, B.; Lee, K.H.; Dechaphunkul, A.; Imamura, F.; Nogami, N.; Kurata, T.; et al. Osimertinib in Untreated EGFR-Mutated Advanced Non–Small-Cell Lung Cancer. *N. Engl. J. Med.* **2017**. [CrossRef] [PubMed]
249. Millett, R.L.; Elkon, J.M.; Tabbara, I.A. Directed Therapies in Anaplastic Lymphoma Kinase-rearranged Non-small Cell Lung Cancer. *Anticancer Res.* **2018**, *38*, 4969–4975. [CrossRef] [PubMed]
250. Pasquini, G.; Giaccone, G. C-MET inhibitors for advanced non-small cell lung cancer. *Expert Opin. Investig. Drugs* **2018**, *27*, 363–375. [CrossRef] [PubMed]
251. Hirsch, F.R.; Scagliotti, G.V.; Mulshine, J.L.; Kwon, R.; Curran, W.J.; Wu, Y.-L.; Paz-Ares, L. Lung cancer: Current therapies and new targeted treatments. *Lancet* **2017**, *389*, 299–311. [CrossRef]
252. Montero, J.; Letai, A. Why do BCL-2 inhibitors work and where should we use them in the clinic? *Cell Death Differ.* **2018**, *25*, 56–64. [CrossRef] [PubMed]
253. Kale, J.; Osterlund, E.J.; Andrews, D.W. BCL-2 family proteins: Changing partners in the dance towards death. *Cell Death Differ.* **2018**, *25*, 65–80. [CrossRef] [PubMed]
254. Hata, A.N.; Yeo, A.; Faber, A.C.; Lifshits, E.; Chen, Z.; Cheng, K.A.; Walton, Z.; Sarosiek, K.A.; Letai, A.; Heist, R.S.; et al. Failure to induce apoptosis via BCL-2 family proteins underlies lack of efficacy of combined MEK and PI3K inhibitors for KRAS-mutant lung cancers. *Cancer Res.* **2014**, *74*, 3146–3156. [CrossRef] [PubMed]
255. Kim, E.Y.; Jung, J.Y.; Kim, A.; Chang, Y.S.; Kim, S.K. ABT-737 Synergizes with Cisplatin Bypassing Aberration of Apoptotic Pathway in Non-small Cell Lung Cancer. *Neoplasia* **2017**, *19*, 354–363. [CrossRef] [PubMed]
256. Chiappori, A.A.; Kolevska, T.; Spigel, D.R.; Hager, S.; Rarick, M.; Gadgeel, S.; Blais, N.; Von Pawel, J.; Hart, L.; Reck, M.; et al. A randomized phase II study of the telomerase inhibitor imetelstat as maintenance therapy for advanced non-small-cell lung cancer. *Ann. Oncol.* **2015**, *26*, 354–362. [CrossRef] [PubMed]
257. Williams, S.C.P. Small nanobody drugs win big backing from pharma. *Nat. Med.* **2013**, *19*, 1355–1356. [CrossRef] [PubMed]
258. Frink, R.E.; Peyton, M.; Schiller, J.H.; Gazdar, A.F.; Shay, J.W.; Minna, J.D. Telomerase inhibitor imetelstat has preclinical activity across the spectrum of non-small cell lung cancer oncogenotypes in a telomere length dependent manner. *Oncotarget* **2016**, *7*, 31639–31651. [CrossRef] [PubMed]
259. Liu, W.; Yin, Y.; Wang, J.; Shi, B.; Zhang, L.; Qian, D.; Li, C.; Zhang, H.; Wang, S.; Zhu, J.; et al. Kras mutations increase telomerase activity targeting telomerase is a promising therapeutic strategy for Kras-mutant, NSCLC. *Oncotarget* **2017**, *8*, 179–190. [CrossRef] [PubMed]
260. Housman, G.; Byler, S.; Heerboth, S.; Lapinska, K.; Longacre, M.; Snyder, N.; Sarkar, S. Drug resistance in cancer: An overview. *Cancers* **2014**, *6*, 1769–1792. [CrossRef] [PubMed]
261. Galluzzi, L.; Vitale, I.; Aaronson, S.A.; Abrams, J.M.; Adam, D.; Agostinis, P.; Alnemri, E.S.; Altucci, L.; Amelio, I.; Andrews, D.W.; et al. Molecular mechanisms of cell death: Recommendations of the Nomenclature Committee on Cell Death 2018. *Cell Death Differ.* **2018**, *25*, 486–541. [CrossRef] [PubMed]
262. Mantovani, A.; Sica, A. Macrophages, innate immunity and cancer: Balance, tolerance, and diversity. *Curr. Opin. Immunol.* **2010**, *22*, 231–237. [CrossRef] [PubMed]
263. Herbst, R.S.; Soria, J.-C.; Kowanetz, M.; Fine, G.D.; Hamid, O.; Gordon, M.S.; Sosman, J.A.; McDermott, D.F.; Powderly, J.D.; Gettinger, S.N.; et al. Predictive correlates of response to the anti-PD-L1 antibody MPDL3280A in cancer patients. *Nature* **2014**, *515*, 563–567. [CrossRef] [PubMed]

264. Garon, E.B.; Rizvi, N.A.; Hui, R.; Leighl, N.; Balmanoukian, A.S.; Eder, J.P.; Patnaik, A.; Aggarwal, C.; Gubens, M.; Horn, L.; et al. Pembrolizumab for the treatment of non-small-cell lung cancer. *N. Engl. J. Med.* **2015**, *372*, 2018–2028. [CrossRef] [PubMed]
265. Herbst, R.S.; Baas, P.; Kim, D.-W.; Felip, E.; Pérez-Gracia, J.L.; Han, J.-Y.; Molina, J.; Kim, J.-H.; Arvis, C.D.; Ahn, M.-J.; et al. Pembrolizumab versus docetaxel for previously treated, PD-L1-positive, advanced non-small-cell lung cancer (KEYNOTE-010): A randomised controlled trial. *Lancet* **2016**, *387*, 1540–1550. [CrossRef]
266. Reck, M.; Rodríguez-Abreu, D.; Robinson, A.G.; Hui, R.; Csőszi, T.; Fülöp, A.; Gottfried, M.; Peled, N.; Tafreshi, A.; Cuffe, S.; et al. Pembrolizumab versus Chemotherapy for PD-L1–Positive Non–Small-Cell Lung Cancer. *N. Engl. J. Med.* **2016**, *375*, 1823–1833. [CrossRef] [PubMed]
267. Curran, M.A.; Montalvo, W.; Yagita, H.; Allison, J.P. PD-1 and CTLA-4 combination blockade expands infiltrating T cells and reduces regulatory T and myeloid cells within B16 melanoma tumors. *Proc. Natl. Acad. Sci. USA* **2010**, *107*, 4275–4280. [CrossRef] [PubMed]
268. Hellmann, M.D.; Rizvi, N.A.; Goldman, J.W.; Gettinger, S.N.; Borghaei, H.; Brahmer, J.R.; Ready, N.E.; Gerber, D.E.; Chow, L.Q.; Juergens, R.A.; et al. Nivolumab plus ipilimumab as first-line treatment for advanced non-small-cell lung cancer (CheckMate 012): Results of an open-label, phase 1, multicohort study. *Lancet Oncol.* **2017**, *18*, 31–41. [CrossRef]
269. Le, D.T.; Uram, J.N.; Wang, H.; Bartlett, B.R.; Kemberling, H.; Eyring, A.D.; Skora, A.D.; Luber, B.S.; Azad, N.S.; Laheru, D.; et al. PD-1 Blockade in Tumors with Mismatch-Repair Deficiency. *N. Engl. J. Med.* **2015**, *372*, 2509–2520. [CrossRef] [PubMed]
270. McGranahan, N.; Furness, A.J.S.; Rosenthal, R.; Ramskov, S.; Lyngaa, R.; Saini, S.K.; Jamal-Hanjani, M.; Wilson, G.A.; Birkbak, N.J.; Hiley, C.T.; et al. Clonal neoantigens elicit T cell immunoreactivity and sensitivity to immune checkpoint blockade. *Science* **2016**, *351*, 1463–1469. [CrossRef] [PubMed]
271. Lou, Y.; Diao, L.; Cuentas, E.R.P.; Denning, W.L.; Chen, L.; Fan, Y.H.; Byers, L.A.; Wang, J.; Papadimitrakopoulou, V.A.; Behrens, C.; et al. Epithelial-Mesenchymal Transition Is Associated with a Distinct Tumor Microenvironment Including Elevation of Inflammatory Signals and Multiple Immune Checkpoints in Lung Adenocarcinoma. *Clin. Cancer Res.* **2016**, *22*, 3630–3642. [CrossRef] [PubMed]
272. Koyama, S.; Akbay, E.A.; Li, Y.Y.; Aref, A.R.; Skoulidis, F.; Herter-Sprie, G.S.; Buczkowski, K.A.; Liu, Y.; Awad, M.M.; Denning, W.L.; et al. STK11/LKB1 Deficiency Promotes Neutrophil Recruitment and Proinflammatory Cytokine Production to Suppress T-cell Activity in the Lung Tumor Microenvironment. *Cancer Res.* **2016**, *76*, 999–1008. [CrossRef] [PubMed]
273. Speiser, D.E.; Ho, P.-C.; Verdeil, G. Regulatory circuits of T cell function in cancer. *Nat. Rev. Immunol.* **2016**, *16*, 599–611. [CrossRef] [PubMed]
274. Ruffell, B.; Chang-Strachan, D.; Chan, V.; Rosenbusch, A.; Ho, C.M.T.; Pryer, N.; Daniel, D.; Hwang, E.S.; Rugo, H.S.; Coussens, L.M. Macrophage IL-10 blocks CD8+ T cell-dependent responses to chemotherapy by suppressing IL-12 expression in intratumoral dendritic cells. *Cancer Cell* **2014**, *26*, 623–637. [CrossRef] [PubMed]
275. Flavell, R.A.; Sanjabi, S.; Wrzesinski, S.H.; Licona-Limón, P. The polarization of immune cells in the tumour environment by TGFβ. *Nat. Rev. Immunol.* **2010**, *10*, 554–567. [CrossRef] [PubMed]
276. Choi, S.; Kim, H.-R.; Leng, L.; Kang, I.; Jorgensen, W.L.; Cho, C.-S.; Bucala, R.; Kim, W.-U. Role of macrophage migration inhibitory factor in the regulatory T cell response of tumor-bearing mice. *J. Immunol.* **2012**, *189*, 3905–3913. [CrossRef] [PubMed]
277. Zhao, Q.; Kuang, D.-M.; Wu, Y.; Xiao, X.; Li, X.-F.; Li, T.-J.; Zheng, L. Activated CD69+ T Cells Foster Immune Privilege by Regulating IDO Expression in Tumor-Associated Macrophages. *J. Immunol.* **2012**, *188*, 1117–1124. [CrossRef] [PubMed]
278. Hughes, R.; Qian, B.-Z.; Rowan, C.; Muthana, M.; Keklikoglou, I.; Olson, O.C.; Tazzyman, S.; Danson, S.; Addison, C.; Clemons, M.; et al. Perivascular M2 Macrophages Stimulate Tumor Relapse after Chemotherapy. *Cancer Res.* **2015**, *75*, 3479–3491. [CrossRef] [PubMed]
279. Olson, O.C.; Kim, H.; Quail, D.F.; Foley, E.A.; Joyce, J.A. Tumor-Associated Macrophages Suppress the Cytotoxic Activity of Antimitotic Agents. *Cell Rep.* **2017**, *19*, 101–113. [CrossRef] [PubMed]
280. De Palma, M.; Lewis, C.E. Macrophage regulation of tumor responses to anticancer therapies. *Cancer Cell* **2013**, *23*, 277–286. [CrossRef] [PubMed]

281. Arlauckas, S.P.; Garris, C.S.; Kohler, R.H.; Kitaoka, M.; Cuccarese, M.F.; Yang, K.S.; Miller, M.A.; Carlson, J.C.; Freeman, G.J.; Anthony, R.M.; et al. In vivo imaging reveals a tumor-associated macrophage-mediated resistance pathway in anti-PD-1 therapy. *Sci. Transl. Med.* **2017**, *9*. [CrossRef] [PubMed]
282. Noman, M.Z.; Desantis, G.; Janji, B.; Hasmim, M.; Karray, S.; Dessen, P.; Bronte, V.; Chouaib, S. PD-L1 is a novel direct target of HIF-1α, and its blockade under hypoxia enhanced MDSC-mediated T cell activation. *J. Exp. Med.* **2014**, *211*, 781–790. [CrossRef] [PubMed]
283. Gordon, S.R.; Maute, R.L.; Dulken, B.W.; Hutter, G.; George, B.M.; McCracken, M.N.; Gupta, R.; Tsai, J.M.; Sinha, R.; Corey, D.; et al. PD-1 expression by tumour-associated macrophages inhibits phagocytosis and tumour immunity. *Nature* **2017**, *545*, 495–499. [CrossRef] [PubMed]
284. Russo, G.L.; Moro, M.; Sommariva, M.; Cancila, V.; Boeri, M.; Centonze, G.; Ferro, S.; Ganzinelli, M.; Gasparini, P.; Huber, V.; et al. Antibody-Fc/FcR Interaction on Macrophages as a Mechanism for Hyperprogressive Disease in Non-Small Cell Lung Cancer Subsequent to PD-1/PD-L1 Blockade. *Clin. Cancer Res.* **2018**. [CrossRef] [PubMed]

3

Lung Cancer Screening, towards a Multidimensional Approach: Why and How?

Jonathan Benzaquen [1,2], Jacques Boutros [1], Charles Marquette [1,2,*], Hervé Delingette [3] and Paul Hofman [2,4]

1 Department of Pulmonary Medicine and Oncology, Université Côte d'Azur, CHU de Nice, FHU OncoAge, 06100 Nice, France; benzaquen.j@chu-nice.fr (J.B.); boutros.j@chu-nice.fr (J.B.)
2 Institute of Research on Cancer and Ageing (IRCAN), Université Côte d'Azur, FHU OncoAge, CNRS, INSERM, 06107 Nice, France; hofman.p@chu-nice.fr
3 Asclepios Project Team, Sophia Antipolis-Mediterranee Research Centre, Université Côte d'Azur, FHU OncoAge, Inria, 06902 Sophia Antipolis, France; herve.delingette@inria.fr
4 Laboratory of Clinical and Experimental Pathology and Biobank BB-0033-00025, Université Côte d'Azur, FHU OncoAge, CHU de Nice, 06001 Nice, France
* Correspondence: marquette.c@chu-nice.fr

Abstract: Early-stage treatment improves prognosis of lung cancer and two large randomized controlled trials have shown that early detection with low-dose computed tomography (LDCT) reduces mortality. Despite this, lung cancer screening (LCS) remains challenging. In the context of a global shortage of radiologists, the high rate of false-positive LDCT results in overloading of existing lung cancer clinics and multidisciplinary teams. Thus, to provide patients with earlier access to life-saving surgical interventions, there is an urgent need to improve LDCT-based LCS and especially to reduce the false-positive rate that plagues the current detection technology. In this context, LCS can be improved in three ways: (1) by refining selection criteria (risk factor assessment), (2) by using Computer Aided Diagnosis (CAD) to make it easier to interpret chest CTs, and (3) by using biological blood signatures for early cancer detection, to both spot the optimal target population and help classify lung nodules. These three main ways of improving LCS are discussed in this review.

Keywords: lung cancer; artificial intelligence; screening

---

1. Introduction

Lung cancer (LC) is the leading cause of death from cancer, but early-stage treatment improves LC prognosis. The National Lung Screening Trial (NLST) demonstrated that annual LC screening (LCS) with low-dose computed tomography (LDCT) reduced mortality by 20% compared to controls [1] (Table 1). More recently, the Dutch–Belgian NELSON lung cancer screening trial presented in September 2018 at the International Association for the Study of Lung Cancer (IASLC) 19th World Conference on Lung Cancer (WCLC) in Toronto, Canada, showed reduced mortality by more than 25% in the LDCT arm compared to the control arm [2] (Table 1). Based on the NLST results, the United States Preventive Services Task Force (UPSTF) issued recommendations for LCS of people meeting the NLST criteria. The Centers for Medicare & Medicaid Services (CMS) decided to provide coverage for LCS in smokers aged 55 to 77 years with more than a 30-pack-years smoking history and who had not quit within the last 15 years [3,4]. Low-dose computed tomography is now the cornerstone of LCS in North America and Australia. Given the confirmatory results of the NELSON screening trial [2], it can be assumed that LDCT screening will be approved in Europe and that health authorities will very soon provide coverage for LDCT-based LCS [5,6], as for breast cancer (mammography) and colon cancer (colonoscopy). However, despite Medicare and Medicaid coverage, the take-up of LCS in the US remains very low (i.e., below 4%) [7–9]. The reasons for such a low take-up of LCS include: (1) patients not wanting screening (fatalism mentality in the elderly, stigma associated with LC, poor lifestyle choice); (2) patients' awareness (i.e., less than breast cancer screening); (3) physicians not referring (difficult recall of smoking history, controversies among primary care societies, controversies among health agencies); and (4) a high false-positive rate requiring cumbersome follow-up [8–10]. Among these reasons, some are related to the practicality of LCS. In this respect, the need for repeated imaging and downstream diagnostic evaluations related to a high false-positive rate of LDCT (ranging from 26 to 58%) [1,7] is responsible for needless anxiety of patients and their family. In the Veterans Health Affairs (VHA) study, up to 52% of the screened patients who did not have LC required downstream diagnostic procedures [7].

Table 1. Summary of the National Lung Screening Trial (NLST) and the NELSON trials.

	NLST	NELSON
Country	USA	BE/NL
Enrollment	2002–2004	2003–NR
Number of Centers	33	4
Number of screens Screening planned at years	 1, 2 and 3	3 1, 2 and 4
Comparison	LDCT vs. Xray	LDCT vs. usual care
Population Age Smoking (pack-years) Sex Years since quit Patients Screened, *n* Planned follow-up, y	 55–74 ≥30 both (male 59%) ≤15 26,722 vs. 26,732 >7	 50–69 (50–75) >15 * men ° (male 84%) ≤10 7907 vs. 7915 10
Nodule Size warranting Follow-up	2011 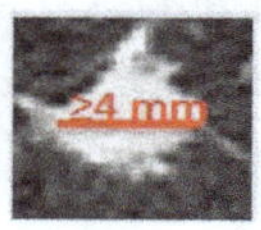	2009 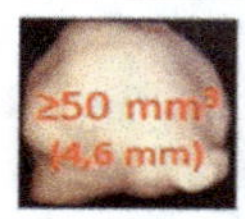 + VDT 2014 ≥100 mm^3 (≥5 mm) + VDT
LC diagnosed at screening, %	1.02	0.9
5 mm Reduction of LC mortality	20%	26% [a]

*, ≥15 cigarettes/day for 25 years or ≥10 cigarettes/day for 30 years; °, both in Belgium; VDT, volume doubling time; [a], in men.

The global shortage of radiologists facing a growing and aging population in Europe will quickly overload existing LC clinics and multidisciplinary teams. In addition, the high rate of false-positive results will lead to cumbersome follow-up and surveillance of incidental pulmonary nodules. Thus, there is urgent need to improve LDCT-based LCS, and especially to reduce the false-positive rate that plagues the current detection technology, to provide patients earlier access to life-saving intervention.

2. Lung Cancer Screening Can Be Improved

Lung cancer screening can be improved in several ways: (1) refine selection criteria (risk factor assessment); (2) use Computer-Aided Diagnosis (CAD) to make it easier to interpret chest CTs; (3) use biomarkers to detect early-stage LC, to spot the optimal target population or to help classify lung nodules; and (4) use highly sensitive bronchoscopic techniques to enhance the detection rate of central airway lesions.

2.1. Refine Selection Criteria to Improve the Effectiveness and Efficiency of Lung Cancer Screening

The following terms must be defined here: 1) screening effectiveness, which is the number needed to screen (NNS) per LC death prevented, and 2) screening efficiency, which is the number of false-positive results and downstream diagnostic procedures per LC death prevented (a surrogate of harm-to-benefit ratio).

Risk-based selection improved LCS effectiveness by 17% as compared to UPSTF screening criteria [11]. A similar conclusion was drawn by Caverly et al., who relied on the Bach risk model [12,13] in the VHA study and found an NNS per LC death prevented ranging from 687 in the highest risk quintile to 6903 in the lowest risk quintile [12]. Risk-based selection can also improve the LCS efficiency. In the VHA study, although the harm (overall rates of false positives requiring tracking or requiring downstream evaluations) did not differ between low- and high-risk quintiles, LCS was much more efficient in the high-risk quintile [7,12].

2.2. Use Computer Aided Diagnosis for Low-Dose Computed Tomography Interpretation to Facilitate Lung Cancer Screening and Lessen the False-Positive Rate

The interpretation of LDCT may be difficult in the setting of LCS. The simple algorithm design should be based on two questions surrounding the key lesion detected with LDCT (i.e., lung nodule): (1) "Does this individual have a nodule?" If the answer is "no", then he/she will be given an appointment for the next screening round; (2) if the answer is yes, then the second question is "Is this nodule cancerous?" Depending on its features, the nodule will be classified as malignant (M), benign (B), or indeterminate (I) (Figure 1). Figure 2 exemplifies the range of difficulties encountered by physicians of LC clinics in the setting of LCS. Lung cancer screening takes time when relying on LDCT alone. Indeed, most decision-making algorithms for lung nodules advocate a repeat CT to study the volume-doubling time (VDT), a datum which, combined with the morphology of the nodule, has the most determinant weight to decide whether or not to go to invasive procedures including surgery [14].

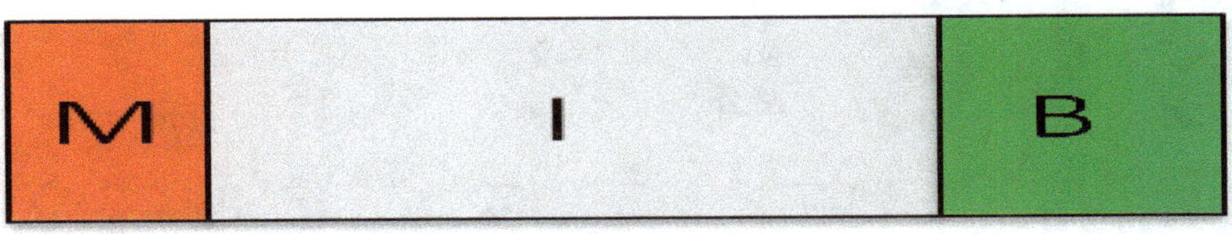

Figure 1. "I" nodules, the "grey zone" of lung cancer screening.

To exemplify the stress and anxiety generated by the discovery of a lung nodule, one can look at the VHA experience in which 56% of the nonmalignant nodules required tracking and took an average of more than a year for the patient to be reassured (or not) of the nature of their nodule.

Deep convolutional neural networks (CNNs) have been successfully developed in the field of medical image analysis over the past five years and can be specifically trained for lung nodule detection and reduction of false positivity. CAD systems for LCS involve two steps: (1) detection of pulmonary nodules (which often includes lung segmentation, nodule detection, and segmentation); and (2) diagnosis of their malignancy based on the analysis of a set of features, such as volume, shape, VDT, and density gradient of each nodule (Figure 3). Currently, there are many studies about the first step, but few about the second step [15,16]. Convolutional neural networks are trained on publicly available databases (Table 2) and then tested on different datasets.

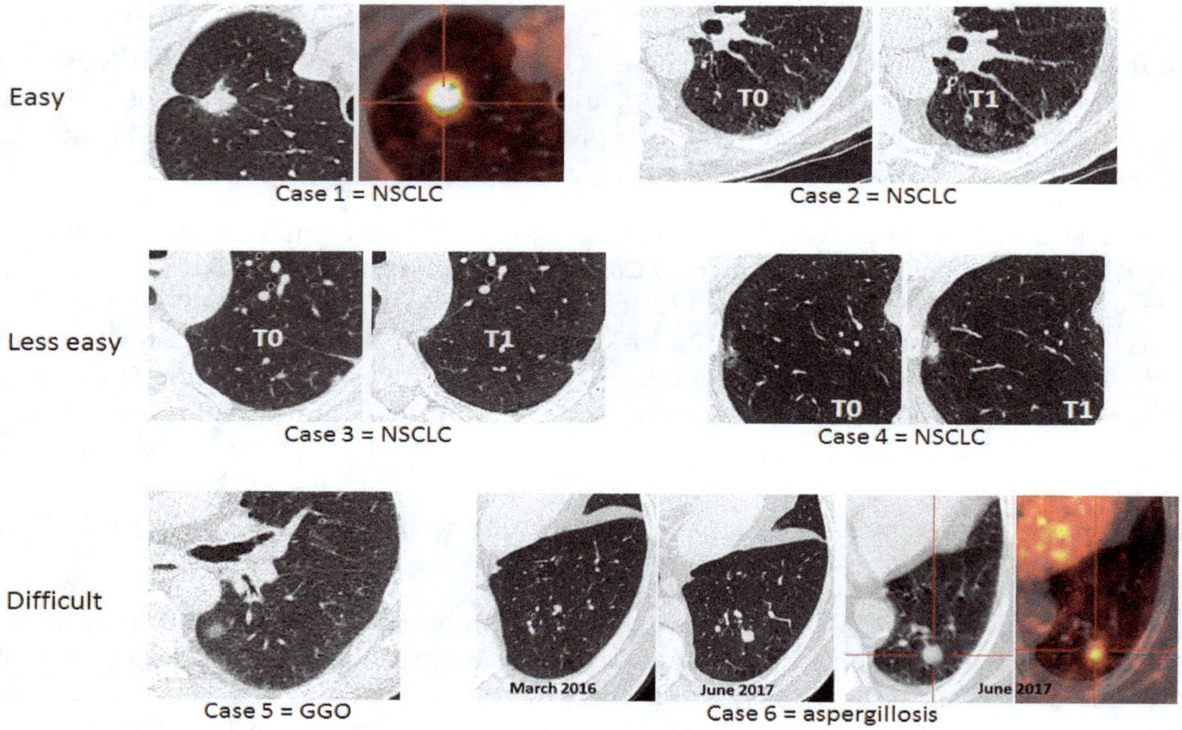

Figure 2. Six lung cancer screening cases illustrating to what extent interpretation of low-dose computed tomography may be difficult. NSCLC: non-small cell lung cancer; GGO: ground glass opacities.

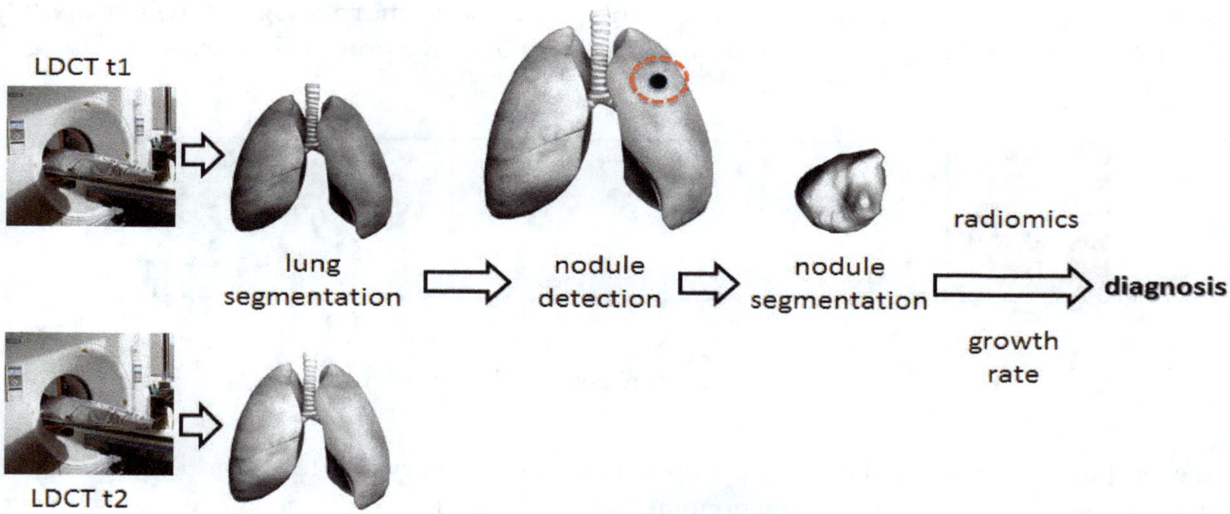

Figure 3. Architecture of computer-aided diagnosis systems for lung cancer screening. t1: first screening round. t2: follow-up.

Table 2. Publicly available databases for lung cancer screening.

	Kaggle	Luna16	NLST	COPDG Gene	LTRC
Number	1397	888	>1000	>1000	>1000
Date			2002–2004 to 2009	Start 2008	
Available without registration	Yes	Yes	No	No	No
COPD * cases				Yes	Yes
Ground truth	Cancer/no cancer one year after the CT scan	x, y, z coordinates and diameter of nodules			
Image data	Yes	Yes	Yes	Yes	Yes
Cohort level	"high-risk patient"		Age 55–74 >30 years smoking history <15 years since quitting	Age 45–80 >10 pack-years smoking history	"Most donor subjects have interstitial fibrotic lung disease or COPD" Average age 60
Individual level			Questionnaire: living condition, family history. Cancer diagnosis: location/tumor size	Subject phenotype: living condition, gender, medical history, comorbidities, physical characteristics ...	Clinical and pathological diagnoses, pulmonary function tests, living condition, exercises tests ...
Biological data			Lung tissues	SNP genotype	Blood and lung tissues

* Chronic obstructive pulmonary disease (COPD); CT: computed tomography; SNP: single nucleotide polymorphisms.

Training databases include: (1) chest CTs with annotated nodules, such as the Lung Nodule Analysis 2016 (LUNA16) dataset, which is a collection of 888 axial CT scans of the patients' chest cavities taken from the Lung Image Database Consortium image collection (LIDC/IDRI) database [17]; in total, 1186 nodules were annotated across 601 patients; and (2) chest CTs labeled as "with cancer" if the associated patient was diagnosed with cancer within one year of the scan, and "without cancer" otherwise. Once trained, the CNN output provided a probability of malignancy between 0 and 1 (Figure 4).

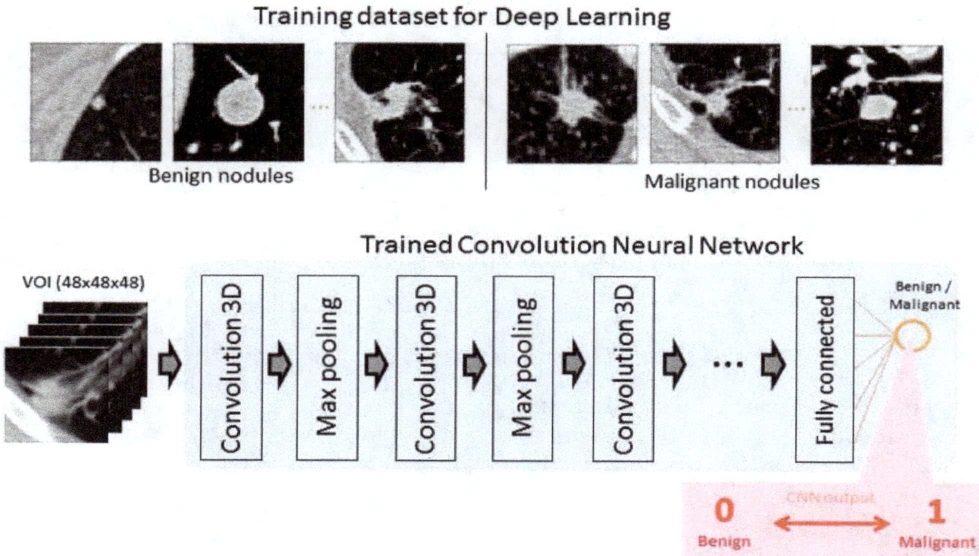

Figure 4. Training CNN for lung cancer screening.

The 2017 Kaggle Data Science Bowl was a critical milestone in support of the National Cancer Institute Cancer Moonshot by convening the data science and medical communities to develop LCS algorithms [18]. Using a dataset of 2101 high-resolution lung scans provided by the National Cancer Institute and labeled as "with" or "without cancer", the 1972 competing teams have developed algorithms to accurately determine when lesions in the lungs were cancerous. Liao et al. won this 2017 Data Science Bowl by proposing the first volumetric end-to-end 3D CNN for 3D lung nodule detection and characterization with an AUC of 87% on the blinded test set [19].

2.3. *Use Blood Biomarkers in the Setting of Lung Cancer Screening*

Different tumor-derived components can be detected and isolated from blood samples, including circulating tumor cells (CTCs), circulating cell-free tumor DNA (cftDNA), cell-free tumor RNA (cftRNA), exosomes, and tumor-educated platelets (TEP) [20,21] (Figure 5). These components can be used as biomarkers: (1) to detect early stage LC; (2) to spot the optimal target population for LCS; or (3) to help classify indeterminate lung nodules.

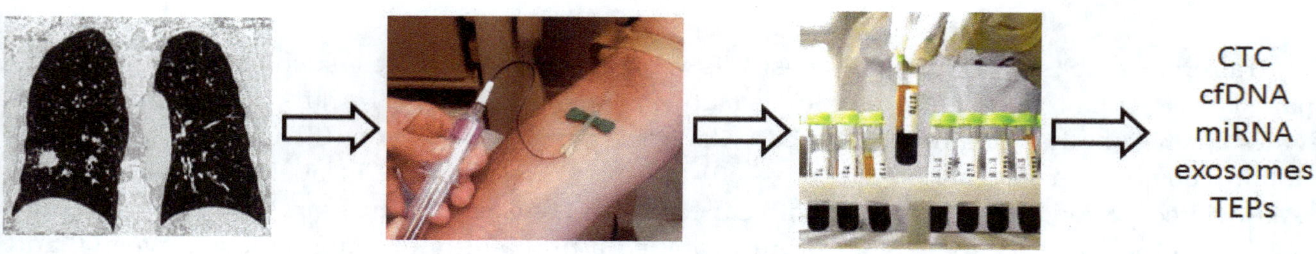

Figure 5. Tumor-derived components that can be used in the setting of lung cancer screening. TEP: tumor-educated platelets; miRNA: microRNA.

2.3.1. Biomarkers to Detect Early-Stage Lung Cancer

We previously showed that in high-risk patients (i.e., Chronic Obstructive Pulmonary Disease (COPD) and heavy smokers), circulating tumor cells (CTCs) detected with the isolation by size of epithelial tumor cell (ISET) technique (RARECELLS, Paris, France) could be detected in patients with COPD without clinically detectable LC up to four years before LC was identified on LDCT [22]. The CTCs detected had a heterogeneous expression of epithelial and mesenchymal markers, and some specific antigens (such as TTF1), which were similar to the corresponding phenotype of the lung tumor [23]. No CTCs were detected in control smoking and nonsmoking healthy individuals. From these preliminary results, we demonstrated for the first time that in high-risk patients, CTCs can be detected very early in the course of LC. We therefore launched a national prospective cohort study (the AIR study) to assess the role of CTCs in LCS in a high-risk population, that is, patients with COPD, heavy smokers, and >55-year-old patients (NCT02500693) [24].

In addition to CTCs, a more or less complex signature of the plasma microRNA (miRNA) has been shown to be associated with localized or metastatic LC [25–27]. More recently, studies have been performed on populations with a high risk of developing LC but without a known cancer. In particular, Sozzi et al. identified a signature of plasma microRNAs that showed an excellent predictive value for LC in a high-risk population [28]. In this latter study, the authors showed that the addition of a 24-microRNA signature classifier (MSC) to LDCT could raise LC detection sensitivity to 98% [28].

Montani et al. identified an LC-predictive signature of 13 microRNAs for high-risk individuals with a sensitivity of 77.8% and a negative predictive value greater than 99%, similar to LDCT test performance, suggesting the eventuality to use first miRNA tests in this population of patients [29].

In addition to CTC and miRNA, Cohen et al. described the CancerSEEK test, which utilizes combined assays for genetic alterations (mutation present in plasma circulating tumor DNA) and protein biomarkers. Not only does this test have the capacity to identify the presence of stage I to III cancers of the ovary, liver, stomach, pancreas, esophagus, colo-rectum, lung, or breast, but also to localize the organ of origin of these cancers [30].

Although still exploratory, gene expression profiling in the respiratory epithelium may help assess LC risk in the setting of detection of early-stage LC. Indeed, there is some evidence that nontumor adjacent cells share some molecular characteristics with tumor cells. In this context, it has been recently demonstrated that most genetic alterations expressed in smoker patients are not only found in bronchial but also in the nasal epithelium [31]. Thus, LC-associated gene expression assessment in nontumor respiratory epithelium may represent a promising field of development to optimize LC risk evaluation and, thus, to better understand its pathogenesis [31].

2.3.2. Biomarkers to Identify High-Risk Individuals and to Spot the Optimal Target Population for Lung Cancer Screening

Several markers were investigated in large prospective LCS programs, such as the Continuous Observation of Smoking Subjects (COSMOS) and the Multicenter Italian Lung Detection (MILD) trial; in interventional programs, such as the Carotene and Retinol Efficacy Trial (CARET); and in observational cohorts, such as the European Prospective Investigation into Cancer and Nutrition (EPIC) and the Northern Sweden Health and Disease Study (NSHDS) [28,29,32]. The miRNA signature [28,29] and serum proteins [32] were evaluated and performed well in determining a risk score for developing LC.

Other investigations, such as methylation of free plasma DNA, are potential options for identifying individuals at high risk of developing LC [33–38] but still need to be evaluated in validation studies.

2.3.3. Biomarkers to Help Classify Indeterminate Lung Nodules

Appropriate management of indeterminate lung nodules is one of the key factors of success in LCS implementation. Several biological signatures have been studied or are under investigation to help classify indeterminate lung nodules. Among them, plasma protein biomarkers combined with clinical risk factors (age, smoking history, nodule diameter, nodule edge characteristics, and nodule location) in an "integrated classifier" performed well in identifying benign nodules among nodules classified as indeterminate [39].

The presence of serum antibodies to a panel of seven LC-associated antigens distinguished malignant from benign nodules in a prospective registry [40]. In this study, patients harboring a 4–20 mm lung nodule with a positive antibodies panel test (EarlyCDT-Lung Test, (ECLS), Oncimmune, De Sotto, MO, USA) had a twofold increased relative risk to develop an LC than patients with a negative test [40]. A combined strategy using ECLS test and risk model integration showed a high specificity (>92%) and a positive predictive value of >70% for LC detection. The capacity of this tumor-associated antigen test, combined with LDCT, to reduce the incidence of late-stage LC at presentation is presently being investigated in a randomized controlled trial [41]. This interventional study includes 12,000 Scottish patients, aged 50–75 years, current or former smokers (with at least 20 pack-years or with less than 20 pack-years plus a family history of LC), tested with ECLS, X-ray chest, and CT scan, and with a follow-up of 24 months [41].

Other immune biological signatures, such as C4d-specific antibodies, have been investigated to diagnose indeterminate lung nodules and showed equivocal results [42].

Finally, a prespecified miRNA signature showed its ability to distinguish LC from the large majority of benign LDCT-detected pulmonary nodules. The combination of MSC/LDCT could reduce LC false-positive rate detection fivefold (19.7% vs. 3.7% for LDCT and MSC/LDCT, respectively) [28].

2.4. Highly Sensitive Bronchoscopic Techniques to Enhance the Detection Rate of Central Airway Lesions

Low-dose computed tomography has a very low detection rate for central airway lesions that are more commonly squamous cell carcinomas (SqCC) and for preinvasive lesions. Therefore, enhancing LDCT detection rate using bronchoscopic techniques, such as autofluorescence bronchoscopy (AFB), narrow band imaging, or high magnification bronchovideoscopy, can be promising [43]. Some authors have incorporated endoscopic techniques in LCS strategies. McWilliams et al. showed promising results when combining sputum atypia with LDCT and AFB [44,45]. The benefit of combining AFB with LDCT in LCS was not confirmed in the large-scale trial performed by Tremblay et al. [46] in which AFB detected too few CT-occult cancers, and thus failed to show any benefit in high-LC-risk patient screening. Furthermore, due to the decreasing incidence of SqCC, and its precursors, that is, dysplasias and SqCC in situ, relative to adenocarcinoma, and in the absence of a clear survival benefit to detecting precancerous central airway lesions, AFB does not seem to have a place in today's LCS strategies [47].

3. Deep Learning for Early Cancer Detection

As yet, in the setting of early cancer diagnosis, deep learning has essentially been applied to chest imaging interpretation. However, the complexity of the approach of deep learning techniques can now be considered, as soon as one simultaneously analyzes parameters that appear to be completely independent. For instance, when developing their CancerSEEK test, Cohen et al. used supervised machine learning to predict the underlying cancer type. The input algorithm took into account the circulating tumor DNA (ctDNA) and protein biomarker levels as well as the gender of the patient [29].

4. Conclusions

It can be reasonably assumed that very soon, European health authorities will provide coverage for LDCT-based LCS. This, added to the global shortage of radiologists, will result in a large number of anxious patients with "indeterminate lung nodules" overloading lung clinics, waiting for repeat chest imaging and invasive tests to obtain a definite answer.

In this context, we strongly believe that there is room for using, as a first reading approach, a CNN-driven LDCT with a predefined detection threshold to label all "nodule-free" examinations as reassuring, and then to incorporate the trilogy of chest imaging, risk factors, and biological signatures into machine learning algorithms to classify the nodules that have been detected according to the level of suspicion. For health care professionals, CNNs are often considered as a black box. Thus, to avoid this pitfall, one will also have to demystify the decision tree and to report on the respective weight of each clinical, radiological, and biological input that led to nodule classification (Figure 6).

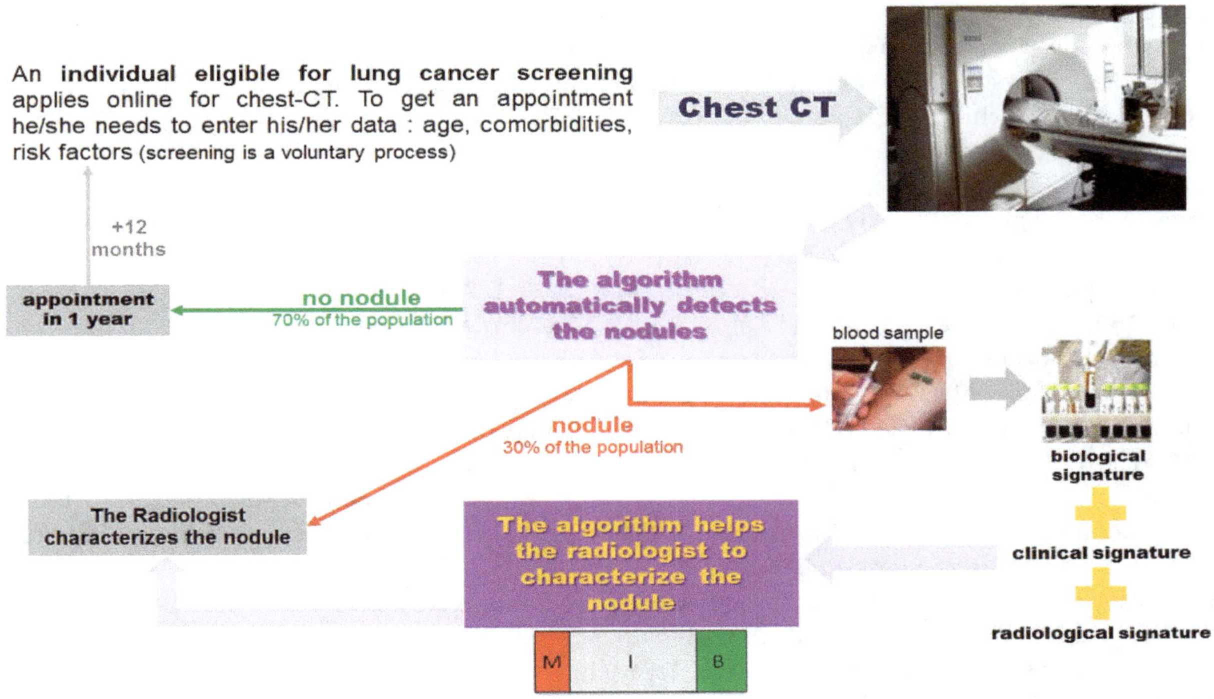

Figure 6. Workflow of lung cancer screening.

References

1. National Lung Screening Trial Research Team; Aberle, D.R.; Adams, A.M.; Berg, C.D.; Black, W.C.; Clapp, J.D.; Fagerstrom, R.M.; Gareen, I.F.; Gatsonis, C.; Marcus, P.M.; et al. Reduced lung-cancer mortality with low-dose computed tomographic screening. *N. Engl. J. Med.* **2011**, *365*, 395–409. [CrossRef] [PubMed]
2. De Koning, H.J.; Van Der Aalst, C.M.; Ten Haaf, K.; Oudkerk, M. PL02.05. Effects of Volume CT Lung Cancer Screening: Mortality Results of the NELSON Randomised-Controlled Population Based Trial. *J. Thorac. Oncol.* **2018**, *13*, S185. [CrossRef]
3. Moyer, V.A.; On behalf of U.S. Preventive Services Task Force. Screening for lung cancer: U.S. preventive services task force recommendation statement. *Ann. Intern. Med.* **2014**, *160*, 330–338. [CrossRef] [PubMed]
4. CMS.gov. Available online: https://www.cms.gov/medicare-coverage-database/details/nca-decision-memo.aspx?NCAId=274 (accessed on 3 February 2019).
5. Oudkerk, M.; Devaraj, A.; Vliegenthart, R.; Henzler, T.; Prosch, H.; Heussel, C.P.; Bastarrika, G.; Sverzellati, N.; Mascalchi, M.; Delorme, S.; et al. European position statement on lung cancer screening. *Lancet Oncol.* **2017**, *18*, e754–e766. [CrossRef]
6. IASLC. Available online: https://www.iaslc.org/news/iaslc-issues-statement-lung-cancer-screening-low-dose-computed-tomography?fbclid=IwAR3LdKR99ek3D2cGKlII4fA8s7IcaW6jhefdxHSYVPJAgkYn1ER8RW0MWOk (accessed on 3 February 2019).
7. Kinsinger, L.S.; Anderson, C.; Kim, J.; Larson, M.; Chan, S.H.; King, H.A.; Rice, K.L.; Slatore, C.G.; Tanner, N.T.; Pittman, K.; et al. Implementation of lung cancer screening in the Veterans Health Administration. *JAMA Intern. Med.* **2017**, *177*, 399–406. [CrossRef]
8. Pham, D.; Bhandari, S.; Oechsli, M.; Pinkston, C.M.; Kloecker, G.H. Lung cancer screening rates: Data from the lung cancer screening registry. *J. Clin. Oncol.* **2018**, *36*, 6504. [CrossRef]
9. Tonge, J.E.; Atack, M.; Crosbie, P.A.; Barber, P.V.; Booton, R.; Colligan, D. "To know or not to know ... ?" Push and pull in ever smokers lung screening uptake decision-making intentions. *Health Expect.* **2018**, *13*, S968. [CrossRef]

10. Haute Autorité de Santé. Available online: https://www.has-sante.fr/portail/jcms/c_2001613/fr/pertinence-du-depistage-du-cancer-broncho-pulmonaire-en-france-point-de-situation-sur-les-donnees-disponibles-analyse-critique-des-etudes-controlees-randomisees (accessed on 3 February 2019).
11. Katki, H.A.; Kovalchik, S.A.; Berg, C.D.; Cheung, L.C.; Chaturvedi, A.K. Development and validation of risk models to select ever-smokers for ct lung cancer screening. *JAMA J. Am. Med. Assoc.* **2016**, *315*, 2300–2311. [CrossRef]
12. Caverly, T.J.; Fagerlin, A.; Wiener, R.S.; Slatore, C.G.; Tanner, N.T.; Yun, S.; Hayward, R. Comparison of Observed Harms and Expected Mortality Benefit for Persons in the Veterans Health Affairs Lung Cancer Screening Demonstration Project. *JAMA Intern. Med.* **2018**, *178*, 426–428. [CrossRef]
13. Bach, P.B.; Elkin, E.B.; Pastorino, U.; Kattan, M.W.; Mushlin, A.I.; Begg, C.B.; Parkin, D.M. Benchmarking lung cancer mortality rates in current and former smokers. *Chest* **2004**, *126*, 1742–1749. [CrossRef]
14. Wood, D.E.; Kazerooni, E.A.; Baum, S.L.; Eapen, G.A.; Ettinger, D.S.; Hou, L.; Jackman, D.M.; Klippenstein, D.; Kumar, R.; Lackner, R.P.; et al. Lung cancer screening, version 3.2018. *JNCCN J. Natl. Compr. Cancer Netw.* **2018**, *16*, 412–441. [CrossRef] [PubMed]
15. El-Baz, A.; Beache, G.M.; Gimel'Farb, G.; Suzuki, K.; Okada, K.; Elnakib, A.; Soliman, A.; Abdollahi, B. Computer-aided diagnosis systems for lung cancer: Challenges and methodologies. *Int. J. Biomed. Imaging* **2013**, *2013*, 942353. [CrossRef] [PubMed]
16. Murphy, A.; Skalski, M.; Gaillard, F. The utilisation of convolutional neural networks in detecting pulmonary nodules: A review. *Br. J. Radiol.* **2018**, *91*, 20180028. [CrossRef] [PubMed]
17. Armato, S.G., 3rd; McLennan, G.; Bidaut, L.; McNitt-Gray, M.F.; Meyer, C.R.; Reeves, A.P.; Zhao, B.; Aberle, D.R.; Henschke, C.I.; Hoffman, E.A.; et al. The Lung Image Database Consortium (LIDC) and Image Database Resource Initiative (IDRI): A completed reference database of lung nodules on CT scans. *Med. Phys.* **2011**, *38*, 915–931. [CrossRef] [PubMed]
18. Kaggle. Kaggle Data Science Bowl 2017. 2017. Available online: https://www.kaggle.com/www.kaggle.com (accessed on 3 February 2019).
19. Liao, F.; Liang, M.; Li, Z.; Hu, X.; Song, S. Evaluate the Malignancy of Pulmonary Nodules Using the 3D Deep Leaky Noisy-or Network. *IEEE Trans. Cybern.* **2017**, *14*, 1–12.
20. Santarpia, M.; Liguori, A.; D'Aveni, A.; Karachaliou, N.; Gonzalez-Cao, M.; Daffinà, M.G.; Lazzari, C.; Altavilla, G.; Rosell, R. Liquid biopsy for lung cancer early detection. *J. Thorac. Dis.* **2018**, *10*, S882–S897. [CrossRef] [PubMed]
21. Hofman, P. Liquid biopsy for early detection of lung cancer. *Curr. Opin. Oncol.* **2017**, *29*, 73–78. [CrossRef]
22. Ilie, M.; Hofman, V.; Long-Mira, E.; Selva, E.; Vignaud, J.M.; Padovani, B.; Mouroux, J.; Marquette, C.H.; Hofman, P. "Sentinel" circulating tumor cells allow early diagnosis of lung cancer in patients with Chronic obstructive pulmonary disease. *PLoS ONE* **2014**, *9*, e111597. [CrossRef]
23. Hofman, V.J.; Ilie, M.; Hofman, P.M. Detection and characterization of circulating tumor cells in lung cancer: Why and how? *Cancer Cytopathol.* **2016**, *124*, 380–387. [CrossRef]
24. Leroy, S.; Benzaquen, J.; Mazzetta, A.; Marchand-Adam, S.; Padovani, B.; Israel-Biet, D.; Pison, C.; Chanez, P.; Cadranel, J.; Mazières, J.; et al. Circulating tumour cells as a potential screening tool for lung cancer (the AIR study): Protocol of a prospective multicentre cohort study in France. *BMJ Open* **2017**, *7*, e018884. [CrossRef]
25. Wozniak, M.B.; Scelo, G.; Muller, D.C.; Mukeria, A.; Zaridze, D.; Brennan, P. Circulating MicroRNAs as Non-Invasive Biomarkers for Early Detection of Non-Small-Cell Lung Cancer. *PLoS ONE* **2015**, *10*, e0125026. [CrossRef] [PubMed]
26. Sanfiorenzo, C.; Ilie, M.I.; Belaid, A.; Barlési, F.; Mouroux, J.; Marquette, C.H.; Brest, P.; Hofman, P. Two Panels of Plasma MicroRNAs as Non-Invasive Biomarkers for Prediction of Recurrence in Resectable NSCLC. *PLoS ONE* **2013**, *8*, e54596. [CrossRef] [PubMed]
27. Boeri, M.; Verri, C.; Conte, D.; Roz, L.; Modena, P.; Facchinetti, F.; Calabro, E.; Croce, C.M.; Pastorino, U.; Sozzi, G. MicroRNA signatures in tissues and plasma predict development and prognosis of computed tomography detected lung cancer. *Proc. Natl. Acad. Sci. USA* **2011**, *108*, 3713–3718. [CrossRef] [PubMed]
28. Sozzi, G.; Boeri, M.; Rossi, M.; Verri, C.; Suatoni, P.; Bravi, F.; Roz, L.; Conte, D.; Grassi, M.; Sverzellati, N.; et al. Clinical utility of a plasma-based miRNA signature classifier within computed tomography lung cancer screening: A correlative MILD trial study. *J. Clin. Oncol.* **2014**, *32*, 768–773. [CrossRef] [PubMed]

29. Montani, F.; Marzi, M.J.; Dezi, F.; Dama, E.; Carletti, R.M.; Bonizzi, G.; Bertolotti, R.; Bellomi, M.; Rampinelli, C.; Maisonneuve, P.; et al. MiR-test: A blood test for lung cancer early detection. *J. Natl. Cancer Inst.* **2015**, *107*, djv063. [CrossRef]
30. Cohen, J.D.; Li, L.; Wang, Y.; Thoburn, C.; Afsari, B.; Danilova, L.; Douville, C.; Javed, A.A.; Wong, F.; Mattox, A.; et al. Detection and localization of surgically resectable cancers with a multi-analyte blood test. *Science* **2018**, *359*, 926–930. [CrossRef] [PubMed]
31. Billatos, E.; Vick, J.L.; Lenburg, M.E.; Spira, A.E. The airway transcriptome as a biomarker for early lung cancer detection. *Clin. Cancer Res.* **2018**, *24*, 2984–2992. [CrossRef] [PubMed]
32. Guida, F.; Sun, N.; Bantis, L.E.; Muller, D.C.; Li, P.; Taguchi, A.; Dhillon, D.; Kundnani, D.L.; Patel, N.J.; Yan, Q.; et al. and the Integrative Analysis of Lung Cancer Etiology and Risk (INTEGRAL) Consortium for Early Detection of Lung Cancer. Assessment of Lung Cancer Risk on the Basis of a Biomarker Panel of Circulating Proteins. *JAMA Oncol.* **2018**, *4*, e182078. [CrossRef] [PubMed]
33. Jiang, T.; Ren, S.; Zhou, C. Role of circulating-tumor DNA analysis in non-small cell lung cancer. *Lung Cancer* **2015**, *90*, 128–134. [CrossRef] [PubMed]
34. Lehmann-Werman, R.; Neiman, D.; Zemmour, H.; Moss, J.; Magenheim, J.; Vaknin-Dembinsky, A.; Rubertsson, S.; Nellgård, B.; Blennow, K.; Zetterberg, H.; et al. Identification of tissue-specific cell death using methylation patterns of circulating DNA. *Proc. Natl. Acad. Sci. USA* **2016**, *113*, E1826–E1834. [CrossRef] [PubMed]
35. Tomasetti, M.; Amati, M.; Neuzil, J.; Santarelli, L. Circulating epigenetic biomarkers in lung malignanciesFrom early diagnosis to therapy. *Lung Cancer* **2017**, *107*, 65–72. [CrossRef] [PubMed]
36. Levine, M.E.; Hosgood, H.D.; Chen, B.; Absher, D.; Assimes, T.; Horvath, S. DNA methylation age of blood predicts future onset of lung cancer in the women's health initiative. *Aging* **2015**, *7*, 690–700. [CrossRef] [PubMed]
37. Warton, K.; Samimi, G. Methylation of cell-free circulating DNA in the diagnosis of cancer. *Front. Mol. Biosci.* **2015**, *2*, 13. [CrossRef] [PubMed]
38. Hulbert, A.; Jusue-Torres, I.; Stark, A.; Chen, C.; Rodgers, K.; Lee, B.; Griffin, C.; Yang, A.; Huang, P.; Wrangle, J.; et al. Early detection of lung cancer using DNA promoter hypermethylation in plasma and sputum. *Clin. Cancer Res.* **2017**, *23*, 1998–2005. [CrossRef] [PubMed]
39. Silvestri, G.A.; Tanner, N.T.; Kearney, P.; Vachani, A.; Massion, P.P.; Porter, A.; Springmeyer, S.C.; Fang, K.C.; Midthun, D.; Mazzone, P.J. and PANOPTIC Trial Team. Assessment of Plasma Proteomics Biomarker's Ability to Distinguish Benign from Malignant Lung Nodules: Results of the PANOPTIC (Pulmonary Nodule Plasma Proteomic Classifier) Trial. *Chest* **2018**, *154*, 491–500. [CrossRef] [PubMed]
40. Massion, P.P.; Healey, G.F.; Peek, L.J.; Fredericks, L.; Sewell, H.F.; Murray, A.; Robertson, J.F.R. Autoantibody Signature Enhances the Positive Predictive Power of Computed Tomography and Nodule-Based Risk Models for Detection of Lung Cancer. *J. Thorac. Oncol.* **2017**, *12*, 578–584. [CrossRef] [PubMed]
41. Sullivan, F.M.; Farmer, E.; Mair, F.S.; Treweek, S.; Kendrick, D.; Jackson, C.; Robertson, C.; Briggs, A.; McCowan, C.; Bedford, L.; et al. Detection in blood of autoantibodies to tumour antigens as a case-finding method in lung cancer using the EarlyCDT®-Lung Test (ECLS): Study protocol for a randomized controlled trial. *BMC Cancer* **2017**, *17*, 187. [CrossRef] [PubMed]
42. Ajona, D.; Okrój, M.; Pajares, M.J.; Agorreta, J.; Lozano, M.D.; Zulueta, J.J.; Verri, C.; Roz, L.; Sozzi, G.; Pastorino, U.; et al. Complement C4d-specific antibodies for the diagnosis of lung cancer. *Oncotarget* **2018**, *9*, 6346–6355. [CrossRef]
43. Andolfi, M.; Potenza, R.; Capozzi, R.; Liparulo, V.; Puma, F.; Yasufuku, K. The role of bronchoscopy in the diagnosis of early lung cancer: A review. *J. Thorac. Dis.* **2016**, *8*, 3329–3337. [CrossRef]
44. McWilliams, A.; Mayo, J.; MacDonald, S.; leRiche, J.C.; Palcic, B.; Szabo, E. Lung Cancer Screening. *Am. J. Respir. Crit. Care Med.* **2003**, *168*, 1167–1173. [CrossRef]
45. McWilliams, A.M.; Mayo, J.R.; Ahn, M.I.; MacDonald, S.L.S.; Lam, S.C. Lung cancer screening using multi-slice thin-section computed tomography and autofluorescence bronchoscopy. *J. Thorac. Oncol.* **2006**, *1*, 61–68. [CrossRef] [PubMed]

46. Tremblay, A.; Taghizadeh, N.; McWilliams, A.M.; MacEachern, P.; Stather, D.R.; Soghrati, K.; Puksa, S.; Goffin, J.R.; Yasufuku, K.; Amjadi, K.; et al. Low Prevalence of High-Grade Lesions Detected with Autofluorescence Bronchoscopy in the Setting of Lung Cancer Screening in the Pan-Canadian Lung Cancer Screening Study. *Chest* **2016**, *150*, 1015–1022. [CrossRef] [PubMed]
47. Epelbaum, O.; Aronow, W.S. Autofluorescence bronchoscopy for lung cancer screening: A time to reflect. *Ann. Transl. Med.* **2016**, *4*. [CrossRef] [PubMed]

4

MicroRNAs and Long Non-Coding RNAs and their Hormone-Like Activities in Cancer

Barbara Pardini [1,2,3,*] **and George A. Calin** [1,4,5,*]

1 Department of Experimental Therapeutics, The University of Texas MD Anderson Cancer Center, Houston, 1515 Holcombe Boulevard, Unit 422, Houston, TX 77030, USA
2 Department of Medical Sciences, University of Turin, Turin 10126, Italy
3 Italian Institute for Genomic Medicine (IIGM), Turin 10126, Italy
4 Center for RNA Interference and Non-Coding RNAs, The University of Texas MD Anderson Cancer Center, Houston, TX 77030, USA
5 Department of Leukemia, The University of Texas MD Anderson Cancer Center, Houston, TX 77030, USA
* Correspondence: BPardini@mdanderson.org (B.P.); gcalin@mdanderson.org (G.A.C.)

Abstract: Hormones are messengers circulating in the body that interact with specific receptors on the cell membrane or inside the cells and regulate, at a distal site, the activities of specific target organs. The definition of hormone has evolved in the last years. Hormones are considered in the context of cell–cell communication and mechanisms of cellular signaling. The best-known mechanisms of this kind are chemical receptor-mediated events, the cell–cell direct interactions through synapses, and, more recently, the extracellular vesicle (EV) transfer between cells. Recently, it has been extensively demonstrated that EVs are used as a way of communication between cells and that they are transporters of specific messenger signals including non-coding RNAs (ncRNAs) such as microRNAs (miRNAs) and long non-coding RNAs (lncRNAs). Circulating ncRNAs in body fluids and extracellular fluid compartments may have endocrine hormone-like effects because they can act at a distance from secreting cells with widespread consequences within the recipient cells. Here, we discuss and report examples of the potential role of miRNAs and lncRNAs as mediator for intercellular communication with a hormone-like mechanism in cancer.

Keywords: non-coding RNAs; microRNAs; long non-coding RNAs; hormones; hormone-like action

---

1. Introduction

The term "hormone" was first introduced in 1905 by Starling, referring to the discovery of secretin [1]. A hormone is a chemical messenger (in general, a peptide or a steroid) produced by the endocrine glands and circulating in the body to regulate the activities of specific target organs at a distal site [2,3]. The mode of action of hormones requires an interaction of these chemical messengers with specific receptors located on the cell membrane or inside the cell. The binding hormone-receptor generates a signaling cascade that modifies cellular activity [4]. The definition of hormones is quite restrictive since not all hormones are originated from endocrine glands, with many of them acting locally via autocrine/paracrine regulation. Specialized cells in various other organs also secrete hormones in response to specific biochemical signals from a wide range of regulatory systems. Serum/calcium concentration, for instance, affects parathyroid hormone synthesis while serum glucose concentration affects insulin synthesis. In addition, since the outputs of the stomach and exocrine pancreas become the input of the small intestine, the small intestine itself secretes hormones to stimulate/inhibit the stomach and pancreas in accordance to how busy it is, in a regulated feedback known more generally as "diffuse endocrine system" [5]. In a broader view, hormones are considered in the cell–cell communication context and in mechanisms of cellular signaling [2,3]. The best-known mechanisms of this kind are chemical receptor-mediated events, the cell–cell direct interactions through synapses, and, more recently, the extracellular vesicle (EV) transfer between cells [6]. EVs are small membrane-enclosed structures produced by different mechanisms that can be secreted from almost all cell types [7,8] in a process evolutionary conserved from bacteria to humans [9]. Each cell type is able to turn on EV biogenesis depending on the physiological states and, also, the EV cargo components can be highly regulated [10]. EVs, such as exosomes and microvesicles, represent the way donor cells communicate with recipient cells and influence their gene expression [11]. In the last years, it has been extensively demonstrated that EVs are used as a way of communication between cells and that they are transporters of specific messenger signals. EVs are, in fact, enriched for specific proteins (as for example cytokines), lipids, messenger RNAs (mRNA), and non-coding RNAs (ncRNAs), such as microRNAs (miRNAs) and long non-coding RNAs (lncRNAs) [6,8,12]. The nature and abundance of EV content are related to the specific cell type, and are influenced by the physiopathological state of the donor cell [13]. The cell–cell communication mediated by RNAs included in EVs has been described for the first time by Valadi et al. in 2007: exosomes carried miRNAs and other RNAs from one cell to another and, when released in the target cell, were able to interact with the gene expression machinery to modify the gene expression profile of the recipient cell [6].

EVs result as an alternative mode of communication between neighboring and distant cells. Respect to conventional mechanisms of cell communication, EVs differ because of specific temporal and spatial properties and mostly because of the potentiality to group multiple signals together [14].

2. miRNAs and Their Hormone-Like Activity in Cancer

The advances in high-throughput sequencing technology and bioinformatics have revolutionized ncRNA discovery [15]. Mammalian genomes are highly transcribed and the majority of the transcripts do not code for proteins. However, this high rate of transcription is not done in an indiscriminate way: the cellular repertoire of ncRNAs includes small housekeeping RNAs (such as ribosomal RNAs (rRNAs) and transfer RNAs (tRNAs)), as well as miRNAs and lncRNAs [16].

miRNAs are a class of single-stranded ncRNAs that play a critical role in the negative regulation of gene expression at post-transcriptional level [17]. Thousands of miRNAs have been identified in all eukaryotes and, so far, the latest version of miRBase (release 22 March 2018) accounts for over 38,000 miRNA gene loci in 271 species. In animal cells, miRNAs pair, in a complementary manner, with the 3′UTR of target mRNAs, inhibiting their translation or inducing their degradation [17]. miRNAs are crucial regulators in a wide range of biological processes but they are also implicated in human diseases, including cancer [16,18–20]. There are several lines of evidence that miRNAs are involved in endocrinology. It has been demonstrated that miRNAs can regulate directly genes encoding hormones or other enzymes involved in hormone maturation and metabolism. miRNAs can also target hormone antagonists or receptors indirectly modifying the hormone-mediated cell signaling transmission [21,22] or could be regulated by hormones either at the level of miRNA transcription and processing [23–25]. For instance, miR-21 and miR-181-b1 genes are expressed after *STAT3* induction, which is activated by interleukin 6 (IL-6) [26]. Moreover, miR-21 is repressed by thyroid hormone (TH) and this downregulation regulates *GRHL3*, a transcriptional inhibitor of type 3 iodothyronine deiodinase (D3) which, in turn, inactivates TH [27].

Recently, the role of miRNAs as mediators for intercellular communication with a hormone-like mechanism has also been established. miRNAs can work as autocrine, paracrine, and endocrine messengers. In fact, the classic mechanism of action of a miRNA is to be transcribed by a cell and induce local signaling on that same cell (autocrine signaling, Figure 1A). On the other hand, a miRNA can also transmit local signaling between nearby cells (paracrine signaling, Figure 1B) [8]. In cancer, the intercellular signaling mediated by miRNAs has been related to the tumor microenvironment (TME) setting or pre-metastatic niche induction [28–30]. An example of this kind of signaling in cancer is the one in which tumor-derived EVs containing miRNAs can directly modify tumor cell invasiveness and motility through modification of the TME [31,32]. Moreover, it has been observed that the ectopic expression of miR-409 in normal prostate fibroblasts conferred a cancer-associated stroma-like phenotype. The release of this miRNA via EVs was able to promote tumorigenesis and epithelial-to-mesenchymal transition (EMT) through repression of Ras suppressor 1 (*RUS1*) and stromal antigen 2 (*STAG2*), well-known tumor suppressors [33]. The discovery of miRNAs in extracellular fluids or loaded in EVs, such as exosomes, is the main evidence that miRNAs may act as paracrine and endocrine interactors [11,34]. EVs containing miRNAs can either work locally or distally via transport within the circulatory system. Moreover, miRNAs circulating within bodily fluids and extracellular fluid compartments may have an endocrine hormone-like effect because they can reach cells that are distant from the secreting cell, modifying their gene expression (Figure 1C) [34,35]. Once released, the EVs containing miRNAs can interact with a recipient cell, deliver its cargo to the cytosol, and modulate the phenotype of the target cell [36]. There is evidence that demonstrates that miRNAs in EVs can be taken up into neighboring or distant cells and modulate the function of those recipient cells in many physiological and pathological conditions [37–39]. For example, Le et al. demonstrated, in vitro and in vivo, that murine and human metastatic breast cancer cells release miR-200 family miRNAs to nonmetastatic cells via EVs. The transfer of these molecules altered gene expression in the recipient cells (which were lung cancer cells in the in vivo experiments) and promoted mesenchymal-to-epithelial transition [40]. Interestingly, the exosomal miRNA cargo occurs non-randomly and, also, the recipient cells are finely targeted, enforcing the idea of specific function for a single miRNA on a specific target [6,16]. miRNA species that are transported via EVs do not reflect the miRNA expression profiling of the donor cells [41,42] and, interestingly, several studies demonstrated that cancer patients have elevated levels of tumor-derived exosomes in plasma or serum compared with healthy controls [43–45]. The secretion of tumor-specific miRNAs via exosomes indicates the importance of this mechanism in influencing the surrounding microenvironment [34].

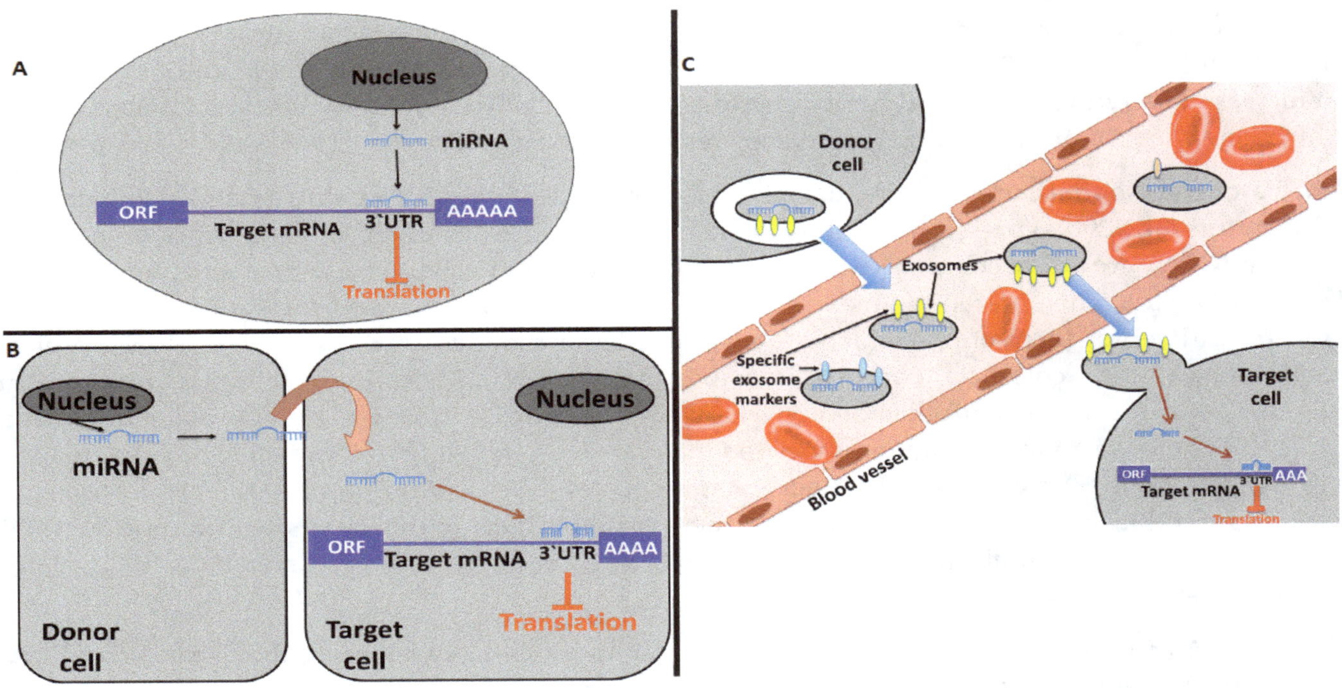

Figure 1. MicroRNAs (miRNAs) working in a hormone-like fashion. (**A**) Autocrine communication: a miRNA produced by a cell binds to autocrine receptors of the same cell inducing a local signaling. (**B**) Paracrine communication: a miRNA produced by a cell transmit a local signaling between nearby cells. (**C**) Endocrine communication: an extracellular vesicle (EV)-embedded miRNA is the mediator of distant signaling.

Functional interactions between cancer cells and the TME are mediated by small molecules such as cytokines and growth factors [46]. In addition, cancer cells may also transfer important functional information through paracrine communication via EVs [47]. EV cargo may actually influence the stroma by activating molecular pathways that differ from those mediated by soluble factors [8]. Therefore, tumor-derived EVs can alter the physiology of surrounding cells and distant non-tumor cells to facilitate cancer dissemination and growth [31].

The TME (which includes extracellular matrix, cancer-associated fibroblasts, tumor-associated macrophages, immune cells, and others) plays a crucial role in all steps of carcinogenesis [48]. Several examples of this biological information transfer between malignant cells and TME components via EV-transported miRNAs have been reviewed in a recent work by Bayraktar et al. [8]. For instance, Baroni et al. [49] found that in cancer-associated fibroblasts from triple-negative breast cancer patients, miR-9 was upregulated when compared with normal fibroblasts. Moreover, miR-9 was released by tumor cells and transferred via exosomes to normal fibroblasts recipients which, as a consequence, overexpressed this miRNA and increased their motility. Therefore, high expression of miR-9 in fibroblasts affects breast cancer progression [49]. Another example was described in the work of Chen et al. in which it was found that miR-940, released in exosomes by ovarian cancer cells, targeted tumor-associated macrophages and promoted tumor growth via the CD206 and CD163 pathways [50].

The assumption that a miRNA might work as a hormone or with a hormone-like mechanism implicates the possibility of the existence of a protein receptor for miRNAs (defined as miRceptor by [34]) and miRNA–protein interaction. The first study demonstrating miRNA–protein binding was published in 2010 by Eiring et al., where the authors provided evidence of steric binding between miR-328 and hnRNPE2 in blast crisis of chronic myelogenous leukemia. This "decoy activity" of miRNA prevents hnRNPE2 binding to *CEBPA* mRNA, thus restoring *C/EBPα* expression that further and directly enhances miR-328 transcription [51].

In 2012, it was demonstrated that EVs containing miR-21 and miR-29a released by non-small cell lung cancer cell lines were targeting tumor-associated macrophages and, more specifically, the human toll-like receptor 8 (*TLR8*), triggering the downstream pathway. As a result, authors observed an increased secretion of IL-6 and tumor necrosis factor-α (TNFα) by tumor-associated macrophages, which determines a pro-tumoral inflammatory response promoting cancer growth and metastasis [52].

Patel and Gooderham observed that IL-6 triggers the IL-6R/STAT3 pathway and also increases miR-21 and miR-29b expression in colorectal cancer cells. The authors proposed a model in which these miRNAs are released via exosomes and reach immune cells, where they interact with the TLR8 miRceptor. This interaction may induce an increase of IL-6 in a feed-forward loop involving miRNA–miRceptor interactions which are responsible for the increased secretion of IL-6, a typical phenomenon in the colorectal cancer microenvironment [53]. Interestingly, a similar mechanism has also been found in neuroblastoma. Endovesicular miR-21, released by neuroblastoma cells, binds to *TLR8* in surrounding tumor-associated macrophages, inducing in these cells the upregulation and the release in EVs of miR-155. Macrophage-derived EVs containing miR-155 are transferred back to neuroblastoma cells where miR-155 acts on its target, telomeric repeat-binding factor 1 (*TERF1*, a telomerase inhibitor). The silencing of *TERF1* induces increased resistance to cisplatin in neuroblastoma cells [54].

miRNAs released by exosomes and working in a hormone-like fashion could also be an optimal therapeutic target in the case of tumor drug resistance [55]. Wei et al., for example, demonstrated the role of exosomal miR-221/222 in the resistance to tamoxifen in breast cancer cells [56]. In another study, it was demonstrated that cancer-associated fibroblasts released exosomes containing miR-21, miR-378e, and miR-143-3p, that were able to induce stemness and epithelial–mesenchymal transition phenotypes in breast cancer cell lines [57].

An intriguing aspect that could be bound to the hormone-like action of miRNAs has been raised by Zhang et al. in 2012 [58] and reinforced by Zhou et al. in 2015 [59]. In these works, researchers demonstrated the possibility that miRNAs derived from plants could potentially travel, through food, from plants to animals via the gastrointestinal tract and access host cellular targets, where they work as bioactive compounds able to influence recipients' physiopathological conditions. The authors proposed that epithelial cells in the intestine could absorb plant-derived miRNAs contained in food and include them into EVs to protect them from degradation and facilitate their release into the blood stream. These "exogenous miRNAs" then seem to be able to reach organs and tissues via circulation and modulate gene expression. The evidence supporting this theory has been summarized in a recent review by Li et al. [60]. This sort of plant–animal communication, named cross-kingdom transmission, is still source of debate in the scientific community. In fact, there is a large amount of evidence contradicting this cross-kingdom communication hypothesis (also widely reviewed by [60]). The main concern is the mechanisms by which exogenous miRNAs can bypass and survive in the gastrointestinal tract, to enter the bloodstream and ultimately reach specific targets. This "exogenous post-transcriptional regulation" could be another factor influencing the development in special cases of diseases, such as cancer, inserting additional levels of complication into an already complicated scenario. If validated, this hypothesis may expand the current knowledge on dietary bioactive compounds and their biological actions once internalized in the organism [60,61].

3. Long Non-Coding RNAs Acting as Hormones

miRNAs are the most studied species of ncRNAs but, in the last years, the attention of researchers has also been focused on other ncRNAs whose functions are still not well described. A special mention should be made for lncRNAs, since their biological roles and mechanisms of action are not yet completely understood, especially in the context of carcinogenesis [62]. Assigning molecular, cellular, and physiological functions to lncRNAs is among the greatest challenges of the next decade, and there is now increased attention on their biological functions in hormonal signaling systems [63–66].

lncRNAs are defined as non-protein coding RNA transcripts larger than 200 nucleotides, but this definition is quite vague since a universal scheme does not exist [62,67]. The working definition for lncRNAs includes all RNA molecules longer than 200 nucleotides, having little coding potential, transcribed by PolII, capped, spliced, and polyadenylated [63]. The expression of lncRNAs is dependent on the cellular, tissue, and metabolic context. As a consequence, there are specific lncRNAs associated with specific cellular processes that may be inferred by their differential pattern of expression in tissues but also in different developmental time points or under specific stimuli [61,63,68]. It is a common belief that lncRNAs are mostly involved in transcriptional regulation and, therefore, reside principally in the nucleus. However, several lncRNAs act, or are even exclusively localized, within the cytoplasm by working as post-transcriptional regulators in interaction with miRNAs, mRNAs, or proteins [69–72]. Interestingly, the EV cargo may be enriched in lncRNAs [10,73,74], as observed in plasma exosomes of patients with castration-resistant prostate cancer [75] and in renal cancer [76]. The scenario is even more complicated due to a large number of lncRNAs that have been implicated in competing endogenous RNA (ceRNA) mechanisms. This is possible since lncRNAs can function as sponges, able to bind and reduce the targeted effects of miRNAs on mRNAs [77,78].

lncRNA have been recognized as having endocrine, paracrine, and autocrine regulatory functions in a way similar to the one already described for miRNAs [74]. In fact, they can have an autocrine hormone-like behavior since they can modulate cellular activity directly by controlling transcription. For example, they can interact with hormone-encoding genes or hormone antagonists/receptors, indirectly modifying the cell signaling transmission [79]. Steroid receptor RNA activator (*SRA*) was among the first lncRNA to be associated to hormone receptor pathways and acting with a hormone-like mechanism. *SRA* is expressed in tissues specifically targeted by steroid hormone, and it works as a co-activator of the steroid receptor to facilitate ligand-dependent transactivation [80]. Additionally, *SRA* can interact with co-repressors of nuclear receptors [81]. Different expression patterns of *SRA* have been observed in breast cancer cell lines [82], demonstrating that its hormone receptor-associated activity may be crucial in breast tumorigenesis.

Growth arrest-specific 5 (*GAS5*) is another interesting example of multifunctional lncRNAs. It works as a multiple nuclear receptor decoy, forming an RNA stem–loop structure that mimics nuclear receptor DNA response elements. For example, it interacts with glucocorticoid DNA binding domain working as a decoy for glucocorticoid receptor response element [83]. As a consequence, the glucocorticoid receptor is liberated from its sites of transcriptional activity. Therefore, the overexpression of *GAS5* blocks cell growths and induces apoptosis in adherent human cell lines. On the other hand, its reduced expression has been observed in human breast cancer cell lines, indicating a possible involvement of this lncRNA in breast carcinogenesis [84].

lncRNAs can also travel via EVs to nearby or distant cells, where they can induce specific phenotypical changes in a paracrine and endocrine way [31]. The most interesting examples in cancer apply to drug resistance, angiogenesis promotion, and tumorigenesis induction [74].

The ability of tumor cells to disseminate the drug-resistant phenotype via exosomes has been recognized mainly through transferring of miRNAs and drug-efflux pumps [85]. However, there is substantial evidence supporting a role for lncRNAs embedded in exosomes in this mechanism. Expression levels of exosomal lncRNAs are greatly different from those of the donor cells, and there is evidence that lncRNAs are not randomly secreted in EVs [86,87].

The role of EVs and lncRNAs in tumor progression and aggressiveness has been demonstrated in several studies reviewed by Andaloussi et al. [55]. The lncRNA called metastasis-associated lung adenocarcinoma transcript (*MALAT1*) regulates alternative splicing and gene expression [88,89] contributing to lung cancer metastasis [90]. In addition, high levels of *MALAT1* have been detected in serum exosomes from non-small cell lung cancer patients and connected with the promotion of cell proliferation and migration of this cancer [91].

Notably, Qu and collaborators demonstrated, in an elegant way, that lncRNA activated in renal cell carcinoma with sunitinib resistance (*lncARSR*) is correlated with poor response to sunitinib, a drug used for the treatment of advanced renal cell carcinoma. The resistance to the drug was directly induced by *lncARSR* that works as a ceRNA for miR-34/miR-449 to facilitate the expression of specific genes implicated in the sunitinib resistance. Most interestingly, the authors found that *lncARSR* is incorporated into exosomes and transmitted to sensitive cells for the dissemination of the resistance in a hormone-like fashion. The transmission of resistance is not only between tumor cells but also involves endothelial cells, implicating that the exosome-mediated communication is also between tumor and stromal cells [76]. The exosomal secretion of lncRNAs is highly selective and different between normal and cancer cells or between sensitive and resistant cells, therefore, identifying cellular molecules responsible for RNA secretion may help in finding a strategy to block this cell-specific mechanism [76].

Lang and collaborators found that glioma cells were enriched in POU class 3 homeobox 3 (*POUF3*) lncRNA. These cells were able to release *POUF3* into the exosomes and target the surrounding normal tissue, inducing cell proliferation, migration, and angiogenesis in an in vivo model [92].

In the last years, another lncRNA, the colon cancer-associated transcript 2 (*CCAT2*), attracted the attention of researchers because of its dysregulation in cancer [65,66,93,94]. Notably, *CCAT2* has been demonstrated to work in a hormone-like fashion [95]. Our group demonstrated an important role of *CCAT2* in regulating *MYC*, miR-17-5p, and miR-20a [96]. Interestingly, *CCAT2* interacts with these targets through TCF7L2 enhancing the WNT signaling activity. However, it has been demonstrated that *CCAT2* is itself a WNT downstream target. Therefore, in colon cancer, there is a feedback loop mechanism between *MYC*, *WNT*, and *CCAT2* [96]. Moreover, *CCAT2* released in exosomes by glioma cells has also been found to be responsible of angiogenesis induction and apoptosis inhibition in endothelial cells [92]. The pro-angiogenesis phenotype of endothelial cells can be induced also by *H19*, another important lncRNA in carcinogenesis. Conigliaro et al. found that CD90+ liver cancer cells can reprogram endothelial cells by releasing *H19*-enriched exosomes [97].

4. Conclusions

In conclusion, there is an increasing interest in circulating ncRNAs as mediators of cell–cell communication and regulators of gene expression in recipient cells. The concept that an ncRNA might function as a hormone (i.e., mediating cells communication) is a challenge for the research community, and the current knowledge is still insufficient for clarifying this topic. Understanding the role of exogenous ncRNAs that could work as messengers in inter-individual and cross-species molecular communication is one of the next scientific targets for researchers. There is high potential for clinical applications not only as diagnostic or prognostic biomarkers but also as therapeutics [98]. Given the rapid and extensive progress made in the field of ncRNAs in the last decade, in the near future, researchers will be able to address these challenges.

References

1. Bayliss, W.M.; Starling, E.H. On the relation of enterokinase to trypsin. *J. Physiol.* **1905**, *32*, 129–136. [CrossRef] [PubMed]
2. Henderson, J. Ernest Starling and 'Hormones': An historical commentary. *J. Endocrinol.* **2005**, *184*, 5–10. [CrossRef] [PubMed]
3. Litwack, G. Hormones and transport systems. Preface. *Vitam. Horm.* **2015**, *98*, xvii–xviii. [CrossRef]
4. White, A. The interaction of enzymes and hormones. *Pediatrics* **1960**, *26*, 476–481.
5. Ameri, P.; Ferone, D. Diffuse Endocrine System, Neuroendocrine Tumors and Immunity: What's New? *Neuroendocrinology* **2012**, *95*, 267–276. [CrossRef] [PubMed]
6. Valadi, H.; Ekstrom, K.; Bossios, A.; Sjostrand, M.; Lee, J.J.; Lotvall, J.O. Exosome-mediated transfer of mRNAs and microRNAs is a novel mechanism of genetic exchange between cells. *Nat. Cell Biol.* **2007**, *9*, 654–659. [CrossRef] [PubMed]
7. Raposo, G.; Stoorvogel, W. Extracellular vesicles: Exosomes, microvesicles, and friends. *J. Cell Biol.* **2013**, *200*, 373–383. [CrossRef]
8. Bayraktar, R.; Van Roosbroeck, K.; Calin, G.A. Cell-to-cell communication: MicroRNAs as hormones. *Mol. Oncol.* **2017**, *11*, 1673–1686. [CrossRef] [PubMed]
9. Van Niel, G.; D'Angelo, G.; Raposo, G. Shedding light on the cell biology of extracellular vesicles. *Nat. Rev. Mol. Cell Biol.* **2018**, *19*, 213–228. [CrossRef]
10. Colombo, M.; Raposo, G.; Thery, C. Biogenesis, secretion, and intercellular interactions of exosomes and other extracellular vesicles. *Annu. Rev. Cell Dev. Biol.* **2014**, *30*, 255–289. [CrossRef]
11. Cortez, M.A.; Bueso-Ramos, C.; Ferdin, J.; Lopez-Berestein, G.; Sood, A.K.; Calin, G.A. MicroRNAs in body fluids–the mix of hormones and biomarkers. *Nat. Rev. Clin. Oncol.* **2011**, *8*, 467–477. [CrossRef] [PubMed]
12. Colombo, M.; Moita, C.; van Niel, G.; Kowal, J.; Vigneron, J.; Benaroch, P.; Manel, N.; Moita, L.F.; Thery, C.; Raposo, G. Analysis of ESCRT functions in exosome biogenesis, composition and secretion highlights the heterogeneity of extracellular vesicles. *J. Cell Sci.* **2013**, *126*, 5553–5565. [CrossRef] [PubMed]
13. Kalra, H.; Drummen, G.P.; Mathivanan, S. Focus on Extracellular Vesicles: Introducing the Next Small Big Thing. *Int. J. Mol. Sci.* **2016**, *17*, 170. [CrossRef] [PubMed]
14. Gangoda, L.; Boukouris, S.; Liem, M.; Kalra, H.; Mathivanan, S. Extracellular vesicles including exosomes are mediators of signal transduction: Are they protective or pathogenic? *Proteomics* **2015**, *15*, 260–271. [CrossRef] [PubMed]
15. Cieslik, M.; Chinnaiyan, A.M. Cancer transcriptome profiling at the juncture of clinical translation. *Nat. Rev. Genet.* **2018**, *19*, 93–109. [CrossRef]
16. Anfossi, S.; Babayan, A.; Pantel, K.; Calin, G.A. Clinical utility of circulating non-coding RNAs—An update. *Nat. Rev. Clin. Oncol.* **2018**, *15*, 541–563. [CrossRef] [PubMed]

17. Gebert, L.F.R.; MacRae, I.J. Regulation of microRNA function in animals. *Nat. Rev. Mol. Cell Biol.* **2019**, *20*, 21–37. [CrossRef] [PubMed]
18. Munker, R.; Calin, G.A. MicroRNA profiling in cancer. *Clin. Sci. (Lond.)* **2011**, *121*, 141–158. [CrossRef]
19. Sevignani, C.; Calin, G.A.; Nnadi, S.C.; Shimizu, M.; Davuluri, R.V.; Hyslop, T.; Demant, P.; Croce, C.M.; Siracusa, L.D. MicroRNA genes are frequently located near mouse cancer susceptibility loci. *Proc. Natl. Acad. Sci. USA* **2007**, *104*, 8017–8022. [CrossRef] [PubMed]
20. Shah, M.Y.; Ferrajoli, A.; Sood, A.K.; Lopez-Berestein, G.; Calin, G.A. microRNA Therapeutics in Cancer—An Emerging Concept. *EBioMedicine* **2016**, *12*, 34–42. [CrossRef]
21. Inui, M.; Martello, G.; Piccolo, S. MicroRNA control of signal transduction. *Nat. Rev. Mol. Cell Biol.* **2010**, *11*, 252–263. [CrossRef] [PubMed]
22. Wang, H.; Gou, X.; Jiang, T.; Ouyang, J. The effects of microRNAs on glucocorticoid responsiveness. *J. Cancer Res. Clin. Oncol.* **2017**, *143*, 1005–1011. [CrossRef] [PubMed]
23. Abramov, R.; Fu, G.; Zhang, Y.; Peng, C. Expression and regulation of miR-17a and miR-430b in zebrafish ovarian follicles. *Gen. Comp. Endocrinol.* **2013**, *188*, 309–315. [CrossRef] [PubMed]
24. Sen, A.; Prizant, H.; Light, A.; Biswas, A.; Hayes, E.; Lee, H.J.; Barad, D.; Gleicher, N.; Hammes, S.R. Androgens regulate ovarian follicular development by increasing follicle stimulating hormone receptor and microRNA-125b expression. *Proc. Natl. Acad. Sci. USA* **2014**, *111*, 3008–3013. [CrossRef] [PubMed]
25. McFall, T.; McKnight, B.; Rosati, R.; Kim, S.; Huang, Y.; Viola-Villegas, N.; Ratnam, M. Progesterone receptor A promotes invasiveness and metastasis of luminal breast cancer by suppressing regulation of critical microRNAs by estrogen. *J. Biol. Chem.* **2018**, *293*, 1163–1177. [CrossRef]
26. Iliopoulos, D.; Jaeger, S.A.; Hirsch, H.A.; Bulyk, M.L.; Struhl, K. STAT3 activation of miR-21 and miR-181b-1 via PTEN and CYLD are part of the epigenetic switch linking inflammation to cancer. *Mol. Cell.* **2010**, *39*, 493–506. [CrossRef]
27. Di Girolamo, D.; Ambrosio, R.; De Stefano, M.A.; Mancino, G.; Porcelli, T.; Luongo, C.; Di Cicco, E.; Scalia, G.; Vecchio, L.D.; Colao, A.; et al. Reciprocal interplay between thyroid hormone and microRNA-21 regulates hedgehog pathway-driven skin tumorigenesis. *J. Clin. Investig.* **2016**, *126*, 2308–2320. [CrossRef]
28. Aucher, A.; Rudnicka, D.; Davis, D.M. MicroRNAs Transfer from Human Macrophages to Hepato-Carcinoma Cells and Inhibit Proliferation. *J. Immunol.* **2013**, *191*, 6250–6260. [CrossRef]
29. Bovy, N.; Blomme, B.; Freres, P.; Dederen, S.; Nivelles, O.; Lion, M.; Carnet, O.; Martial, J.A.; Noel, A.; Thiry, M.; et al. Endothelial exosomes contribute to the antitumor response during breast cancer neoadjuvant chemotherapy via microRNA transfer. *Oncotarget* **2015**, *6*, 10253–10266. [CrossRef]
30. Nishida-Aoki, N.; Ochiya, T. Interactions between cancer cells and normal cells via miRNAs in extracellular vesicles. *Cell. Mol. Life Sci.* **2015**, *72*, 1849–1861. [CrossRef]
31. Tkach, M.; Thery, C. Communication by Extracellular Vesicles: Where We Are and Where We Need to Go. *Cell* **2016**, *164*, 1226–1232. [CrossRef] [PubMed]
32. Sung, B.H.; Ketova, T.; Hoshino, D.; Zijlstra, A.; Weaver, A.M. Directional cell movement through tissues is controlled by exosome secretion. *Nat. Commun.* **2015**, *6*, 7164. [CrossRef] [PubMed]
33. Josson, S.; Gururajan, M.; Sung, S.Y.; Hu, P.; Shao, C.; Zhau, H.E.; Liu, C.; Lichterman, J.; Duan, P.; Li, Q.; et al. Stromal fibroblast-derived miR-409 promotes epithelial-to-mesenchymal transition and prostate tumorigenesis. *Oncogene* **2015**, *34*, 2690–2699. [CrossRef] [PubMed]
34. Fabbri, M. MicroRNAs and miRceptors: A new mechanism of action for intercellular communication. *Philos. Trans. R. Soc. Lond. B Biol. Sci.* **2018**, *373*. [CrossRef] [PubMed]
35. Zhang, Y.J.; Liu, D.Q.; Chen, X.; Li, J.; Li, L.M.; Bian, Z.; Sun, F.; Lu, J.W.; Yin, Y.A.; Cai, X.; et al. Secreted Monocytic miR-150 Enhances Targeted Endothelial Cell Migration. *Mol. Cell* **2010**, *39*, 133–144. [CrossRef]
36. Huang-Doran, I.; Zhang, C.Y.; Vidal-Puig, A. Extracellular Vesicles: Novel Mediators of Cell Communication In Metabolic Disease. *Trends Endocrinol. Metab.* **2017**, *28*, 3–18. [CrossRef]
37. Ying, W.; Riopel, M.; Bandyopadhyay, G.; Dong, Y.; Birmingham, A.; Seo, J.B.; Ofrecio, J.M.; Wollam, J.; Hernandez-Carretero, A.; Fu, W.; et al. Adipose Tissue Macrophage-Derived Exosomal miRNAs Can Modulate In Vivo and In Vitro Insulin Sensitivity. *Cell* **2017**, *171*, 372–384.e12. [CrossRef]
38. Zhang, Y.; Shi, L.; Mei, H.; Zhang, J.; Zhu, Y.; Han, X.; Zhu, D. Inflamed macrophage microvesicles induce insulin resistance in human adipocytes. *Nutr. Metab. (Lond.)* **2015**, *12*, 21. [CrossRef] [PubMed]

39. Costa-Silva, B.; Aiello, N.M.; Ocean, A.J.; Singh, S.; Zhang, H.; Thakur, B.K.; Becker, A.; Hoshino, A.; Mark, M.T.; Molina, H.; et al. Pancreatic cancer exosomes initiate pre-metastatic niche formation in the liver. *Nat. Cell Biol.* **2015**, *17*, 816–826. [CrossRef] [PubMed]
40. Le, M.T.N.; Hamar, P.; Guo, C.Y.; Basar, E.; Perdigao-Henriques, R.; Balaj, L.; Lieberman, J. miR-200-containing extracellular vesicles promote breast cancer cell metastasis. *J. Clin. Investig.* **2014**, *124*, 5109–5128. [CrossRef] [PubMed]
41. Pigati, L.; Yaddanapudi, S.C.; Iyengar, R.; Kim, D.J.; Hearn, S.A.; Danforth, D.; Hastings, M.L.; Duelli, D.M. Selective release of microRNA species from normal and malignant mammary epithelial cells. *PLoS ONE* **2010**, *5*, e13515. [CrossRef]
42. Anfossi, S.; Fu, X.; Nagvekar, R.; Calin, G.A. MicroRNAs, Regulatory Messengers Inside and Outside Cancer Cells. *Adv. Exp. Med. Biol.* **2018**, *1056*, 87–108. [CrossRef] [PubMed]
43. Jin, X.C.; Chen, Y.F.; Chen, H.B.; Fei, S.R.; Chen, D.D.; Cai, X.N.; Liu, L.; Lin, B.C.; Su, H.F.; Zhao, L.H.; et al. Evaluation of Tumor-Derived Exosomal miRNA as Potential Diagnostic Biomarkers for Early-Stage Non-Small Cell Lung Cancer Using Next-Generation Sequencing. *Clin. Cancer Res.* **2017**, *23*, 5311–5319. [CrossRef]
44. Matsumura, T.; Sugimachi, K.; Iinuma, H.; Takahashi, Y.; Kurashige, J.; Sawada, G.; Ueda, M.; Uchi, R.; Ueo, H.; Takano, Y.; et al. Exosomal microRNA in serum is a novel biomarker of recurrence in human colorectal cancer. *Br. J. Cancer* **2015**, *113*, 275–281. [CrossRef]
45. Sugimachi, K.; Matsumura, T.; Hirata, H.; Uchi, R.; Ueda, M.; Ueo, H.; Shinden, Y.; Iguchi, T.; Eguchi, H.; Shirabe, K.; et al. Identification of a bona fide microRNA biomarker in serum exosomes that predicts hepatocellular carcinoma recurrence after liver transplantation. *Br. J. Cancer* **2015**, *112*, 532–538. [CrossRef] [PubMed]
46. Schoepp, M.; Strose, A.J.; Haier, J. Dysregulation of miRNA Expression in Cancer Associated Fibroblasts (CAFs) and Its Consequences on the Tumor Microenvironment. *Cancers* **2017**, *9*, 54. [CrossRef]
47. Mulcahy, L.A.; Pink, R.C.; Carter, D.R. Routes and mechanisms of extracellular vesicle uptake. *J. Extracell. Vesicles* **2014**, *3*. [CrossRef] [PubMed]
48. Berindan-Neagoe, I.; Calin, G.A. Molecular pathways: MicroRNAs, cancer cells, and microenvironment. *Clin. Cancer Res.* **2014**, *20*, 6247–6253. [CrossRef]
49. Baroni, S.; Romero-Cordoba, S.; Plantamura, I.; Dugo, M.; D'Ippolito, E.; Cataldo, A.; Cosentino, G.; Angeloni, V.; Rossini, A.; Daidone, M.G.; et al. Exosome-mediated delivery of miR-9 induces cancer-associated fibroblast-like properties in human breast fibroblasts. *Cell Death Dis.* **2016**, *7*, e2312. [CrossRef] [PubMed]
50. Chen, X.; Ying, X.; Wang, X.; Wu, X.; Zhu, Q. Exosomes derived from hypoxic epithelial ovarian cancer deliver microRNA-940 to induce macrophage M2 polarization. *Oncol. Rep.* **2017**, *38*, 522–528. [CrossRef]
51. Eiring, A.M.; Harb, J.G.; Neviani, P.; Garton, C.; Oaks, J.J.; Spizzo, R.; Liu, S.; Schwind, S.; Santhanam, R.; Hickey, C.J.; et al. miR-328 functions as an RNA decoy to modulate hnRNP E2 regulation of mRNA translation in leukemic blasts. *Cell* **2010**, *140*, 652–665. [CrossRef]
52. Fabbri, M.; Paone, A.; Calore, F.; Galli, R.; Gaudio, E.; Santhanam, R.; Lovat, F.; Fadda, P.; Mao, C.; Nuovo, G.J.; et al. MicroRNAs bind to Toll-like receptors to induce prometastatic inflammatory response. *Proc. Natl. Acad. Sci. USA* **2012**, *109*, E2110–E2116. [CrossRef]
53. Patel, S.A.; Gooderham, N.J. IL6 Mediates Immune and Colorectal Cancer Cell Cross-talk via miR-21 and miR-29b. *Mol. Cancer Res.* **2015**, *13*, 1502–1508. [CrossRef]
54. Challagundla, K.B.; Wise, P.M.; Neviani, P.; Chava, H.; Murtadha, M.; Xu, T.; Kennedy, R.; Ivan, C.; Zhang, X.; Vannini, I.; et al. Exosome-mediated transfer of microRNAs within the tumor microenvironment and neuroblastoma resistance to chemotherapy. *J. Natl. Cancer Inst.* **2015**, *107*. [CrossRef] [PubMed]
55. EL Andaloussi, S.; Mager, I.; Breakefield, X.O.; Wood, M.J. Extracellular vesicles: Biology and emerging therapeutic opportunities. *Nat. Rev. Drug Discov.* **2013**, *12*, 347–357. [CrossRef] [PubMed]
56. Wei, Y.; Lai, X.; Yu, S.; Chen, S.; Ma, Y.; Zhang, Y.; Li, H.; Zhu, X.; Yao, L.; Zhang, J. Exosomal miR-221/222 enhances tamoxifen resistance in recipient ER-positive breast cancer cells. *Breast Cancer Res. Treat.* **2014**, *147*, 423–431. [CrossRef]
57. Donnarumma, E.; Fiore, D.; Nappa, M.; Roscigno, G.; Adamo, A.; Iaboni, M.; Russo, V.; Affinito, A.; Puoti, I.; Quintavalle, C.; et al. Cancer-associated fibroblasts release exosomal microRNAs that dictate an aggressive phenotype in breast cancer. *Oncotarget* **2017**, *8*, 19592–19608. [CrossRef] [PubMed]

58. Zhang, L.; Hou, D.; Chen, X.; Li, D.; Zhu, L.; Zhang, Y.; Li, J.; Bian, Z.; Liang, X.; Cai, X.; et al. Exogenous plant MIR168a specifically targets mammalian LDLRAP1: Evidence of cross-kingdom regulation by microRNA. *Cell Res.* **2012**, *22*, 107–126. [CrossRef]
59. Zhou, Z.; Li, X.; Liu, J.; Dong, L.; Chen, Q.; Kong, H.; Zhang, Q.; Qi, X.; Hou, D.; Zhang, L.; et al. Honeysuckle-encoded atypical microRNA2911 directly targets influenza A viruses. *Cell Res* **2015**, *25*, 39–49. [CrossRef]
60. Li, Z.; Xu, R.; Li, N. MicroRNAs from plants to animals, do they define a new messenger for communication? *Nutr. Metab. (Lond.)* **2018**, *15*, 68. [CrossRef]
61. Xie, W.; Weng, A.; Melzig, M.F. MicroRNAs as New Bioactive Components in Medicinal Plants. *Planta Med.* **2016**, *82*, 1153–1162. [CrossRef] [PubMed]
62. Wilusz, J.E.; Sunwoo, H.; Spector, D.L. Long noncoding RNAs: Functional surprises from the RNA world. *Genes Dev.* **2009**, *23*, 1494–1504. [CrossRef] [PubMed]
63. Sun, M.; Kraus, W.L. From Discovery to Function: The Expanding Roles of Long Non-Coding RNAs in Physiology and Disease. *Endocr. Rev.* **2015**. [CrossRef]
64. Ferdin, J.; Nishida, N.; Wu, X.; Nicoloso, M.S.; Shah, M.Y.; Devlin, C.; Ling, H.; Shimizu, M.; Kumar, K.; Cortez, M.A.; et al. HINCUTs in cancer: Hypoxia-induced noncoding ultraconserved transcripts. *Cell Death Differ.* **2013**, *20*, 1675–1687. [CrossRef] [PubMed]
65. Redis, R.S.; Vela, L.E.; Lu, W.; Ferreira de Oliveira, J.; Ivan, C.; Rodriguez-Aguayo, C.; Adamoski, D.; Pasculli, B.; Taguchi, A.; Chen, Y.; et al. Allele-Specific Reprogramming of Cancer Metabolism by the Long Non-coding RNA CCAT2. *Mol. Cell* **2016**, *61*, 640. [CrossRef] [PubMed]
66. Shah, M.Y.; Ferracin, M.; Pileczki, V.; Chen, B.; Redis, R.; Fabris, L.; Zhang, X.; Ivan, C.; Shimizu, M.; Rodriguez-Aguayo, C.; et al. Cancer-associated rs6983267 SNP and its accompanying long noncoding RNA CCAT2 induce myeloid malignancies via unique SNP-specific RNA mutations. *Genome Res.* **2018**, *28*, 432–447. [CrossRef]
67. Djebali, S.; Davis, C.A.; Merkel, A.; Dobin, A.; Lassmann, T.; Mortazavi, A.; Tanzer, A.; Lagarde, J.; Lin, W.; Schlesinger, F.; et al. Landscape of transcription in human cells. *Nature* **2012**, *489*, 101–108. [CrossRef]
68. Wu, W.; Wagner, E.K.; Hao, Y.; Rao, X.; Dai, H.; Han, J.; Chen, J.; Storniolo, A.M.; Liu, Y.; He, C. Tissue-specific Co-expression of Long Non-coding and Coding RNAs Associated with Breast Cancer. *Sci. Rep.* **2016**, *6*, 32731. [CrossRef]
69. Zhao, J.; Ohsumi, T.K.; Kung, J.T.; Ogawa, Y.; Grau, D.J.; Sarma, K.; Song, J.J.; Kingston, R.E.; Borowsky, M.; Lee, J.T. Genome-wide identification of polycomb-associated RNAs by RIP-seq. *Mol. Cell* **2010**, *40*, 939–953. [CrossRef]
70. Gong, C.; Maquat, L.E. lncRNAs transactivate STAU1-mediated mRNA decay by duplexing with 3′ UTRs via Alu elements. *Nature* **2011**, *470*, 284–288. [CrossRef]
71. Wang, P.; Xue, Y.; Han, Y.; Lin, L.; Wu, C.; Xu, S.; Jiang, Z.; Xu, J.; Liu, Q.; Cao, X. The STAT3-binding long noncoding RNA lnc-DC controls human dendritic cell differentiation. *Science* **2014**, *344*, 310–313. [CrossRef]
72. Long, Y.; Wang, X.; Youmans, D.T.; Cech, T.R. How do lncRNAs regulate transcription? *Sci. Adv.* **2017**, *3*, eaao2110. [CrossRef]
73. Yanez-Mo, M.; Siljander, P.R.; Andreu, Z.; Zavec, A.B.; Borras, F.E.; Buzas, E.I.; Buzas, K.; Casal, E.; Cappello, F.; Carvalho, J.; et al. Biological properties of extracellular vesicles and their physiological functions. *J. Extracell. Vesicles* **2015**, *4*, 27066. [CrossRef]
74. Dragomir, M.; Chen, B.; Calin, G.A. Exosomal lncRNAs as new players in cell-to-cell communication. *Transl. Cancer Res.* **2018**, *7*, S243–S252. [CrossRef] [PubMed]
75. Huang, X.; Yuan, T.; Liang, M.; Du, M.; Xia, S.; Dittmar, R.; Wang, D.; See, W.; Costello, B.A.; Quevedo, F.; et al. Exosomal miR-1290 and miR-375 as prognostic markers in castration-resistant prostate cancer. *Eur. Urol.* **2015**, *67*, 33–41. [CrossRef]
76. Qu, L.; Ding, J.; Chen, C.; Wu, Z.J.; Liu, B.; Gao, Y.; Chen, W.; Liu, F.; Sun, W.; Li, X.F.; et al. Exosome-Transmitted lncARSR Promotes Sunitinib Resistance in Renal Cancer by Acting as a Competing Endogenous RNA. *Cancer Cell* **2016**, *29*, 653–668. [CrossRef] [PubMed]
77. Cesana, M.; Cacchiarelli, D.; Legnini, I.; Santini, T.; Sthandier, O.; Chinappi, M.; Tramontano, A.; Bozzoni, I. A long noncoding RNA controls muscle differentiation by functioning as a competing endogenous RNA. *Cell* **2011**, *147*, 358–369. [CrossRef] [PubMed]

78. Salmena, L.; Poliseno, L.; Tay, Y.; Kats, L.; Pandolfi, P.P. A ceRNA hypothesis: The Rosetta Stone of a hidden RNA language? *Cell* **2011**, *146*, 353–358. [CrossRef] [PubMed]
79. Fatica, A.; Bozzoni, I. Long non-coding RNAs: New players in cell differentiation and development. *Nat. Rev. Genet.* **2014**, *15*, 7–21. [CrossRef] [PubMed]
80. Lanz, R.B.; McKenna, N.J.; Onate, S.A.; Albrecht, U.; Wong, J.; Tsai, S.Y.; Tsai, M.J.; O'Malley, B.W. A steroid receptor coactivator, SRA, functions as an RNA and is present in an SRC-1 complex. *Cell* **1999**, *97*, 17–27. [CrossRef]
81. Hatchell, E.C.; Colley, S.M.; Beveridge, D.J.; Epis, M.R.; Stuart, L.M.; Giles, K.M.; Redfern, A.D.; Miles, L.E.; Barker, A.; MacDonald, L.M.; et al. SLIRP, a small SRA binding protein, is a nuclear receptor corepressor. *Mol. Cell* **2006**, *22*, 657–668. [CrossRef]
82. Cooper, C.; Guo, J.; Yan, Y.; Chooniedass-Kothari, S.; Hube, F.; Hamedani, M.K.; Murphy, L.C.; Myal, Y.; Leygue, E. Increasing the relative expression of endogenous non-coding Steroid Receptor RNA Activator (SRA) in human breast cancer cells using modified oligonucleotides. *Nucleic Acids Res.* **2009**, *37*, 4518–4531. [CrossRef]
83. Mayama, T.; Marr, A.K.; Kino, T. Differential Expression of Glucocorticoid Receptor Noncoding RNA Repressor Gas5 in Autoimmune and Inflammatory Diseases. *Horm. Metab. Res.* **2016**, *48*, 550–557. [CrossRef] [PubMed]
84. Mourtada-Maarabouni, M.; Pickard, M.R.; Hedge, V.L.; Farzaneh, F.; Williams, G.T. GAS5, a non-protein-coding RNA, controls apoptosis and is downregulated in breast cancer. *Oncogene* **2009**, *28*, 195–208. [CrossRef]
85. Sousa, D.; Lima, R.T.; Vasconcelos, M.H. Intercellular Transfer of Cancer Drug Resistance Traits by Extracellular Vesicles. *Trends Mol. Med.* **2015**, *21*, 595–608. [CrossRef] [PubMed]
86. Chen, M.; Xu, R.; Ji, H.; Greening, D.W.; Rai, A.; Izumikawa, K.; Ishikawa, H.; Takahashi, N.; Simpson, R.J. Transcriptome and long noncoding RNA sequencing of three extracellular vesicle subtypes released from the human colon cancer LIM1863 cell line. *Sci. Rep.* **2016**, *6*, 38397. [CrossRef] [PubMed]
87. Koldemir, O.; Ozgur, E.; Gezer, U. Accumulation of GAS5 in exosomes is a marker of apoptosis induction. *Biomed. Rep.* **2017**, *6*, 358–362. [CrossRef] [PubMed]
88. Tripathi, V.; Ellis, J.D.; Shen, Z.; Song, D.Y.; Pan, Q.; Watt, A.T.; Freier, S.M.; Bennett, C.F.; Sharma, A.; Bubulya, P.A.; et al. The nuclear-retained noncoding RNA MALAT1 regulates alternative splicing by modulating SR splicing factor phosphorylation. *Mol. Cell* **2010**, *39*, 925–938. [CrossRef] [PubMed]
89. Yang, L.; Lin, C.; Liu, W.; Zhang, J.; Ohgi, K.A.; Grinstein, J.D.; Dorrestein, P.C.; Rosenfeld, M.G. ncRNA- and Pc2 methylation-dependent gene relocation between nuclear structures mediates gene activation programs. *Cell* **2011**, *147*, 773–788. [CrossRef] [PubMed]
90. Schmidt, L.H.; Spieker, T.; Koschmieder, S.; Schaffers, S.; Humberg, J.; Jungen, D.; Bulk, E.; Hascher, A.; Wittmer, D.; Marra, A.; et al. The long noncoding MALAT-1 RNA indicates a poor prognosis in non-small cell lung cancer and induces migration and tumor growth. *J. Thorac. Oncol.* **2011**, *6*, 1984–1992. [CrossRef] [PubMed]
91. Zhang, R.; Xia, Y.; Wang, Z.; Zheng, J.; Chen, Y.; Li, X.; Wang, Y.; Ming, H. Serum long non coding RNA MALAT-1 protected by exosomes is up-regulated and promotes cell proliferation and migration in non-small cell lung cancer. *Biochem. Biophys. Res. Commun.* **2017**, *490*, 406–414. [CrossRef] [PubMed]
92. Lang, H.L.; Hu, G.W.; Zhang, B.; Kuang, W.; Chen, Y.; Wu, L.; Xu, G.H. Glioma cells enhance angiogenesis and inhibit endothelial cell apoptosis through the release of exosomes that contain long non-coding RNA CCAT2. *Oncol. Rep.* **2017**, *38*, 785–798. [CrossRef] [PubMed]
93. Redis, R.S.; Sieuwerts, A.M.; Look, M.P.; Tudoran, O.; Ivan, C.; Spizzo, R.; Zhang, X.; de Weerd, V.; Shimizu, M.; Ling, H.; et al. CCAT2, a novel long non-coding RNA in breast cancer: Expression study and clinical correlations. *Oncotarget* **2013**, *4*, 1748–1762. [CrossRef] [PubMed]
94. Ozawa, T.; Matsuyama, T.; Toiyama, Y.; Takahashi, N.; Ishikawa, T.; Uetake, H.; Yamada, Y.; Kusunoki, M.; Calin, G.; Goel, A. CCAT1 and CCAT2 long noncoding RNAs, located within the 8q.24.21 'gene desert', serve as important prognostic biomarkers in colorectal cancer. *Ann. Oncol.* **2017**, *28*, 1882–1888. [CrossRef] [PubMed]
95. Fosselteder, J.; Calin, G.A.; Pichler, M. Long non-coding RNA CCAT2 as a therapeutic target in colorectal cancer. *Expert Opin. Ther. Targets* **2018**, *22*, 973–976. [CrossRef]

96. Ling, H.; Spizzo, R.; Atlasi, Y.; Nicoloso, M.; Shimizu, M.; Redis, R.S.; Nishida, N.; Gafa, R.; Song, J.; Guo, Z.; et al. CCAT2, a novel noncoding RNA mapping to 8q24, underlies metastatic progression and chromosomal instability in colon cancer. *Genome Res.* **2013**, *23*, 1446–1461. [CrossRef] [PubMed]
97. Conigliaro, A.; Costa, V.; Lo Dico, A.; Saieva, L.; Buccheri, S.; Dieli, F.; Manno, M.; Raccosta, S.; Mancone, C.; Tripodi, M.; et al. CD90+ liver cancer cells modulate endothelial cell phenotype through the release of exosomes containing H19 lncRNA. *Mol. Cancer* **2015**, *14*, 155. [CrossRef]
98. Bullock, M.D.; Silva, A.M.; Kanlikilicer-Unaldi, P.; Filant, J.; Rashed, M.H.; Sood, A.K.; Lopez-Berestein, G.; Calin, G.A. Exosomal Non-Coding RNAs: Diagnostic, Prognostic and Therapeutic Applications in Cancer. *Noncoding RNA* **2015**, *1*, 53–68. [CrossRef]

5

Non-Smoking-Associated Lung Cancer: A Distinct Entity in Terms of Tumor Biology, Patient Characteristics and Impact of Hereditary Cancer Predisposition

Elisabeth Smolle [1] and Martin Pichler [2,*]

[1] Division of Pulmonology, Department of Internal Medicine, Medical University Graz, 8036 Graz, Austria; elisabeth.smolle@medunigraz.at
[2] Department of Experimental Therapeutics, Division of Medicine, The UT MD Anderson Cancer Center, Houston, TX 77030, USA
* Correspondence: mart.pichler@gmx.net

Abstract: Non-small cell lung cancer (NSCLC) in non-, and especially in never-smoking patients is considered a biologically unique type of lung cancer, since risk factors and tumorigenic conditions, other than tobacco smoke, come into play. In this review article, we comprehensively searched and summarized the current literature with the aim to outline what exactly triggers lung cancer in non-smokers. Changes in the tumor microenvironment, distinct driver genes and genetic pathway alterations that are specific for non-smoking patients, as well as lifestyle-related risk factors apart from tobacco smoke are critically discussed. The data we have reviewed highlights once again the importance of personalized cancer therapy, i.e., careful molecular and genetic assessment of the tumor to provide tailored treatment options with optimum chances of good response—especially for the subgroups of never-smokers.

Keywords: non-small cell lung cancer; non-smoker; tumor microenvironment; targeted treatment

---

1. Introduction

Lung cancer is the second most common incident cancer diagnosis in men, and the fourth most common cancer diagnosis in women, accounting for most cancer-related deaths in both men and women, with 1.7 million global deaths a year [1–3]. More than 85% of lung cancer cases are related to a positive history of smoking (i.e., smoking-related or smoking-associated lung cancer). Smoking leads to an accumulation of genetic alterations in oncogenes and tumor suppressor genes ultimately causing cancer [4]. Previous reports and literature reviews have addressed the topic of lung cancer in non- and never-smokers [5–12], and here we aim at providing a more updated review by going into detail also with molecular, immunological and genetic aspects. In Asian countries the proportion of never-smoking lung cancer patients is generally higher (up to 15%) [8]. Epidemiologic studies show that never-smoking lung cancer patients are more often female, show an adenocarcinoma (AC) histologic subtype and are often of East Asian ethnicity. Within the last decade, genome-wide studies clearly indicated that the underlying tumor biology in lung cancers of non-smokers (meaning never-smokers and patients with a negligible history of smoking and small likelihood that the tumor was smoking-related) differs dramatically from smoking-related lung cancer, featuring a different pattern of molecular alterations [10,13–17]. Another interesting finding in non-smoker lung cancer is the fact that patients are significantly younger, have a better prognosis and respond to treatment better than smokers with lung cancer [5,7,9,18]. The main reason for the favorable outcome in non-smokers is the occurrence of certain molecular subtypes (oncogene-addicted lung cancer), enabling the specific treatment with Previous epidermal growth factor receptor-tyrosine kinase inhibitors (EGFR-TKIs) or other agents [19,20]. Such genetic alterations and patterns of mutation that are specific for lung cancer have primarily been outlined for AC, whereas no genetic mutations have been linked to squamous cell carcinoma (SCC) specifically, especially not for non-smokers [4].

Generally spoken, environmental tobacco smoke at home or at the workplace [21], radon [22], cooking oil vapor [23], indoor coal burning, hormonal replacement therapy [20], exposure to asbestos/heavy metals [6], infectious factors and air pollution have been linked to lung carcinogenesis in non-smokers [24,25].

It has also been proposed that lung cancer in smokers versus non-smokers is characterized by a distinct tumor microenvironment [26]. Tobacco smoke causes DNA damage in cells of the bronchial epithelium which causes dysfunction in the immune system of the lung. Immune cells that infiltrate the tumor are likely to influence survival, and possibly response to treatment. However, the role of the tumor microenvironment with a special emphasis on immune cells has not been widely studied yet [26]. In the next sections, we will highlight and discuss the knowledge of distinct molecular and epidemiological differences between lung cancer in never-smokers with a special emphasis and separation between different lung cancer histology.

2. Squamous Cell Carcinoma in Non- or Never-Smokers

In 2017, Park and colleagues performed a study to identify potential genetic alterations specific for squamous cell carcinoma (SCC) in non-smokers [4]. For that purpose, an Array comparative genomic hybridization (ArrayCGH) analysis was conducted in 19 patients suffering from SCC. Previous CGH analyses have shown that amplification of chromosome 3q25-qter frequently occurs in SCC [27]. Among the 19 SCC patients that were studied by Park et al., there were eight non-smokers compared to 11 smokers. Sixteen gene regions were significantly altered, according to ArrayCGH. Three gain (5p15.33, 8q24.21, and 11q13.3) and four loss regions (4q35.2, 9p21.3, 10q23.31, and 15q11.2) were found, that also overlapped with data from The Cancer Genome Atlas (TCGA) which contains data on copy number variations in SCC [28]. The investigators identified 15 genes within the significantly altered regions, that have also been reported in the Cancer Gene Census (*ATM, CCND1, CDKN2A, DUX4L1, EZH2, FOXP1, LRIG3, MEN1, MITF, NRG1, NUMA1, PTEN, TERT, WHSC1L1, and WRN*) [29]. The proto-oncogene *GAB2* (11q14.1) was found to be frequently amplified in non-smoking patients [4]. To secure this finding, protein expression of GAB2 was investigated by means of immunohistochemistry, and the protein was also found to be upregulated in tissues of non-smokers as compared to smokers (37.5% vs. 9.0%, $p = 0.007$) [4]. Thus, *GAB2* amplification is likely to contribute to SCC development in the subgroup of non-smokers, and may also serve as a biomarker in the near future.

An interesting case report of a non-smoker female patient with SCC of the lung favors a genomics-, proteomics- and metabolomics-based approach to treatment, highlighting the importance of personalized medicine especially in non-smoking individuals [30]. The Caucasian female patient developed SCC in the absence of smoking, and with no history of asbestos exposure. The patient's father, who was a smoker, died from lung cancer at age 63; apart from that, no family history of cancer was known. The tumor was surgically removed shortly after diagnosis, and at pathologic examination the SCC featured a unique, mainly perialveolar and perivascular growth pattern. There was positive immunostaining for p63 and cytokeratin (CK) 5/6, whereas CK7, thyroid transcription factor 1, synaptophysin and chromogranin were all negative. Ki67 proliferation marker immunostaining showed 20 percent positive cells [30]. Interestingly, this patient had undergone surgical resection of a SCC of the head and neck region two years prior to diagnosis of the lung SCC. According to in-depth pathological assessment it was stated that these two tumors were two distinct entities of SCC, and that the lung tumor was not recurrent disease of the head and neck SCC. The patient is still alive two years after the lung tumor resection, and four years after the resection of the SCC at the neck. In this special case, analysis of certain somatic driver mutations was carried out. A predominance of

C>T transitions in tumoral lung tissue was found, not corresponding to the specific cancer signature usually correlating with tobacco smoking (characterized by an abundance of C>A transversions). Pathway analysis showed that mutations in the SCC tissue predominantly affected genes involved in extracellular matrix organization ($p = 0.005$), transmembrane transport of small molecules ($p = 0.010$) and collagen formation ($p = 0.034$). Mutations in these pathways have previously been reported in a study on whole exome sequencing in lung cancer [31]. Interestingly, in this case no mutations in the most frequent lung cancer driver genes, namely *EGFR, KRAS, AKT* and *ROS1* were present in the tumor sample, and neither was the *EML4-ALK* fusion gene [30]. The authors then used a combination of next generations sequencing (NGS) techniques to test the hypothesis that in this case of a never-smoking female, the lung carcinoma was of oligogenic origin. Among the 11 germline-mutated cancer-related genes, two (*ACACA* and *DEPTOR*) are known to be associated with common driver genes: *ACACA* is associated with *BRCA1*, and *DEPTOR* with *EGFR*. One particular missense variant in the *ACACA* gene (c.C1948T, p.Arg650Trp (NM_198837.1, exon 16)) has been predicted as deleterious, leading to a loss of function of Acetyl-CoA carboxylase alpha which is a crucial enzyme for long-chain fatty acid synthesis [32]. The authors of this case report conclude that both primary SCC tumors which the patient developed were triggered by a special oligogenic germline signature consisting of at least 11 mutations, two of them leading to the activation of mTOR and *BRCA1* [30]. A proteomic/genomic/metabolomic sequencing approach is thus particularly useful to find personalized treatment strategies and accurate estimations of prognosis, especially in patients that lack common risk factors for a certain cancer species, e.g. tobacco smoking for lung cancer. However, it must be pointed out that this report has a clear limitation, because tissue from only one individual was analyzed. In the future, more sequencing data of tissue samples from never-smoker lung cancer patients would be of use to find out more about genetic patterns in this special subgroup of patients.

In another interesting study, the effect of the programmed death 1 (PD-1)-receptor targeting checkpoint inhibitor nivolumab in never-smokers with advanced squamous non-small cell lung cancer was investigated [33]. Data on the general response to immunotherapy in non-smokers is controversial: some studies have shown better response rates, whilst other analyses showed that never-smokers seem to benefit less from immunotherapy than smokers. In this study, the authors aimed to analyze a cohort of never-smokers with advanced SCC in-depth with respect to their response to nivolumab. Nivolumab was administered in 371 patients at a dosage of 3 mg/kg every 2 weeks for a maximum of 24 months, and safety was monitored [33]. Among the cohort there were 31 never-smokers (8%). The objective response rate, disease-control rate, and the median overall survival were 23%, 45%, and 12.1 months (95% confidence interval: 3.7–20.4), respectively, in never-smokers, and 18%, 47%, and 7.9 months (95% confidence interval: 6.2–9.6), respectively, in the whole population analyzed. Any-grade and grade 3–4 treatment-related adverse events (AE) were reported in 12 (39%) and 3 (10%) never-smokers, respectively, and in 109 (29%) and 21 (6%) patients of the total group, respectively. Treatment had to be discontinued due to side effects in 4 non-smokers, and in 26 patients overall [33]. Summing up this report, in the pre-treated never-smokers suffering from advanced SCC, safety and efficacy of nivolumab treatment were similar and consistent to the overall study population as well as to previous reports on nivolumab. According to this analysis, there is no evidence that never-smokers might benefit less from nivolumab as compared to smokers.

3. Adenocarcinoma in Non- or Never-Smokers: Patient Characteristics

Starting again with a case report, we discuss an article about a never-smoker female lung cancer patient with multifocal lung AC, where morphological and genetic heterogeneity was assessed [34]. The patient presented with three lung nodules occurring at different time points, which were surgically removed. Unfortunately, the patient relapsed, and was subsequently treated with an EGFR-directed tyrosine kinase inhibitor (TKI), since *EGFR* exon 21 mutation had been detected. Progression free survival upon treatment with the TKI lasted for three months and was continued for six months, until clinical progression [34]. Tumor samples were then analyzed by means of a 30-gene NGS-gene panel, allowing for the evaluation of intra- and inter-tumor heterogeneity. Interestingly, the three lung tumors were confirmed independently according to NGS. The synchronous tumor samples featured different molecular profiles. Identical *EGFR*, *PIK3CA* and *TP53* mutations were found in one of the three primary tumors and in the metastasis that occurred later [34]. The patient in this case report may have a certain genetic cancer predisposition, which may explain the independent lung ACs, limited response to treatment and the fact that she was a never-smoker. In a review article by Okazaki et al., it was stated that genes commonly associated with the metabolic syndrome overlapped with genes frequently mutated in AC in never smokers [35]. Moreover, the incidence of AC is obviously increasing worldwide, and generally AC is more prevalent in never-smokers than any other histologic lung cancer type. All these findings lead to further questions, e.g. whether lung AC is a different disease than non-AC lung cancers, why there is an obvious female predisposition and what prevention strategies exist [35].

Recently, Li and colleagues conducted an integrative analysis where they included 11 lung cancer gene-expression datasets that provide data from 1111 lung AC and 200 samples of adjacent normal tissue [26]. According to this study, distinct pathways were altered in ever-smokers, and different pathways in never-smokers. Never-smokers had a better outcome as well. In the course of this study, compositional patterns of 21 types of immune cells in lung AC were characterized, revealing complex and multilayered associations between the composition of immune cell subtypes and clinical outcome [26]. Two subsets of immune cells, namely mast cells and CD4+ memory T cells were found to have completely opposite associations with outcome in resting, as compared to activated status. Resting mast cells (defined by not having undergone degranulation), which were found to be decreased in numbers in tumor samples, compared with adjacent normal tissue, were predictors of a favorable outcome, but macrophages, activated mast cells (mast cells after degranulation) and activated CD4+ memory T cells that were enriched in the carcinoma samples predicted a poor prognosis [26]. Differences in the composition of immune cell types were found in never- and ever-smokers: there were more resting mast cells in never-smokers, and more resting CD4+ memory T cells as well, these being associated with a better outcome. In ever-smokers, there were more activated mast cells and CD4+ cells, which correlated with a generally worse prognosis. What's more, a variety of chemokines and associated chemokine receptors (e.g., the CKCL11-CXCR1 axis) were selectively mutated in smoking-associated lung cancers, and these alterations also correlated with the status switch of immune cells from resting to the activated form. Taken together, these findings indicate unique changes in the lung cancer microenvironment that are caused by tobacco smoke, altering the intrinsic immune system of the bronchi. It is thus very likely that certain patterns of immune cell dysfunction lead to a worse prognosis especially in lung cancer patients who continue smoking [26].

The role of metabolic syndrome in lung AC, especially in non-smoking patients, is currently under intensive exploration: Yang and colleagues did a survey on body mass index (BMI) and waist circumference in a prospectively studied population of women aged 55–69 years, who were followed up for 13 years. It was significant ($p < 0.15$) that patients with lung cancer had higher waist circumferences [36]. According to another investigation where the pattern of adiponectin quantitative trait loci (QTLs) in association with gene expression correlation was analyzed, genes related to metabolic syndrome were found also to contribute to cancer formation [37]. *EGFR*, *VTL1A*, *TNFRSF10C*, *C3ORF21* and hyper-methylation of *TNFSF10C*, *BHLHB5*, and *BOLL* are involved in both lung AC formation and pathways related to metabolic syndrome, according to genome wide association studies (GWAS) [5,35]. The link between the metabolic syndrome and lung AC in non-smokers is also supported by Mazieres and colleagues who examined 140 female AC patients, amongst them 63 never-smokers and 77 former or current smokers [38]. In never-smokers, histology showed lipidic features (lipid droplets inside cancer cells; not to be confounded with a lepidic growth pattern of NSCLC) significantly more often (60.3% vs. 37.7%, $p = 0.008$) as compared to smokers. It is common knowledge that obesity, a predominantly sedentary lifestyle, too much alcohol consumption and a diet high in—especially saturated fatty acids - lead to metabolic syndrome but is also associated with a higher incidence of malignant disease in general [39,40]. A frequent complication of metabolic syndrome is type-2 diabetes, which increases the risk of lung cancer, most of all for females (relative risk for women with diabetes = 1.14) [41].

4. Physical Inactivity

Cannioto et al. investigated the association of physical inactivity with lung cancer [42]. Since it has been proven for many types of malignant disease that lifetime inactivity goes along with an increased cancer risk, the authors wanted to show whether this holds true also for lung cancer, independently of other risk factors such as smoking. In this hospital-based, case-control study, data from 660 lung cancer patients and 1335 matched controls, who did not suffer from any malignant disease, were analyzed [42]. Multivariate logistic regression analysis was used to assess the association between a primarily sedentary lifestyle and the risk of lung cancer. Furthermore, Cox proportional hazard models were utilized for a calculation on how closely lifetime physical inactivity and mortality among lung cancer patients is related. Not surprisingly, a significant positive correlation of physical inactivity and lung cancer risk was observed [Odds ratio (OR) = 2.23, 95% confidence interval (CI): 1.77–2.81]. Among never-smokers (OR = 3.00, 95% CI: 1.33–6.78) and former smokers (OR = 3.00, 95% CI: 1.33–6.78) the association was significant as well. The authors also described a significant positive correlation between lifetime physical inactivity and the mortality from lung cancer [Hazard ratio (HR) = 1.40, 95% CI: 1.14–1.71]; here the association remained significant also for the non-smoking patients [42]. A different study published in 2017 also evaluated the impact of physical activity on lung cancer risk. It has already been shown in numerous studies that regular physical activity decreases lung cancer risk; the risk reduction has been reported to range from 20 to 50% when the most active study participants were compared to the least active individuals [43]. Being either underweight or obese also increases lung cancer risk, following a nonlinear inverted U-shaped relation [43]. It has to be kept in mind though, that an active lifestyle and regular exercise often means less likelihood to engage in smoking. Thus, Patel and colleagues especially stratified for smoking status when investigating physical activity and lung cancer; also because smokers tend to be not only less active, but on average also have a lower body-mass-index as compared to non-smokers. Data of 162679 men and women from the American Cancer Society Cancer Prevention Study-II Nutrition Cohort were analyzed, who were all free of cancer at enrollment in this study (1992–1993) [44]. Baseline physical activity (MET-hours per week; none, 0.1 to < 8.75; 8.75–17.4; >17.5 MET-hours/week), baseline body mass index and waist circumference were assessed in relation to lung cancer risk [43]. Risk stratification for smoking history, years since quitting among former smokers and adjustment for other possible confounders was carried out. During the follow-up time of 2,384,546-person years, 4669 men and women were diagnosed with lung cancer (453 never smokers, 1452 current smokers and 2764 ex-smokers) [43]. Interestingly, physical activity was not associated with lung cancer risk in this large analysis within any of the smoking strata, except in former smokers who quit less than 10 years ago (RR = 0.77; 95% CI 0.67–0.90 for >17.5 MET hours/week). BMI was inversely associated with lung cancer risk in a similar way, also in the former-smoking group who quit <10 years (RR = 0.68; 95% CI 0.55–0.84 for >30 kg/m2). The authors clearly conclude that—although evidently protective against a variety of cancer subtypes—physical activity may not lower the risk for lung cancer [43].

5. Asbestos and Radon

Although uncommon causes of lung cancer per se, occupational carcinogens and radon can sometimes contribute to lung carcinogenesis. In the literature, no data on this topic addressing specifically the non-smoking population, can be found—most probably due to the fact that most cases of lung cancer where occupational carcinogens also play a role, do occur in individuals who smoked as well. A study has been done on the occurrence of radioactive radon gas, generated from uranium and thorium in underlying rocks and seeps, in Norwegian buildings [45]. Radon gas and its decay products emit radiation that promotes lung carcinogenesis, and in people exposed to radon, this is considered the second most important risk factor for lung cancer, directly after tobacco smoke. In Norway, average radon concentrations in buildings are higher than in most industrialized countries. Hassfjell et al. have estimated the radon-related risk of lung cancer in Norway, using data from the largest pooled European analysis of case-control studies, combined with the largest set of data on radon concentration measurements in Norwegian homes. According to this data, it was calculated that radon gas contributes to about 12% of all cases of lung cancer annually in Norway; meaning that in the year 2015 for instance, in 373 cases of lung cancer radon was a contributory factor [45]. However, the authors clearly state that in most lung cancer cases, former or current tobacco smoking was still the main risk factor.

Asbestos is an occupational carcinogen that also endorses lung cancer formation, though asbestos is usually known for causing pleural mesothelioma. Accumulating evidence has highlighted the role of epigenetic deregulation caused by asbestos exposure, and thus in 2017 Kettunen et al. did a genome-wide DNA-methylation analysis, investigating the impact of asbestos on DNA methylation [46]. The researchers used "Illumina HumanMethylation450K BeadChip" for methylation analysis in 28 samples of lung cancer tissue. Also, in this study, the majority of patients investigated were smokers [46]. Differentially methylated regions (DMR), as well as differentially methylated CpGs (DVMC) were identified, with individual CpGs being evaluated in-depth by pyrosequencing in an independent series of 91 NSCLC samples and corresponding normal lung tissue. *BEND4, ZSCAN31* and *GPR135* were found to be significantly hypermethylated in asbestos-associated NSCLS. DMRs in the genes *RARB, GPR135,* and DVMCs in the genes *NPTN, NRG2* and *GLTs5D2* (amongst others) were significantly associated with asbestos exposure (comparing exposed vs. not-exposed tumors). The authors of this study also compared DVMCs related to asbestos or positive smoking history, and found that 96% of the elements were unique to either of the exposures, suggesting that the methylation pattern is strongly influenced by the specific risk factor. This data suggests, that epigenetic changes may be influenced by environmental risk factors very strongly, and that asbestos causes different changes than tobacco smoke alone [46]. Another interesting analysis aimed at outlining altered micro RNA (miRNA) expression in NSCLC upon exposure to asbestos [47]. Generally, it is known that altered miRNA expression is an early step in carcinogenesis when occupational and environmental carcinogens come into play. The authors sought to identify an asbestos-related profile of miRNA changes, able to discern asbestos-induced NSCLC from cancer with a different etiology. Four groups of patients were included in this study: those with asbestos-related NSCLC, asbestos-unrelated NSCLC, subjects with malignant pleural mesothelioma, and healthy individuals. Four serum miRNAs (miR-126, miR-205, miR-222 and miR-520g) were significantly associated with asbestos-related NSCLC, or mesothelioma [47]. Increased expression of miR-126 and miR-222 are both involved in major cancer-promoting pathways. The authors suggest that epigenetic changes caused by asbestos, as well as cross-talk between cancer- and stroma-cells could lead to the repression of miR-126 which promotes tumor growth, angiogenesis and invasion. It is concluded that miRNAs are potentially involved in asbestos-related malignant disease, influencing specific mechanisms whereby asbestos promotes cancer formation—and these mechanisms may also differ from the conventional tobacco-smoke related ones.

6. Immunological Changes: Tumor Microenvironment in Never-Smokers

In never-smokers, the immunologic homeostasis within the tumor microenvironment seems to be less compromised when compared to ever-smokers [26]. Notably, not all immune cells impact lung carcinogenesis in a similar way: inflammatory cells are recruited into the lung as a result of tobacco smoking. On the one hand these cells are helpful because they are trying to minimize the damage which is done by the carcinogenic substances, on the other hand, however, the immune cells may weaken the bronchial epithelial cells and cause harmful pro-inflammatory and immune reactions [48]. When a tumor arises, the immune cells are also part of the harmful tumor microenvironment and can even contribute to tumor growth, invasion and metastatic spread [49]. This is proven by certain biologicals that have recently been established as targeted treatment options for lung cancer, targeting for instance cytotoxic T-lymphocyte-associated antigen 4 (CTLA-4) (ipilimumab), or PD-1-receptor and PD-1 ligand (PD-L1) which are targeted by nivolumab and atezolizumab [49]. It has been reported according to a study published in 2018, that 17 out of 20 investigated pathways of carcinogenesis, related to immune response, were altered in a different way in AC of never-smokers as compared to ever-smokers [26]. Compositional differences of 14 kinds of immune subsets between tumors and normal samples were reported, and the composition of leukocyte subtypes correlated strongly not only with smoking history, but also with outcome [26]. M0 macrophages and total macrophage count strongly correlated with a poor prognosis. Furthermore, the immune score of CD8+ T cells was associated with a more favorable prognosis. Although it has been shown in ovarian- and breast cancer that CD8+ T cells usually mean a better outcome [50], in lung AC the results were controversial: in stage IV NSCLC patients undergoing chemotherapy, CD8+ T cells also correlated with a better prognosis [51], but some other studies suggested no influence of CD8+ T cells on NSCLC survival whatsoever [52,53]. Numerous studies have already shown how strongly immune reactions are associated with carcinogenesis. Either the immune system is capable to protect against cancer progression, or it can enhance tumor growth, invasion and metastasis by negatively influencing the tumor microenvironment and weakening the surrounding healthy cells. Thus, it is very likely that smoking, which obviously alters the immune system in the bronchi long before carcinogenic effects are observed, allows for specific changes in the cancers of smokers, featuring ultimately a different microenvironment as compared to lung cancers of never-smokers.

7. Anaplastic Lymphoma Tyrosine Kinase -Rearrangement in Lung Adenocarcinoma in Non- and Never-Smokers

Targeted therapy has become a well-established therapeutic tool for the treatment of lung cancer. In tumors featuring anaplastic lymphoma tyrosine kinase (*ALK*)-rearrangement, agents like crizotinib, ceritinib, alectinib, brigatinib and lorlatinib are valid treatment options, hence a correct molecular profiling of newly diagnosed tumors is of great importance [54,55]. Frequently, *ALK* rearrangements result from inversions on chromosome 2p [inv(2)(p21;p23)] which leads to a fusion of *ALK* with the echinoderm microtubule-associated protein-like 4 (*EML4*) gene [56]. The gold standard to evaluate ALK-rearrangement is by fluorescence in situ hybridization (FISH). In a study by Williams and colleagues, the aim was to assess the prevalence of *ALK*-rearrangements in lung AC samples of lifetime non-smokers, as well as long-term ex-smokers (quit > 10 years prior to diagnosis) [57]. According to the literature, *ALK* gene rearrangement is found in 2–5% of all non-small cell lung cancers, being more common in lifetime non-smokers with adenocarcinoma as compared to smokers with adenocarcinoma, or squamous cell carcinoma. However, accurate assessment of *ALK*-rearrangement in long-term ex-smokers has not been done before the year 2016 [57]. The authors enrolled 251 cases of resected lung AC samples, including 79 non-smokers and 172 ex-smokers who had quit smoking for over 10 years [57]. *ALK*-rearrangement was evaluated via FISH, and immunohistochemistry (IHC) as well. Four out of 251 cases featured *ALK*-rearrangement. All of these four were non-smokers. In samples of long-term ex-smokers, no *ALK*-rearrangements were observed [57]. The analysis revealed strong evidence of an increased prevalence of *ALK* gene rearrangement in the non-smoking population, as compared to the general population of lung adenocarcinoma patients. Interestingly, there was no significant difference in *ALK*-rearrangement between the ex-smokers and the general population of patients with resected lung AC. This study confirmed that ALK-rearrangement is more common in non-smoking patients suffering from lung adenocarcinoma. However, the incidence reported in this analysis is uncommonly low (5.1% in non-smokers; 1.6% overall) when compared to previous reports. This is presumably due to the circumstance that most samples were early-stage, resected lung cancers; since it has been shown that *ALK*-rearrangements tend to occur more often in advanced, mainly stage IV, cancers [58].

Overall, the occurrence of the *ALK*-translocation in lung AC of never-smokers clearly indicated that the patho-mechanism is based on a single genetic driver rather than on an accumulation of genetic lesions in a variety of cancer genes, as it is the case in smoking-related AC.

8. Conclusions

The data which we have summarized above indicates that NSCLC in non-, especially in never-smokers, is a distinct tumor entity featuring a different tumor biology and microenvironment as compared to tobacco associated lung carcinomas. We have summarized key findings of the studies mentioned in the table below (Table 1).

From the epidemiological perspective, other risk factors such as metabolic disorders may play a role, as well as germline mutations that lead to cancer formation in certain individuals independent from lifestyle and exposure to carcinogens. The take-home message of this short literature review is the paramount importance of personalized medicine, in-depth molecular assessment and targeted treatment options especially in never-smoking patients suffering from lung cancer, since their tumors differ distinctly in molecular pathology, prognosis and response to treatment in comparison to "conventional" smoking-associated tumors.

Table 1. Non-smoking associated lung cancer—summary of recent findings.

Tumor Type	Patient Characteristics	Aim Of The Study	Methods	Key Findings	Discussion/Conclusion	Reference
Adenocarcinoma (AC)	1111 lung AC and 200 samples of adjacent normal tissue; comparison of smokers vs. non-smokers	Characterization of tumor microenvironment/pattern of tumor-associated immune cells	Online lung cancer data analysis via Gene Expression Omnibus (GEO); to determine the fraction of immune cells in tumors, a linear support vector regression-based method, CIBERSORT, was applied to estimate the relative ratios of 21 leukocyte subtypes	Distinct pathways were altered in lung carcinogenesis in ever-smokers and never-smokers. Never-smoker patients had a better outcome than ever-smoker patients. Mast cells and CD4$^+$ memory T cells were associated with poor outcome when activated compared to the resting form; cigarette smoke induced activation of these immune cells	Tobacco smoke alters the composition of immune cells in lung adenocarcinoma; activation of CD4+ memory T cells and mast cells by smoking may be responsible for the worse outcome in smokers as compared to non-smokers	[26]
AC	1 never-smoker female patient with multifocal lung AC; after surgery the patient underwent treatment with EGFR-TKI	Assessment of morphological and genetic tumorheterogeneity	30-gene next generation sequencing (NGS) panel, allowing for evaluation of intra- and inter-tumoral heterogeneity	The 3 lung tumors were confirmed independent according to NGS; identical *EGFR, PIK3CA* and *TP53* mutations were found in one of the three primary tumors and in the metastasis that occurred later on	In this non-smoker female patient, some type of genetic cancer predispositon is likely, explaining the three genetically independent lung ACs and limited response to treatment	[34]
Lung cancer (any histological type)	Prospectively studied population of women aged 55-69 years, who were followed up for 13 years	Evaluation of the role of metabolic syndrome in lung cancer	Prospective cohort study; focus on body mass index (BMI) and waist circumference	Patients with lung cancer had a significantly higher waist circumference	Abdominal obesity may increase the risk for lung cancer when stratifying for other common risk factors	[36]
AC	140 female AC patients, amongst them 63 never-smokers and 77 former or current smokers	Investigating the link of metabolic disorders and lung AC in never-smokers	Histologic analysis of tumor samples, smoking-associated vs. not smoking-associated tumors	In never-smokers, lipidic histologic differentiation was found significantly more often as compared to smokers	Non-smokers with a sedentary lifestyle, hyperlipidemia and other signs of metabolic disease might be at higher risk for lung cancer as compared to non-smokers without metabolic syndrome	[38]
Lung cancer (any histological type)	660 lung cancer patients and 1335 matched controls who did not suffer from any malignant disease	To determine whether physical inactivity increases lung cancer risk, and whether it increases mortality in case of lung cancer	Case-control study; assessment of the association of inactive lifestyle and risk of lung cancer via multivariate logistic regression analysis; Cox proportional hazard models were used for estimation of the connex of inactivity and mortality from lung cancer	Significant positive correlation of physical inactivity and risk of lung cancer; significant positive correlation between lifetime physical inactivity and lung cancer-related mortality; also significant for non-smoking lung cancer patients	Physical inactivity increases not only the risk of lung cancer but also lung cancer-related mortality	[42]
Lung cancer (any histological type)	Data of 162679 men and women from the American Cancer Society Cancer Prevention Study-II Nutrition Cohort were analyzed, who were all free of cancer at enrollment in this study (1992–1993)	Assessment of the correlation of baseline physical activity and lung cancer incidence over the follow-up period	Baseline physical activity (MET-hours per week; none, 0.1 to <8.75; 8.75-17.4; >17.5 MET-hours/week), BMI and waist circumference were assessed in relation to lung cancer risk	Physical activity was not associated with lung cancer risk, except in former smokers who quit less than 10 years ago (for >17.5 MET hours/week); BMI was inversely associated with lung cancer risk	According to this study, physical activity is not a protective factor regarding the incidence of lung cancer	[43]
AC	Never-smokers and long-term ex-smokers who quit >10 years prior to diagnosis with AC; 251 cases of resected lung AC (79 never-, and 172 ex-smokers)	To assess the prevalence of *ALK*-rearrangements in lung AC samples of lifetime non-smokers, as well as long-term ex-smokers (quit >10 years prior to diagnosis)	*ALK*-rearrangement was evaluated via fluorescence in situ hybridization FISH, and immunohistochemistry (IHC)	strong evidence of increased *ALK* gene rearrangement in the non-smoking population; no significant difference in *ALK*-rearrangement between the ex-smokers and the general population	*ALK*-rearrangement is more common in non-smoking patients	[57]
Squamous cell carcinoma (SCC)	19 patients suffering from SCC (8 non-smokers, 11 smokers)	Evaluation of genetic differences in SCC of smokers, as compared to non-smokers	Array comparative genomic hybridization (ArrayCGH); immunohistochemistry	16 gene regions were significantly altered, according to ArrayCGH in non-smokers compared to smokers; the proto-oncogene *GAB2* (11q14.1) was significantly amplified in non-smoking patients, and the GAB2 protein was upregulated as well	*GAB2* amplification is likely to contribute to SCC development in non-smokers	[4]
SCC	1 non-smoker female patient with SCC and history of a SCC at the neck 2 years prior	To determine germline cancer predisposition in this special case	Assessment of somatic driver mutations via whole exome sequencing	Predominance of C>T transitions in tumoral lung tissue; usually not found in tobacco-smoke-associated lung cancer; no mutations of frequent driver genes of lung cancer were found	In this case a special oligogenic germline signature predisposed for SCC formation; personalized medicine is especially important in non-smoker patients	[30]
SCC	371 patients with SCC; among them were 31 never-smokers	Analyzing the response to nivolumab in SCC patients who are non-smokers	Nivolumab was administered at a dosage of 3 mg/kg every 2 weeks for a maximum of 24 months, and safety was monitored	The objective response rate, disease-control rate and median overall survival were comparable in the smoking vs. the never-smoking group	Safety and effecacy of nivolumab seems to be similar in never-smokers as compared to smokers with SCC	[33]

References

1. Global Burden of Disease Cancer Collaboration. Global, Regional, and National Cancer Incidence, Mortality, Years of Life Lost, Years Lived with Disability, and Disability-Adjusted Life-years for 32 Cancer Groups, 1990 to 2015: A Systematic Analysis for the Global Burden of Disease Study. *JAMA Oncol.* **2017**, *3*, 524–548. [CrossRef] [PubMed]
2. Siegel, R.; Naishadham, D.; Jemal, A. Cancer statistics, 2013. *CA Cancer J. Clin.* **2013**, *63*, 11–30. [CrossRef] [PubMed]
3. Bray, F.; Ferlay, J.; Soerjomataram, I.; Siegel, R.L.; Torre, L.A.; Jemal, A. Global cancer statistics 2018: GLOBOCAN estimates of incidence and mortality worldwide for 36 cancers in 185 countries. *CA Cancer J. Clin.* **2018**, *68*, 394–424. [CrossRef]
4. Park, Y.R.; Bae, S.H.; Ji, W.; Seo, E.J.; Lee, J.C.; Kim, H.R.; Jang, S.J.; Chang-Min, C. GAB2 Amplification in Squamous Cell Lung Cancer of Non-Smokers. *J. Korean Med. Sci.* **2017**, *32*, 1784–1791. [CrossRef] [PubMed]
5. Okazaki, I.; Ishikawa, S.; Ando, W.; Sohara, Y. Lung Adenocarcinoma in Never Smokers: Problems of Primary Prevention from Aspects of Susceptible Genes and Carcinogens. *Anticancer Res.* **2016**, *36*, 6207–6224. [CrossRef]
6. Couraud, S.; Zalcman, G.; Milleron, B.; Morin, F.; Souquet, P.J. Lung cancer in never smokers–a review. *Eur. J. Cancer* **2012**, *48*, 1299–1311. [CrossRef] [PubMed]
7. Sun, S.; Schiller, J.H.; Gazdar, A.F. Lung cancer in never smokers—a different disease. *Nat. Rev. Cancer* **2007**, *7*, 778–790. [CrossRef]
8. Thun, M.J.; Hannan, L.M.; Adams-Campbell, L.L.; Boffetta, P.; Buring, J.E.; Feskanich, D.; Flanders, D.W.; Jee, S.H.; Katanoda, K.; Kolonel, L.N.; et al. Lung cancer occurrence in never-smokers: An analysis of 13 cohorts and 22 cancer registry studies. *PLoS Med.* **2008**, *30*, e185. [CrossRef]
9. Kawaguchi, T.; Takada, M.; Kubo, A.; Matsumura, A.; Fukai, S.; Tamura, A.; Saito, R.; Kawahara, M.; Maruyama, Y. Gender, histology, and time of diagnosis are important factors for prognosis: Analysis of 1499 never-smokers with advanced non-small cell lung cancer in Japan. *J. Thorac. Oncol.* **2010**, *5*, 1011–1017. [CrossRef]
10. Pao, W.; Miller, V.; Zakowski, M.; Doherty, J.; Politi, K.; Sarkaria, I.; Singh, B.; Heelan, R.; Rusch, V.; Fulton, L.; et al. EGF receptor gene mutations are common in lung cancers from "never smokers" and are associated with sensitivity of tumors to gefitinib and erlotinib. *Proc. Natl. Acad. Sci. USA* **2004**, *101*, 13306–13311. [CrossRef]
11. Samet, J.M. Lung Cancer, Smoking, and Obesity: It's Complicated. *J. Natl. Cancer Inst.* **2018**, *110*, 795–796. [CrossRef] [PubMed]
12. Samet, J.M. Tobacco smoking: The leading cause of preventable disease worldwide. *Thorac. Surg. Clin.* **2013**, *23*, 103–112. [CrossRef] [PubMed]
13. Lynch, T.J.; Bell, D.W.; Sordella, R.; Gurubhagavatula, S.; Okimoto, R.A.; Brannigan, B.W.; Harris, P.L.; Haserlat, S.M.; Supko, J.G.; Haluska, F.G.; et al. Activating mutations in the epidermal growth factor receptor underlying responsiveness of non-small-cell lung cancer to gefitinib. *N. Engl. J. Med.* **2004**, *350*, 2129–2139. [CrossRef]
14. Koo, L.C.; Ho, J.H. Worldwide epidemiological patterns of lung cancer in nonsmokers. *Int. J. Epidemiol.* **1990**, *19*, S14–S23. [CrossRef] [PubMed]
15. Nordquist, L.T.; Simon, G.R.; Cantor, A.; Alberts, W.M.; Bepler, G. Improved survival in never-smokers vs current smokers with primary adenocarcinoma of the lung. *Chest* **2004**, *126*, 347–351. [CrossRef] [PubMed]
16. Paez, J.G.; Janne, P.A.; Lee, J.C.; Tracy, S.; Greulich, H.; Gabriel, S.; Herman, P.; Kaye, F.J.; Lindeman, N.; Boggon, T.J.; et al. EGFR mutations in lung cancer: Correlation with clinical response to gefitinib therapy. *Science* **2004**, *304*, 1497–1500. [CrossRef] [PubMed]
17. Malhotra, J.; Malvezzi, M.; Negri, E.; La Vecchia, C.; Boffetta, P. Risk factors for lung cancer worldwide. *Eur. Respir. J.* **2016**, *48*, 889–902. [CrossRef]
18. Lee, D.H.; Lee, J.S.; Wang, J.; Hsia, T.C.; Wang, X.; Kim, J.; Orlando, M. Pemetrexed-Erlotinib, Pemetrexed Alone, or Erlotinib Alone as Second-Line Treatment for East Asian and Non-East Asian Never-Smokers with Locally Advanced or Metastatic Nonsquamous Non-small Cell Lung Cancer: Exploratory Subgroup Analysis of a Phase II Trial. *Cancer Res. Treat.* **2015**, *47*, 616–629.

19. Miller, V.A.; Kris, M.G.; Shah, N.; Patel, J.; Azzoli, C.; Gomez, J.; Krug, L.M.; Pao, W.; Rizvi, N.; Pizzo, B.; et al. Bronchioloalveolar pathologic subtype and smoking history predict sensitivity to gefitinib in advanced non-small-cell lung cancer. *J. Clin. Oncol.* **2004**, *22*, 1103–1109. [CrossRef]
20. Shigematsu, H.; Lin, L.; Takahashi, T.; Nomura, M.; Suzuki, M.; Wistuba, I.I.; Fong, K.M.; Lee, H.; Toyooka, S.; Shimizu, N.; et al. Clinical and biological features associated with epidermal growth factor receptor gene mutations in lung cancers. *J. Natl. Cancer Inst.* **2005**, *97*, 339–346. [CrossRef]
21. Islami, F.; Torre, L.A.; Jemal, A. Global trends of lung cancer mortality and smoking prevalence. *Transl. Lung Cancer Res.* **2015**, *4*, 327–338. [PubMed]
22. Choi, J.R.; Park, S.Y.; Noh, O.K.; Koh, Y.W.; Kang, D.R. Gene mutation discovery research of non-smoking lung cancer patients due to indoor radon exposure. *Ann. Occup. Environ. Med.* **2016**, *28*, 13. [CrossRef] [PubMed]
23. Secretan, B.; Straif, K.; Baan, R.; Grosse, Y.; El Ghissassi, F.; Bouvard, V.; Benbrahim-Tallaa, L.; Guha, N.; Freeman, C.; Galichet, L.; et al. A review of human carcinogens–Part E: Tobacco, areca nut, alcohol, coal smoke, and salted fish. *Lancet Oncol.* **2009**, *10*, 1033–1034. [CrossRef]
24. Cheng, Y.W.; Chiou, H.L.; Sheu, G.T.; Hsieh, L.L.; Chen, J.T.; Chen, C.Y.; Su, J.M.; Lee, H. The association of human papillomavirus 16/18 infection with lung cancer among nonsmoking Taiwanese women. *Cancer Res.* **2001**, *61*, 2799–2803. [PubMed]
25. Liang, H.Y.; Li, X.L.; Yu, X.S.; Guan, P.; Yin, Z.H.; He, Q.C.; Zhou, B.S. Facts and fiction of the relationship between preexisting tuberculosis and lung cancer risk: A systematic review. *Int. J. Cancer* **2009**, *125*, 2936–2944. [CrossRef] [PubMed]
26. Li, X.; Li, J.; Wu, P.; Zhou, L.; Lu, B.; Ying, K.; Chen, E.; Lu, Y.; Liu, P. Smoker and non-smoker lung adenocarcinoma is characterized by distinct tumor immune microenvironments. *Oncoimmunology* **2018**, *7*, e1494677. [CrossRef] [PubMed]
27. Brunelli, M.; Bria, E.; Nottegar, A.; Cingarlini, S.; Simionato, F.; Calio, A.; Eccher, A.; Parolini, C.; Iannucci, A.; Gilioli, E.; et al. True 3q chromosomal amplification in squamous cell lung carcinoma by FISH and aCGH molecular analysis: Impact on targeted drugs. *PLoS ONE* **2012**, *7*, e49689. [CrossRef]
28. Cancer Genome Atlas Research Network. Comprehensive genomic characterization of squamous cell lung cancers. *Nature* **2012**, *489*, 519–525. [CrossRef]
29. Forbes, S.A.; Beare, D.; Gunasekaran, P.; Leung, K.; Bindal, N.; Boutselakis, H.; Ding, M.; Bamford, S.; Cole, C.; Ward, S.; et al. COSMIC: Exploring the world's knowledge of somatic mutations in human cancer. *Nucleic Acids Res.* **2015**, *43*, D805–CD811. [CrossRef]
30. Baldassarri, M.; Fallerini, C.; Cetta, F.; Ghisalberti, M.; Bellan, C.; Furini, S.; Spiga, O.; Crispino, S.; Gotti, G.; Ariani, F. Omic Approach in Non-smoker Female with Lung Squamous Cell Carcinoma Pinpoints to Germline Susceptibility and Personalized Medicine. *Cancer Res. Treat.* **2018**, *50*, 356–365. [CrossRef]
31. Vanni, I.; Coco, S.; Bonfiglio, S.; Cittaro, D.; Genova, C.; Biello, F.; Mora, M.; Rossella, V.; Dal Bello, M.G.; Truini, A.; et al. Whole exome sequencing of independent lung adenocarcinoma, lung squamous cell carcinoma, and malignant peritoneal mesothelioma: A case report. *Medicine (Baltimore)* **2016**, *95*, e5447. [CrossRef] [PubMed]
32. Tong, L. Acetyl-coenzyme A carboxylase: Crucial metabolic enzyme and attractive target for drug discovery. *Cell Mol. Life Sci.* **2005**, *62*, 1784–1803. [CrossRef] [PubMed]
33. Garassino, M.C.; Crino, L.; Catino, A.; Ardizzoni, A.; Cortesi, E.; Cappuzzo, F.; Bordi, P.; Calabrò, L.; Barbieri, F.; Santo, A.; et al. Nivolumab in never-smokers with advanced squamous non-small cell lung cancer: Results from the Italian cohort of an expanded access program. *Tumour Biol.* **2018**, *40*, 1010428318815047. [CrossRef] [PubMed]
34. Bonanno, L.; Calabrese, F.; Nardo, G.; Calistri, D.; Tebaldi, M.; Tedaldi, G.; Polo, V.; Vuljan, S.; Favaretto, A.; Conte, P.; et al. Morphological and genetic heterogeneity in multifocal lung adenocarcinoma: The case of a never-smoker woman. *Lung Cancer* **2016**, *96*, 52–55. [CrossRef] [PubMed]
35. Okazaki, I.; Ishikawa, S.; Sohara, Y. Genes associated with succeptibility to lung adenocarcinoma among never smokers suggest the mechanism of disease. *Anticancer Res.* **2014**, *34*, 5229–5240.

36. Yang, P.; Cerhan, J.R.; Vierkant, R.A.; Olson, J.E.; Vachon, C.M.; Limburg, P.J.; Parker, A.S.; Anderson, K.E.; Sellers, T.A. Adenocarcinoma of the lung is strongly associated with cigarette smoking: Further evidence from a prospective study of women. *Am. J. Epidemiol.* **2002**, *156*, 1114–1122. [CrossRef] [PubMed]
37. Zhang, Y.; Kent, J.W.; Olivier, M.; Ali, O.; Cerjak, D.; Broeckel, U.; Abdou, R.M.; Dyer, T.D.; Comuzzie, A.; Curran, J.E.; et al. A comprehensive analysis of adiponectin QTLs using SNP association, SNP cis-effects on peripheral blood gene expression and gene expression correlation identified novel metabolic syndrome, MetS) genes with potential role in carcinogenesis and systemic inflammation. *BMC Med. Genomics* **2013**, *6*, 14.
38. Mazieres, J.; Rouquette, I.; Lepage, B.; Milia, J.; Brouchet, L.; Guibert, N.; Beau-Faller, M.; Validire, P.; Hofman, P.; Fouret, P. Specificities of lung adenocarcinoma in women who have never smoked. *J. Thorac. Oncol.* **2013**, *8*, 923–929. [CrossRef] [PubMed]
39. Russo, A.; Autelitano, M.; Bisanti, L. Metabolic syndrome and cancer risk. *Eur. J. Cancer* **2008**, *44*, 293–297. [CrossRef]
40. Flegal, K.M.; Graubard, B.I.; Williamson, D.F.; Gail, M.H. Cause-specific excess deaths associated with underweight, overweight, and obesity. *JAMA* **2007**, *298*, 2028–2037. [CrossRef]
41. Lee, J.Y.; Jeon, I.; Lee, J.M.; Yoon, J.M.; Park, S.M. Diabetes mellitus as an independent risk factor for lung cancer: A meta-analysis of observational studies. *Eur. J. Cancer* **2013**, *49*, 2411–2423. [CrossRef] [PubMed]
42. Cannioto, R.; Etter, J.L.; LaMonte, M.J.; Ray, A.D.; Joseph, J.M.; Al Qassim, E.; Eng, K.H.; Moysich, K.B. Lifetime Physical Inactivity is Associated with Lung Cancer Risk and Mortality. *Cancer Treat. Res. Commun.* **2018**, *14*, 37–45. [CrossRef] [PubMed]
43. Patel, A.V.; Carter, B.D.; Stevens, V.L.; Gaudet, M.M.; Campbell, P.T.; Gapstur, S.M. The relationship between physical activity, obesity, and lung cancer risk by smoking status in a large prospective cohort of US adults. *Cancer Causes Control.* **2017**, *28*, 1357–1368. [CrossRef] [PubMed]
44. Calle, E.E.; Rodriguez, C.; Jacobs, E.J.; Almon, M.L.; Chao, A.; McCullough, M.L.; McCullough, M.L.; Feigelson, H.S.; Thun, M.J. The American Cancer Society Cancer Prevention Study II Nutrition Cohort: Rationale, study design, and baseline characteristics. *Cancer* **2002**, *94*, 2490–2501. [CrossRef] [PubMed]
45. Hassfjell, C.S.; Grimsrud, T.K.; Standring, W.J.F.; Tretli, S. Lung cancer incidence associated with radon exposure in Norwegian homes. *Tidsskr. Nor. Laegeforen.* **2017**, *137*, 14–15. [CrossRef]
46. Kettunen, E.; Hernandez-Vargas, H.; Cros, M.P.; Durand, G.; Le Calvez-Kelm, F.; Stuopelyte, K.; Jarmalaite, S.; Salmenkivi, K.; Anttila, S.; Wolff, H.; et al. Asbestos-associated genome-wide DNA methylation changes in lung cancer. *Int. J. Cancer* **2017**, *141*, 2014–2029. [CrossRef] [PubMed]
47. Santarelli, L.; Gaetani, S.; Monaco, F.; Bracci, M.; Valentino, M.; Amati, M.; Rubini, C.; Sabbatini, A.; Pasquini, E.; Zanotta, N.; et al. Four-miRNA Signature to Identify Asbestos-Related Lung Malignancies. *Cancer Epidemiol. Biomarkers Prev.* **2019**, *28*, 119–126. [CrossRef]
48. Goncalves, R.B.; Coletta, R.D.; Silverio, K.G.; Benevides, L.; Casati, M.Z.; da Silva, J.S.; Nociti, F.H., Jr. Impact of smoking on inflammation: Overview of molecular mechanisms. *Inflamm. Res.* **2011**, *60*, 409–424. [CrossRef]
49. Quail, D.F.; Joyce, J.A. Microenvironmental regulation of tumor progression and metastasis. *Nat. Med.* **2013**, *19*, 1423–1437. [CrossRef]
50. Fridman, W.H.; Pages, F.; Sautes-Fridman, C.; Galon, J. The immune contexture in human tumours: Impact on clinical outcome. *Nat. Rev. Cancer* **2012**, *12*, 298–306. [CrossRef]
51. Kawai, O.; Ishii, G.; Kubota, K.; Murata, Y.; Naito, Y.; Mizuno, T.; Aokage, K.; Saijo, N.; Nishiwaki, Y.; Gemma, A.; et al. Predominant infiltration of macrophages and CD8+) T Cells in cancer nests is a significant predictor of survival in stage IV nonsmall cell lung cancer. *Cancer* **2008**, *113*, 1387–1395. [CrossRef] [PubMed]
52. Trojan, A.; Urosevic, M.; Dummer, R.; Giger, R.; Weder, W.; Stahel, R.A. Immune activation status of CD8+ T cells infiltrating non-small cell lung cancer. *Lung Cancer* **2004**, *44*, 143–147. [CrossRef] [PubMed]
53. Hiraoka, K.; Miyamoto, M.; Cho, Y.; Suzuoki, M.; Oshikiri, T.; Nakakubo, Y.; Itoh, T.; Ohbuchi, T.; Kondo, S.; Katoh, H. Concurrent infiltration by CD8+ T cells and CD4+ T cells is a favourable prognostic factor in non-small-cell lung carcinoma. *Br. J. Cancer* **2006**, *94*, 275–280. [CrossRef]
54. Tobin, N.P.; Foukakis, T.; De Petris, L.; Bergh, J. The importance of molecular markers for diagnosis and selection of targeted treatments in patients with cancer. *J. Intern. Med.* **2015**, *278*, 545–570. [CrossRef] [PubMed]

55. Popper, H.H.; Ryska, A.; Timar, J.; Olszewski, W. Molecular testing in lung cancer in the era of precision medicine. *Transl. Lung Cancer Res.* **2014**, *3*, 291–300. [PubMed]

56. Sampsonas, F.; Ryan, D.; McPhillips, D.; Breen, D.P. Molecular testing and personalized treatment of lung cancer. *Curr. Mol. Pharmacol.* **2014**, *7*, 22–32. [CrossRef]

57. Williams, A.S.; Greer, W.; Bethune, D.; Craddock, K.J.; Flowerdew, G.; Xu, Z. ALK+ lung adenocarcinoma in never smokers and long-term ex-smokers: Prevalence and detection by immunohistochemistry and fluorescence in situ hybridization. *Virchows Arch.* **2016**, *469*, 533–540. [CrossRef]

58. Rodig, S.J.; Mino-Kenudson, M.; Dacic, S.; Yeap, B.Y.; Shaw, A.; Barletta, J.A.; Stubbs, H.; Law, K.; Lindeman, N.; Mark, E.; et al. Unique clinicopathologic features characterize ALK-rearranged lung adenocarcinoma in the western population. *Clin. Cancer Res.* **2009**, *15*, 5216–5223. [CrossRef]

6

Targeting the Interplay between Epithelial-to-Mesenchymal-Transition and the Immune System for Effective Immunotherapy

Rama Soundararajan [1,†], Jared J. Fradette [2,†], Jessica M. Konen [2,†], Stacy Moulder [3,†], Xiang Zhang [4,†], Don L. Gibbons [2,†], Navin Varadarajan [5,†], Ignacio I. Wistuba [1,†], Debasish Tripathy [3,†], Chantale Bernatchez [6], Lauren A. Byers [2], Jeffrey T. Chang [7,†], Alejandro Contreras [8], Bora Lim [3], Edwin Roger Parra [1], Emily B. Roarty [2], Jing Wang [9], Fei Yang [1], Michelle Barton [10], Jeffrey M. Rosen [4,†,*] and Sendurai A. Mani [1,†,*]

1 Department of Translational Molecular Pathology, The University of Texas MD Anderson Cancer Center, Houston, TX 77030, USA
2 Department of Thoracic/Head-Neck Medical Oncology, The University of Texas MD Anderson Cancer Center, Houston, TX 77030, USA
3 Department of Breast Medical Oncology, The University of Texas MD Anderson Cancer Center, Houston, TX 77030, USA
4 Department of Molecular and Cellular Biology, Baylor College of Medicine, Houston, TX 77030, USA
5 Department of Chemical and Biomolecular Engineering, University of Houston, Houston, TX 77204, USA
6 Departments of Melanoma Medical Oncology–Research and Translational Molecular Pathology, The University of Texas MD Anderson Cancer Center, Houston, TX 77030, USA
7 Department of Integrative Biology and Pharmacology, The University of Texas Health Sciences Center, Houston, TX 77030, USA
8 Department of Pathology (Anatomical), The University of Texas MD Anderson Cancer Center, Houston, TX 77030, USA
9 Department of Bioinformatics and Computational Biology, The University of Texas MD Anderson Cancer Center, Houston, TX 77030, USA
10 Department of Epigenetics and Molecular Carcinogenesis, The University of Texas MD Anderson Cancer Center, Houston, TX 77030, USA
* Correspondence: jrosen@bcm.edu (J.M.R.); smani@mdanderson.org (S.A.M.)
† These authors contributed equally to this work.

Abstract: Over the last decade, both early diagnosis and targeted therapy have improved the survival rates of many cancer patients. Most recently, immunotherapy has revolutionized the treatment options for cancers such as melanoma. Unfortunately, a significant portion of cancers (including lung and breast cancers) do not respond to immunotherapy, and many of them develop resistance to chemotherapy. Molecular characterization of non-responsive cancers suggest that an embryonic program known as epithelial-mesenchymal transition (EMT), which is mostly latent in adults, can be activated under selective pressures, rendering these cancers resistant to chemo- and immunotherapies. EMT can also drive tumor metastases, which in turn also suppress the cancer-fighting activity of cytotoxic T cells that traffic into the tumor, causing immunotherapy to fail. In this review, we compare and contrast immunotherapy treatment options of non-small cell lung cancer (NSCLC) and triple negative breast cancer (TNBC). We discuss why, despite breakthrough progress in immunotherapy, attaining predictable outcomes in the clinic is mostly an unsolved problem for these tumors. Although these two cancer types appear different based upon their tissues of origin and molecular classification, gene expression indicate that they possess many similarities. Patient tumors exhibit activation of EMT, and resulting stem cell properties in both these cancer types associate with metastasis and resistance to existing cancer therapies. In addition, the EMT transition in both these cancers plays a crucial role in immunosuppression, which exacerbates treatment resistance. To improve cancer-related survival we need to understand and circumvent, the mechanisms through which these tumors become therapy resistant. In this review, we discuss new information and complementary perspectives to inform combination treatment strategies to expand and improve the anti-tumor responses of currently available clinical immune checkpoint inhibitors.

Keywords: CD8 T Cells; immune blockade; NSCLC; reversal of EMT; tumor microenvironment; tumor plasticity; TNBC

---

1. Rethinking Cancer Therapy Development

Over the last decade, pivotal technological and clinical advances have dramatically impacted the survival of some cancer patients. This began with rapid and efficient genomic sequencing that markedly expanded our knowledge beyond the scaffold delivered by the initial Human Genome Project into the realm of tumor-driving mutations, some of which are seen in only a small fraction of cancers. Primarily due to the advancements facilitated by these data, the majority of new oncologic agents approved today are biologically targeted as opposed to cytotoxics.

Among various cancers, non-small cell lung cancer (NSCLC) and triple-negative breast cancer (TNBC) are the first and fourth most common causes of cancer-related mortality in the U.S. [1]. These cancers possess many similarities based on molecular classification and gene expression analyses despite their distinct tissues of origin [2]. Epithelial cells are the heartiest of embryologically derived layers. Topologically, they are external-facing barrier cells that are therefore endowed with protective mechanisms including membrane transport channels, tight junctions, and built-in plasticity mechanisms for adaptive responses to numerous insults even in their benign states—this makes them formidable enemies when they undergo malignant transformation. Targeted therapies for oncogenic aberration in lung (e.g., EGFR and ALK kinase inhibitors) and breast (e.g., HER2 therapies) cancer have improved survival, but have not resulted in cures for all patients. In advanced NSCLC, responsible for the largest number of cancer-caused deaths in the U.S., it has now become standard clinical practice in metastatic disease to obtain genomic sequencing, including for EGFR or ALK gene mutations/rearrangements in order to select drugs that significantly improve survival. Assays for HER2 overexpression and/or gene amplification are standard for every breast cancer case.

As the cost of gene sequencing has dropped, methods of "deeper" sequencing with accuracy to single-cell resolution have been developed. Single-cell sequencing has revealed that tumors are composed of genomically and transcriptionally diverse cells. Clonal selection and adaptive responses lead to drug resistance, immune escape, and tumor dissemination. Single-cell sequencing using topographic spatial information in tissue sections of breast ductal carcinoma and associated metastases revealed the direct genomic lineage between in situ and invasive subpopulations, demonstrating that such diversity is an early phenomenon that allows for pre-invasive selection and likely explains the complex constellation of phenotypes that cancer cells possess from the outset [3–5]. Innovations in both genomics and proteomic analytic techniques, increasingly being applied pre- and post-treatment, have also revealed extensive rewiring of cellular networks associated with tumor progression, metastasis, and drug resistance. These adaptive changes can be mediated by epigenetic modifications or microRNAs (miRNAs), and other pre- and post-transcriptional, post-translational and tumor microenvironmental events [6–8]. Each of these processes represents therapeutic opportunities that can be tested in preclinical models and ultimately in the clinic.

Importantly, interactions of malignant cells with the tumor microenvironment, including immune cells, the vascular system, stromal cells, and stem cells of different lineages contribute to phenotypic plasticity driven by de-differentiation, increased stem-cell behavior, and cells that have undergone the epithelial-mesenchymal transition (EMT) [9]. These events can generate overlapping yet distinct functional compartments that escape natural immunity and subsequent treatment [10–12]. In fact, the characteristics of immunoevasion, energy reprogramming, and "collusion" with the tumor microenvironment are recognized as the next generation of the hallmarks of cancer [13,14]. These interacting traits are part of a multi-dimensional construct that necessitates creative approaches to therapeutic intervention. RECIST (Response Evaluation Criteria in Solid Tumors) is currently used for evaluating objective treatment response for the majority of clinical trials. Clearly, based upon the above discussion RECIST as the sole endpoint for clinical trials is clearly not sufficient as revealed by the extensive intratumoral and microenvironmental heterogeneity observed in both primary and metastatic disease. Instead, better criteria, including the inclusion of the expression and spatial localization of specific biomarkers, both tumor intrinsic and in the microenvironment, and the detailed evaluation of residual disease will be required to develop more efficacious cancer therapies.

2. Tumors Responsive to Immunotherapy

Though immune responses to cancer have been recognized for decades, the general consensus was that most were insufficient to eradicate established cancers due to immune suppression mediated through several mechanisms. Immune checkpoint blockade therapies (ICBT) are revolutionizing and rapidly emerging as a game-changing approach in the treatment of many cancer types. ICBTs are remarkably effective and approved for several cancer types including metastatic melanoma and non-small cell lung cancer [15–17]. The premise of cancer immune checkpoint therapy (ICBT) is that harnessing the patient's natural cancer immune defense system leads these cells to selectively search out and destroy cancer cells [18]. By targeting negative regulators of T cell activity, they unleash anti-tumor immunity.

In September 2014, the anti-PD-1 antibody pembrolizumab was the first agent targeting the PD-1/PD-L1 interaction to receive FDA approval for metastatic melanoma. There are data suggesting that PD-L1 expression on the tumor may be a biomarker predicting response to this class of therapy [19,20]. PD-L1 expression was also seen in 20% of TNBC tumors suggesting that targeting PD-1 or PD-L1 may have therapeutic benefit in TNBC [21]. Single-agent trials of PD-1 or PD-L1 inhibition in TNBC have demonstrated response rates of 5–19%, with some patients experiencing prolonged, durable responses. [22–24]. Some of these studies required ≥1% expression of PD-L1 as an entry criterion, while others did not. Responses have been seen in tumors that lack PD-L1 expression, and thus far, the data do not definitively suggest that PD-L1 expression is required for single agent biologic activity of immune checkpoint inhibitors in TNBC.

Tumor cell killing by cytotoxic chemotherapy like anthracyclines and carboplatins can facilitate immunogenic cell death and facilitate an adaptive immune response [25]. Invigorating tumor-specific T-cell immunity in this setting by inhibiting PD-L1/PD-1 signaling may result in deeper and more durable responses compared to standard chemotherapy alone.

Supporting this hypothesis, a randomized phase III trial of nab-paclitaxel+/− atezolizumab for the first line treatment of metastatic TNBC was the first to show a benefit for immunotherapy [26]. Notably, unlike single agent checkpoint inhibitor trials, benefit was only seen in the group of tumors that expressed PD-L1 within the immune infiltrate and, as such, the combinatorial strategy has been recently FDA approved for unresectable locally advanced or metastatic TNBC patients who have PD-L1 stained tumor-infiltrating immune cells covering at least ≥1% of the tumor area (https://www.fda.gov/Drugs/InformationOnDrugs/ApprovedDrugs/ucm633065.htm).

In lung cancer, immunotherapy has rapidly become a standard part of therapy for patients with advanced cancers, with several anti-PD1 and/or anti-PDL1 drugs approved by the FDA for non-small cell lung cancer (NSCLC). Specifically, patients with metastatic NSCLC and PDL1 tumor proportion score of at least 50% can be treated with front-line single agent pembrolizumab, while patients with PDL1 levels below 50% can receive immunotherapy in combination with chemotherapy (i.e., carboplatin-pemetrexed-pembrolizumab, carboplatin-taxane-pembrlizumab combinations) in the frontline setting or one of three single-agent immunotherapy agents (pembrolizumab, nivolumab, or atezolizumab) in the second-line setting for relapsed disease [27–29]. However, despite the enthusiasm for immunotherapy for lung cancer, many patients do not receive clinical benefit from these agents, and even in those who do respond initially, therapeutic resistance can develop over time.

The renaissance of immunotherapy with the discovery of checkpoints and other modulators of immunity has brought on a new era in cancer therapeutics. In many types of non-epithelial malignancies, immune checkpoint blockade therapy (ICBT) achieves long-term remissions. However, ICBT is often ineffective in lung cancer and is rarely successful for breast cancer, for which this therapy remains investigational [30,31]. In addition to intrinsic resistance to ICBT, acquired resistance, defined as clinical progression after an initial response or prolonged stability, is also seen with targeted or cytotoxic therapy.

3. Role of EMT in Immune Evasion

EMT directly regulates expression of PD-L1 and is associated with several other checkpoint ligands [32,33] (Figure 1). Thus, EMT is expected to induce checkpoint-dependent resistance to anti-tumor immunity. Due to the redundancy of the multiple checkpoints, EMT may render cancer cells non-responsive to therapies targeting one or few checkpoints (e.g., anti-PD-L1 and anti-CTLA4). Due to the limited scope of this review, we are unable to discuss many articles here; however, the reader is referred some notable publications in this context [12,34–38]. Additionally, EMT drives the recruitment of tumor-associated macrophages, which may, in turn, mediate resistance to immunotherapies [39,40]. This may be achieved through direct regulation of cytokinome of cancer cells (e.g., CCL2). The immunosuppression by macrophages, especially the alternatively activated macrophages (M2), has been extensively studied and involves several mechanisms [41]. The tumor suppressive and tumor promoting effects of EMT shift the balance between macrophages and neutrophils. Thus, inhibition of EMT, while overcoming immunosuppression by cancer cells and macrophages, may coincidentally cause accumulation of a type of neutrophils in some tumors defined as myeloid-derived suppressor cells leading to an "escape" pathway from anti-EMT treatment. Therefore, it is important to examine the clinical correlation between EMT and the entire immune microenvironment, including the myeloid cell compartment.

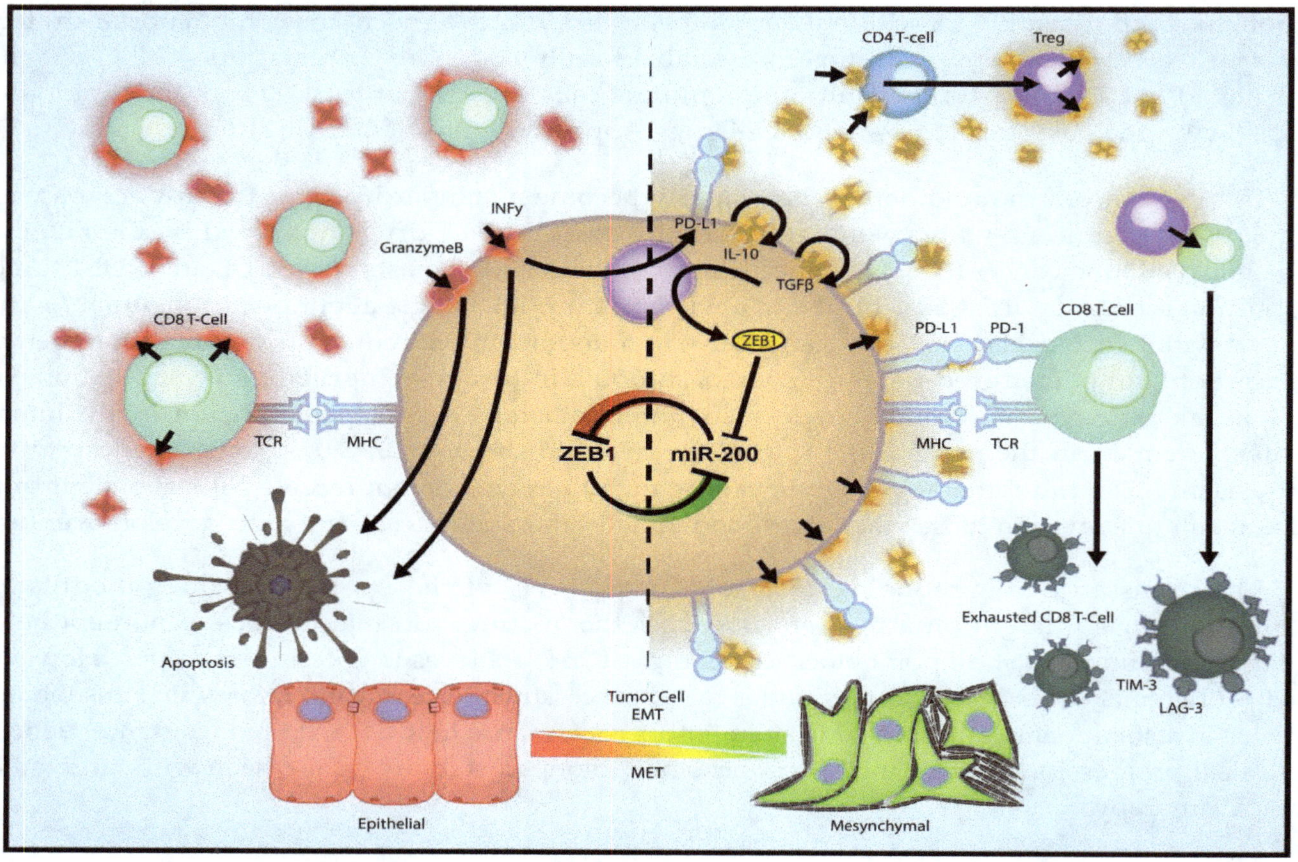

Figure 1. Tumor cell EMT drives multiple parallel pathways of immune suppression. Epithelial tumor cells are more sensitive to the effects of CD8+ effector cytotoxic T cells. Mesenchymal tumor cells, as illustrated by high expression of the transcriptional repressor ZEB1 and concordant suppression of the microRNA-200 family, express increased levels of PD-L1, immune suppressive cytokines (e.g., TGFβ), and enhanced recruitment of immune suppressive cells (e.g., CD4+ T regulatory cells). These EMT-directed changes produce exhaustion of CD8+ T cells or suppress their recruitment into the tumor microenvironment. CD8 T cell: CD8+ effector cytotoxic T cells; Treg: Regulatory T cell.

4. EMT as a Driver of Immune Escape from ICBT

Despite the presence of an immune response, some tumors continue to grow, a process that has been referred to as "immune escape". Tumor cell escape can occur through multiple different mechanisms [42]. Tumor cells themselves promote an immunosuppressive microenvironment by producing suppressive cytokines including TGF-β, VEGF, or indoleamine 2,3-dioxygenase. The tumor microenvironment also contains immune cells such as regulatory T cells and myeloid-derived suppressor cells that function to suppress the immune response. At the individual tumor cell level, alterations leading to decreased immune recognition (such as loss of tumor antigens, downregulation of major histocompatibility complex molecules, or loss of antigen processing function within the tumor cell), or increased resistance to the cytotoxic effects of immunity (such as via induction of anti-apoptotic mechanisms) can promote tumor growth. Finally, tumor cells can upregulate T cell-inhibitory molecules such as PD-L1, which is why activating the immune system for therapeutic benefit in cancer is an area of active investigation. For a more elaborate discussion on this topic, we refer readers to some recent reviews [10,43,44].

We and others have previously described epithelial-mesenchymal transition (EMT) as a frequent mechanism of de novo and acquired therapeutic resistance in mammary tumor cells, as well as all subtypes of NSCLC, including lung cancers with oncogenic driver mutations in EGFR and KRAS [45–48]. Furthermore, we and others have demonstrated that EMT upregulates expression of PD-L1 in murine and human NSCLC and directly leads to CD8+ T cell exhaustion and immunosuppression. To facilitate the study of EMT across large cohorts, our group identified a robust, platform-independent lung cancer EMT gene expression signature valid in lung cancer cell lines and NSCLC patient tumors [45]. The signature was then further refined to develop a patient-based, pan-cancer EMT signature using 1934 patient tumors from multiple solid tumor types including breast, lung, colon, and other common cancers [2]. The Lung EMT and Pan-Cancer EMT signatures are highly correlated with mesenchymal cancers from distinct tumor types showing striking similarities in their molecular profiles. Using the EMT signatures, an individual cancer cell line or tumor can be scored for the degree to which it has undergone EMT. These mRNA-based EMT signature scores are easy to measure, and are highly correlated with other established EMT markers (such as expression of E-cadherin protein) as well as with other factors known to regulate EMT (e.g., miR200 family and the transcription factor ZEB1). The applicability of EMT scores to predict lung cancer has been mirrored in breast cancer patients as well [49]. Residual breast cancers after conventional chemotherapy were shown to exhibit mesenchymal features. In addition to applying the EMT scores in our lung cancer research, we generated EMT scores for multiple TCGA cohorts, which has allowed integrated analyses of the relationships between EMT and other molecular or immune data profiles (i.e., miRNA and methylation profiles, iCLUSTER data) [32,50,51].

In addition to its broad tumor cell-autonomous impact, EMT in breast cancer also profoundly alters the microenvironment landscape, especially immune cell constituents (Figure 1). Macrophages and neutrophils are key modulators of the tumor microenvironment [52,53]. Recent evidence suggests a strong correlation between EMT and a switch from a neutrophil- enriched immune profile to a macrophage-dominant profile. Tumors exhibiting an epithelial-like phenotype tend to have local and systemic accumulation of neutrophils. In contrast, tumors with mesenchymal features are predominantly infiltrated with macrophages that are often but not always polarized to the M2 (alternatively activated) status. These two categories of tumors are defined as a neutrophil-enriched subtype (NES) and a macrophage-enriched subtype (MES), respectively. Inducible expression of miR-200, a master regulator of EMT, shifts the macrophage/neutrophil balance, supporting the causal role of EMT in determining the myeloid cell profile of the tumor microenvironment.

Mechanistically, several transcriptional suppressors regulate EMT, including the two-handed zinc-finger δEF1 family transcription factors ZEB1 and ZEB2 [54–57]. ZEB1/2 binds to E-box regions in the promoters of key epithelial differentiation genes such as E-cadherin, and transcriptionally suppress their expression [58]. ZEB1/2 also regulates the miR-200 family of miRNAs miR-141, 200a/b/c, and 429 that are broadly expressed in normal epithelial cells [59]. miR-200 is a master EMT regulator, governed by a double-negative feedback loop with the ZEB repressors [60–64] and regulated by multiple EMT inducers (e.g., TGFβ) [61,62]. miR-200 loss has been linked to stem-like features and chemoresistance [65,66]. Evidence from several epithelial tumor types, including lung and breast, implicates miR-200 dysregulation in disease progression [64,67,68]. Using the KP mouse model and a panel of human NSCLC cell lines, we have demonstrated that the miR-200/ZEB1 feedback loop is a critical regulatory axis that determines metastatic potential [69,70] by controlling global mRNA changes in an invasive subset of tumor cells, modulating matrix-dependent tumor activation and invasion [70–73].

5. Relationship between CD8 T Cells and EMT, and Impact of EMT on ICBT

In breast cancer, there is a strong correlation between tumor-infiltrating T and B cells and favorable prognostic outcome or therapeutic responses (standard therapies) [18,74–77]. Many standard-of-care therapies require the immune system to exert their effects. The most prominent example is anti-HER2 treatment with trastuzumab, which heavily relies on functional host immunity [78]. Furthermore, it has recently been recognized that the response of some chemotherapy regimens is achieved by their impact on immunosuppressive cells [79–81]. Thus, it appears that the immune system in breast cancer patients retains the potential of fighting cancer. Ongoing clinical trials suggest that although some breast cancer patients may benefit from ICBT [22,82], the percentage is disappointingly low. Possible mechanisms of resistance include low level or ineffective neoantigens [83,84] and/or the enrichment of immunosuppressive cells [85,86], and the elaboration of immunosuppressive cytokines (e.g., IL-10, TGF-β), all of which may result in a scarcity of functional cytotoxic T cells. Therefore, to improve the efficacy of immunotherapy it will be critically important to tackle these potential mechanisms. In the following section, we will focus on the latter: the immunosuppressive microenvironment that prevents anti-tumor immunity.

ICBT enhances anti-tumor responses by increasing the activity of the cytotoxic CD8+ T lymphocyte subpopulations; these cells are key players in the effector functions of adaptive immunity [87]. In addition to secreting chemokines and cytokines, tumor-specific T cells interact through T cell receptors with the major histocompatibility complex (MHC) on antigen-presenting cells, which in turn triggers a signaling cascade resulting in the death of target cells [88,89]. Currently, adoptive T cell-transfer, oncolytic viruses, cancer vaccines, T cell co-stimulatory agonists and monoclonal antibodies are used either alone or in combination with ICBT [90]. Checkpoint regulators of immune activation help maintain immune homeostasis and prevent autoimmunity. However, the immune checkpoint pathways are frequently activated in cancer to suppress the nascent anti-tumor immune response. A combination of immune checkpoint inhibitors namely PD-1 and CTLA-4 can effectively kill cancer cells because they function primarily through complementary mechanisms [91]. When CD8+ T cells recognize self-antigen on tumor cells, they fail to kill cancer cells; this immunological tolerance is a drawback of the ICBT [92]. In addition, CD8+ T cell exhaustion due to chronic exposure to antigens negatively affects the efficacy of ICBT [93].

Tumor cells evade immunosurveillance by altering their phenotype via immunoediting, and it is known that immuno-edited tumors display properties of cells that have undergone EMT [94]. Activated $CD8^+$ T cells, macrophages, and several other immune cell types produce TGF-β, a crucial promoter of EMT [95–97]. We previously demonstrated that two key EMT factors that are also markers of cancer stem cells (CSCs), FOXC2 and Twist, are necessary for the process of breast carcinoma metastasis [57,98]. Early evidence suggested an antitumor response of $CD8^+$ T cells delayed metastasis and eliminated disseminated tumor cells (DTC) of P815 mastocytoma [99]. In a melanoma mouse model, $CD8^+$ T cells are involved in maintaining DTC dormancy in visceral organs like the lungs and the reproductive tract, thereby preventing overt metastasis and limiting disease progression [32]. $CD8^+$ T cells are also known to inhibit tumor growth thus prolonging the survival of experimental mice by selectively targeting cancer stem cells (CSCs) [100]. $CD8^+$ T cell suppression within the tumor microenvironment is dependent on PD-L1 regulation on tumor cells via a pathway involving the microRNA miR-200 and the transcription factor ZEB1; these molecules are the links between EMT, $CD8^+$ T cell exhaustion, and tumor suppression [32]. Furthermore, the inhibition of breast cancer onset and progression is inhibited by $CD8^+$ T cells and natural killer (NK) cells due to increased cytotoxic activity mediated by the protein TIPE2 [101]. Although EMT leads to up-regulation of multiple checkpoint molecules that inhibit T cell-mediated cytotoxicity, it also reduces expression of many adhesion molecules including E-cadherin, which is a known inhibitory ligand of NK cell receptor (KLRG1) [102]. Other well-established NK cell-activating molecules, such as PVR, are also upregulated upon EMT induction [103,104]. It is, therefore, not surprising that EMT may be accompanied by increased sensitivity to NK cell-mediated cytotoxicity [105]. Although the anti-tumor potential of $CD8^+$ T cells is well accepted, the prognostic significance of their intratumoral homing is highly variable across different breast tumor subtypes [106]. The impact of $CD8^+$ T cells in the tumor microenvironment (TME) on tumor epithelial-mesenchymal plasticity, on the interplay with other immune cells, and on associated metastatic traits in breast cancer cells are incompletely understood. Furthermore, it will be critical to clarify how the inflammatory TME and epithelial-mesenchymal plasticity influence CD8+ T cell activity and survival.

6. Impact of Immunosuppressive TME on ICBT

The intertumoral heterogeneity of the immune microenvironment dictates ICBT responses. We profiled the immune compartment in a wide variety of syngeneic triple-negative breast cancer (TNBC) models and discovered two prototypes of the immune microenvironment. In the first prototype, tumors induce systemic accumulation of neutrophils. These neutrophils overexpress multiple immunosuppressive pathways and may represent granulocytic myeloid-derived suppressor cells (gMDSCs). Macrophages co-exist but only constitute a minority of the myeloid cells in the tumor. In the second prototype, there does not appear to be an increase of neutrophils; rather, there is exclusively a local enrichment of tumor macrophages, which often (but not always) polarize toward the immunosuppressive M2 status. We have denoted these two "immunosubtypes" of mammary tumors as NES and MES, respectively. Apparently, NES and MES rely on different types of myeloid cells to escape immunosurveillance (data not shown). Indeed, when initially responsive MES tumors recurred neutrophils or gMDSCs accumulated, suggesting a conversion from MES toward NES or a switch of suppressor cell types. Depletion of neutrophils reduced this acquired ICBT resistance. Thus, immunosuppression may be exerted by different cell types in different tumor contexts.

EMT clearly contributes to the development of different immune microenvironments. Intriguingly, analyses of eight murine models representative of both NES and MES subtypes revealed that EMT contributes to the development of the dichotomous myeloid microenvironment. EMT has been linked to the recruitment of macrophages to the tumor microenvironment via chemokines like CCL2 [39,40]. Previous studies have also demonstrated that EMT drives expression of checkpoint ligands in cancer cells [51]. Taken together, the connection between EMT and cancer cell- or macrophage-mediated immunosuppression has been well established, which makes it an appealing therapeutic target to enhance immunotherapies. Inhibition of EMT, by targeting the EMT signaling pathways using TGF-β1 inhibitors while reverse immunosuppression by cancer cells and macrophages, may coincidentally cause accumulation of neutrophils, which can act as gMDSCs and lead to an alternative immunosuppressive mechanism, independent of checkpoints. Indeed, previous studies using syngeneic lung cancer models already indicate the existence of the dichotomous myeloid cell compartment in this cancer type as well [107]. Preclinical studies demonstrate that gMDSCs promote tumor progression through suppressing anti-tumor immunity [108,109] and promoting tumor-initiating cells (TIC) through the Notch pathway [109]. Interestingly, a recent study suggested that the former activity may depend on endogenous estrogen receptor alpha (ER) signaling [110], raising the possibility that endocrine deprivation therapies could be used for gMDSC elimination [111]. Endocrine deprivation therapies are standard-of-care for ER+ breast cancer.

All these findings suggest that EMT drives a switch of immunosuppression from gMDSC-mediated, checkpoint-independent mechanisms to macrophage/cancer cell-mediated, checkpoint-dependent mechanisms. Consequently, gMDSC accumulation may represent an escape pathway upon EMT inhibition that allows tumors to maintain an immunosuppressive microenvironment. Moreover, estrogen signaling and the Notch pathway mediate the pro-tumor effects of gMDSCs and provide potential therapeutic targets to eliminate these cells, a strategy that may complement anti-EMT treatment and ICBT.

7. Role of Bioinformatics

To identify potential relationships between phenotypic traits of tumors, including EMT and immune cell populations, and cancer outcomes, bioinformatics has long played a critical role. Gene expression profiles reveal the underlying biology of the tumors and can be used to dissect the features that are correlated with responses. A key observation is that signaling events lead to a transcriptional response, even if they are driven upstream by post-translational modifications. Thus, the signature of a pathway can be used to identify the molecular processes associated with clinical events.

Gene expression signatures involving biological processes have been generated using machine learning techniques. In short, the development of signatures is typically framed as a classification problem, where the goal is to identify a set of genes that can distinguish two biological states, such as epithelial or mesenchymal cells. To accomplish this, a training set is generated comprised of gene expression profiles of the two states. Then, differential expression analysis methods, such as DESeq2 [112] or EdgeR [113], are used to identify genes that can differentiate the two states. Finally, machine learning algorithms, such as SIGNATURE [114], can be used to score the expression profiles of new samples to provide a quantitative measure of the similarity to one or the other state.

Based on such approaches, an EMT signature has been linked to several outcomes including responses to chemotherapy [115], targeted therapies [116], patient survival [117,118], recurrence [119], and metastasis [120]. In addition to these outcomes, our studies and others have linked an EMT signature with markers or other evidence of immune modulation such as immune checkpoints [51] or low T cell infiltration in NSCLC [121]. Indeed, an increasing amount of evidence points to an association between EMT and the immune system in human tumors.

Independent of EMT, several bioinformatic analyses have supported the role of immune cells and clinical outcomes [122–130]. This demonstrates the ability of this technology to identify signatures of immune cells in bulk tumor samples. These analyses are enabled by the fact that the gene expression profiles of tumors reflect both the cancer cell and stromal/immune compartments. Although the signature of the immune cells can be seen in the bulk gene expression profiles, methods have been developed that can deconvolute the profiles into the constituent parts, enabling a more accurate quantification of the immune cell types that comprise the tumor [131,132].

One of the limitations of the prior studies is that they provide a limited resolution in quantifying the immune cell types (i.e., how many CD4+ T cells there are), and also in identifying the cell subtypes (i.e., are these Th1, Th2, or other CD4+ T cells). To address these questions, single-cell sequencing technologies that have the have the capacity to profile a range of cell types are rapidly being adopted. While powerful, these technologies have introduced a new bioinformatics challenge. The result of a single-cell RNA-Seq (scRNA-Seq) assay is the generation of transcriptional profiles of a likely heterogeneous immune cell population. Therefore, one step in the processing is to identify the cell types present in the population. While markers for immune cells have long been established for flow cytometry experiments, they are of more limited use in scRNA-Seq profiles due to issues such as drop-out, a phenomenon where a gene is not profiled due to factors including a lack of sensitivity in the assay; or ambiguities in the accepted markers. In the future, to address this, machine learning methods can be applied to identify immune cells from scRNA-Seq profiles. Nevertheless, a recent study has revealed a previously unknown range of T cell activation states within breast tumors [133]. Future studies using single-cell technologies, coupled with increasingly sophisticated bioinformatic analyses, will likely reveal new nuances in the relationships between the immune system, EMT, and cancer. Additional multiplex technologies will allow the spatial localization of these cells.

8. Conclusions

In this review, we have highlighted mechanistic vulnerabilities in mesenchymal tumor cells due to their ability to reprogram the tumor immune microenvironment. Because immunotherapy is rapidly emerging as a game-changing approach in many cancer types, including lung cancer, it will be critical to develop a greater understanding of those patients most likely to benefit and the mechanisms defining primary and acquired resistance. It will also be important to co-target EMT-related vulnerabilities along with the PD-L1/PD-1 immune checkpoint axis, given the large contribution of EMT to resistance mechanisms. Most importantly, the EMT phenotype has a distinct relationship with the immune microenvironment that can potentially be leveraged for a transformative clinical benefit for common epithelial tumors. EMT broadly up-regulates multiple immune checkpoint and inflammatory molecules to produce CD8+ T cell exhaustion, highlighting multiple potential mechanisms for the development of therapeutic resistance to immune therapy in mesenchymal tumors. EMT is a multidimensional process with different axes and these multiple parameters are exploited in malignancy under selective pressures including cytotoxic and biological therapies, hypoxia, energetics, and immune surveillance. As such, there is a pressing clinical need for targeted, biomarker-directed therapies to address both primary and acquired immunotherapy resistance. Incorporation of targeted agents (and validated biomarkers) that modulate immune suppression could expand the patient population that responds to immune checkpoint inhibitors and help address immunotherapy resistance. Studying these questions and integrating information across cancer types, instead of a single cancer, will shed light on combinatorial strategies that may be more generally applicable. Moreover, these comparative studies may also yield new insights since the treatment of cancer as evidenced in recent basket trials now is geared to understanding common vulnerabilities, e.g., mismatch repair deficiencies, as criteria for using ICBT across tumor types.

Acknowledgments: We thank NIH/NCI CCSG P30-CA01667 (L.A.B.), NIH/NCI SPORE P5-CA070907 (L.A.B.), an MD Andersen Cancer Center Physician Scientist Award (L.A.B.), LUNGevity Foundation (L.A.B.), philanthropic contributions to The University of Texas MD Anderson Cancer Center Lung Cancer Moonshot Program (L.A.B.), NIH R37 CA214609-01A1 (D.L.G.), CPRIT-MIRA-RP160652-P3 (D.L.G.), Rexanna's Foundation for Fighting Lung Cancer (D.L.G.), P50 CA070907 from UT Lung SPORE Career Enhancement Award (J.M.K.), NIH/NCI-R01CA200970 (S.A.M.), NIH/NCI-2R01CA155243 (S.A.M.), National Science Foundation-15-597-1605817 (S.A.M.), CPRIT-MIRA-RP160710 (S.A.M., Project-3), CPRIT-IIRA-RP170172 (J.M.R., S.A.M.), Diana Helis Henry and Andrienne Helis Malvin Medical Research Foundation Grant (J.M.R., X.Z.), P50 CA140388 from the National Cancer Institute (University of Texas MD Anderson Prostate Cancer SPORE Career Enhancement Program Award) (R.S.), MD Anderson Institutional Research Grant (R.S.), CPRIT-MIRA-RP180712 (D.T., Core), CPRIT-RP180466 (N.V.), MRA-509800 (N.V.), for financial support.

References

1. Siegel, R.L.; Miller, K.D.; Jemal, A. Cancer Statistics, 2017. *CA Cancer J. Clin.* **2017**, *67*, 7–30. [CrossRef] [PubMed]
2. Mak, M.P.; Tong, P.; Diao, L.; Cardnell, R.J.; Gibbons, D.L.; William, W.N.; Skoulidis, F.; Parra, E.R.; Rodriguez-Canales, J.; Wistuba, I.I.; et al. A Patient-Derived, Pan-Cancer EMT Signature Identifies Global Molecular Alterations and Immune Target Enrichment Following Epithelial-to-Mesenchymal Transition. *Clin. Cancer Res.* **2016**, *22*, 609–620. [CrossRef] [PubMed]
3. Casasent, A.K.; Schalck, A.; Gao, R.; Sei, E.; Long, A.; Pangburn, W.; Casasent, T.; Meric-Bernstam, F.; Edgerton, M.E.; Navin, N.E. Multiclonal Invasion in Breast Tumors Identified by Topographic Single Cell Sequencing. *Cell* **2018**, *172*, 205–217.e212. [CrossRef] [PubMed]
4. Hernandez, L.; Wilkerson, P.M.; Lambros, M.B.; Campion-Flora, A.; Rodrigues, D.N.; Gauthier, A.; Cabral, C.; Pawar, V.; Mackay, A.; A'Hern, R.; et al. Genomic and mutational profiling of ductal carcinomas in situ and matched adjacent invasive breast cancers reveals intra-tumour genetic heterogeneity and clonal selection. *J. Pathol.* **2012**, *227*, 42–52. [CrossRef]
5. Niyomnaitham, S.; Parinyanitikul, N.; Roothumnong, E.; Jinda, W.; Samarnthai, N.; Atikankul, T.; Suktitipat, B.; Thongnoppakhun, W.; Limwongse, C.; Pithukpakorn, M. Tumor mutational profile of triple negative breast cancer patients in Thailand revealed distinctive genetic alteration in chromatin remodeling gene. *PeerJ* **2019**, *7*, e6501. [CrossRef]
6. Fardi, M.; Alivand, M.; Baradaran, B.; Farshdousti Hagh, M.; Solali, S. The crucial role of ZEB2: From development to epithelial-to-mesenchymal transition and cancer complexity. *J. Cell Physiol.* **2019**. [CrossRef] [PubMed]
7. Zhang, L.; Liang, Y.; Li, S.; Zeng, F.; Meng, Y.; Chen, Z.; Liu, S.; Tao, Y.; Yu, F. The interplay of circulating tumor DNA and chromatin modification, therapeutic resistance, and metastasis. *Mol. Cancer* **2019**, *18*, 36. [CrossRef]
8. Schwarzenbacher, D.; Balic, M.; Pichler, M. The role of microRNAs in breast cancer stem cells. *Int. J. Mol. Sci.* **2013**, *14*, 14712–14723. [CrossRef]
9. Markiewicz, A.; Topa, J.; Nagel, A.; Skokowski, J.; Seroczynska, B.; Stokowy, T.; Welnicka-Jaskiewicz, M.; Zaczek, A.J. Spectrum of Epithelial-Mesenchymal Transition Phenotypes in Circulating Tumour Cells from Early Breast Cancer Patients. *Cancers* **2019**, *11*, 59. [CrossRef] [PubMed]

10. Terry, S.; Savagner, P.; Ortiz-Cuaran, S.; Mahjoubi, L.; Saintigny, P.; Thiery, J.P.; Chouaib, S. New insights into the role of EMT in tumor immune escape. *Mol. Oncol.* **2017**, *11*, 824–846. [CrossRef]
11. Akalay, I.; Janji, B.; Hasmim, M.; Noman, M.Z.; Andre, F.; De Cremoux, P.; Bertheau, P.; Badoual, C.; Vielh, P.; Larsen, A.K.; et al. Epithelial-to-mesenchymal transition and autophagy induction in breast carcinoma promote escape from T-cell-mediated lysis. *Cancer Res.* **2013**, *73*, 2418–2427. [CrossRef]
12. Chouaib, S.; Janji, B.; Tittarelli, A.; Eggermont, A.; Thiery, J.P. Tumor plasticity interferes with anti-tumor immunity. *Crit. Rev. Immunol.* **2014**, *34*, 91–102. [CrossRef] [PubMed]
13. Hanahan, D.; Weinberg, R.A. Hallmarks of cancer: The next generation. *Cell* **2011**, *144*, 646–674. [CrossRef]
14. Terry, S.; Chouaib, S. EMT in immuno-resistance. *Oncoscience* **2015**, *2*, 841–842. [CrossRef] [PubMed]
15. Sharma, P.; Allison, J.P. Immune checkpoint targeting in cancer therapy: Toward combination strategies with curative potential. *Cell* **2015**, *161*, 205–214. [CrossRef]
16. Pardoll, D.M. The blockade of immune checkpoints in cancer immunotherapy. *Nat. Rev. Cancer* **2012**, *12*, 252–264. [CrossRef]
17. Topalian, S.L.; Drake, C.G.; Pardoll, D.M. Immune checkpoint blockade: A common denominator approach to cancer therapy. *Cancer Cell* **2015**, *27*, 450–461. [CrossRef]
18. Gentles, A.J.; Newman, A.M.; Liu, C.L.; Bratman, S.V.; Feng, W.; Kim, D.; Nair, V.S.; Xu, Y.; Khuong, A.; Hoang, C.D.; et al. The prognostic landscape of genes and infiltrating immune cells across human cancers. *Nat. Med.* **2015**, *21*, 938–945. [CrossRef] [PubMed]
19. Brahmer, J.R.; Tykodi, S.S.; Chow, L.Q.; Hwu, W.J.; Topalian, S.L.; Hwu, P.; Drake, C.G.; Camacho, L.H.; Kauh, J.; Odunsi, K.; et al. Safety and activity of anti-PD-L1 antibody in patients with advanced cancer. *N. Engl. J. Med.* **2012**, *366*, 2455–2465. [CrossRef]
20. Zhang, M.; Sun, H.; Zhao, S.; Wang, Y.; Pu, H.; Wang, Y.; Zhang, Q. Expression of PD-L1 and prognosis in breast cancer: A meta-analysis. *Oncotarget* **2017**, *8*, 31347–31354. [CrossRef] [PubMed]
21. Mittendorf, E.A.; Philips, A.V.; Meric-Bernstam, F.; Qiao, N.; Wu, Y.; Harrington, S.; Su, X.; Wang, Y.; Gonzalez-Angulo, A.M.; Akcakanat, A.; et al. PD-L1 expression in triple-negative breast cancer. *Cancer Immunol. Res.* **2014**, *2*, 361–370. [CrossRef]
22. Nanda, R.; Chow, L.Q.; Dees, E.C.; Berger, R.; Gupta, S.; Geva, R.; Pusztai, L.; Pathiraja, K.; Aktan, G.; Cheng, J.D.; et al. Pembrolizumab in Patients With Advanced Triple-Negative Breast Cancer: Phase Ib KEYNOTE-012 Study. *J. Clin. Oncol.* **2016**, *34*, 2460–2467. [CrossRef]
23. Dirix, L.Y.; Takacs, I.; Jerusalem, G.; Nikolinakos, P.; Arkenau, H.T.; Forero-Torres, A.; Boccia, R.; Lippman, M.E.; Somer, R.; Smakal, M.; et al. Avelumab, an anti-PD-L1 antibody, in patients with locally advanced or metastatic breast cancer: A phase 1b JAVELIN Solid Tumor study. *Breast Cancer Res. Treat.* **2018**, *167*, 671–686. [CrossRef]
24. Adams, S.; Schmid, P.; Rugo, H.S.; Winer, E.P.; Loirat, D.; Awada, A.; Cescon, D.W.; Iwata, H.; Campone, M.; Nanda, R.; et al. Pembrolizumab Monotherapy for Previously Treated Metastatic Triple-Negative Breast Cancer: Cohort A of the Phase 2 KEYNOTE-086 Study. *Ann. Oncol.* **2018**. [CrossRef]
25. Wang, Y.J.; Fletcher, R.; Yu, J.; Zhang, L. Immunogenic effects of chemotherapy-induced tumor cell death. *Genes Dis.* **2018**, *5*, 194–203. [CrossRef]
26. Schmid, P.; Adams, S.; Rugo, H.S.; Schneeweiss, A.; Barrios, C.H.; Iwata, H.; Dieras, V.; Hegg, R.; Im, S.A.; Shaw Wright, G.; et al. Atezolizumab and Nab-Paclitaxel in Advanced Triple-Negative Breast Cancer. *N. Engl. J. Med.* **2018**. [CrossRef]
27. Reck, M.; Rodriguez-Abreu, D.; Robinson, A.G.; Hui, R.; Csoszi, T.; Fulop, A.; Gottfried, M.; Peled, N.; Tafreshi, A.; Cuffe, S.; et al. Pembrolizumab versus Chemotherapy for PD-L1-Positive Non-Small-Cell Lung Cancer. *N. Engl. J. Med.* **2016**, *375*, 1823–1833. [CrossRef] [PubMed]
28. Langer, C.J.; Gadgeel, S.M.; Borghaei, H.; Papadimitrakopoulou, V.A.; Patnaik, A.; Powell, S.F.; Gentzler, R.D.; Martins, R.G.; Stevenson, J.P.; Jalal, S.I.; et al. Carboplatin and pemetrexed with or without pembrolizumab for advanced, non-squamous non-small-cell lung cancer: A randomised, phase 2 cohort of the open-label KEYNOTE-021 study. *Lancet Oncol.* **2016**, *17*, 1497–1508. [CrossRef]
29. Rittmeyer, A.; Barlesi, F.; Waterkamp, D.; Park, K.; Ciardiello, F.; von Pawel, J.; Gadgeel, S.M.; Hida, T.; Kowalski, D.M.; Dols, M.C.; et al. Atezolizumab versus docetaxel in patients with previously treated non-small-cell lung cancer (OAK): A phase 3, open-label, multicentre randomised controlled trial. *Lancet* **2017**, *389*, 255–265. [CrossRef]

30. Reck, M.; Rabe, K.F. Precision Diagnosis and Treatment for Advanced Non-Small-Cell Lung Cancer. *N. Engl. J. Med.* **2017**, *377*, 849–861. [CrossRef]
31. McArthur, H.L.; Page, D.B. Immunotherapy for the treatment of breast cancer: Checkpoint blockade, cancer vaccines, and future directions in combination immunotherapy. *Clin. Adv. Hematol. Oncol.* **2016**, *14*, 922–933. [PubMed]
32. Chen, L.; Gibbons, D.L.; Goswami, S.; Cortez, M.A.; Ahn, Y.H.; Byers, L.A.; Zhang, X.; Yi, X.; Dwyer, D.; Lin, W.; et al. Metastasis is regulated via microRNA-200/ZEB1 axis control of tumour cell PD-L1 expression and intratumoral immunosuppression. *Nat. Commun.* **2014**, *5*, 5241. [CrossRef]
33. Loi, S.; Dushyanthen, S.; Beavis, P.A.; Salgado, R.; Denkert, C.; Savas, P.; Combs, S.; Rimm, D.L.; Giltnane, J.M.; Estrada, M.V.; et al. RAS/MAPK Activation Is Associated with Reduced Tumor-Infiltrating Lymphocytes in Triple-Negative Breast Cancer: Therapeutic Cooperation Between MEK and PD-1/PD-L1 Immune Checkpoint Inhibitors. *Clin. Cancer Res.* **2016**, *22*, 1499–1509. [CrossRef]
34. Dong, P.; Xiong, Y.; Yue, J.; Hanley, S.J.B.; Watari, H. Tumor-Intrinsic PD-L1 Signaling in Cancer Initiation, Development and Treatment: Beyond Immune Evasion. *Front. Oncol.* **2018**, *8*, 386. [CrossRef]
35. Asgarova, A.; Asgarov, K.; Godet, Y.; Peixoto, P.; Nadaradjane, A.; Boyer-Guittaut, M.; Galaine, J.; Guenat, D.; Mougey, V.; Perrard, J.; et al. PD-L1 expression is regulated by both DNA methylation and NF-kB during EMT signaling in non-small cell lung carcinoma. *Oncoimmunology* **2018**, *7*, e1423170. [CrossRef] [PubMed]
36. Li, F.; Zhu, T.; Yue, Y.; Zhu, X.; Wang, J.; Liang, L. Preliminary mechanisms of regulating PDL1 expression in nonsmall cell lung cancer during the EMT process. *Oncol. Rep.* **2018**, *40*, 775–782. [CrossRef]
37. Kumar, S.; Davra, V.; Obr, A.E.; Geng, K.; Wood, T.L.; De Lorenzo, M.S.; Birge, R.B. Crk adaptor protein promotes PD-L1 expression, EMT and immune evasion in a murine model of triple-negative breast cancer. *Oncoimmunology* **2017**, *7*, e1376155. [CrossRef] [PubMed]
38. Kim, S.; Koh, J.; Kim, M.Y.; Kwon, D.; Go, H.; Kim, Y.A.; Jeon, Y.K.; Chung, D.H. PD-L1 expression is associated with epithelial-to-mesenchymal transition in adenocarcinoma of the lung. *Hum. Pathol.* **2016**, *58*, 7–14. [CrossRef] [PubMed]
39. Low-Marchelli, J.M.; Ardi, V.C.; Vizcarra, E.A.; van Rooijen, N.; Quigley, J.P.; Yang, J. Twist1 induces CCL2 and recruits macrophages to promote angiogenesis. *Cancer Res.* **2013**, *73*, 662–671. [CrossRef]
40. Hsu, D.S.; Wang, H.J.; Tai, S.K.; Chou, C.H.; Hsieh, C.H.; Chiu, P.H.; Chen, N.J.; Yang, M.H. Acetylation of snail modulates the cytokinome of cancer cells to enhance the recruitment of macrophages. *Cancer Cell* **2014**, *26*, 534–548. [CrossRef]
41. Noy, R.; Pollard, J.W. Tumor-associated macrophages: From mechanisms to therapy. *Immunity* **2014**, *41*, 49–61. [CrossRef]
42. Schreiber, R.D.; Old, L.J.; Smyth, M.J. Cancer immunoediting: Integrating immunity's roles in cancer suppression and promotion. *Science* **2011**, *331*, 1565–1570. [CrossRef]
43. Galon, J.; Bruni, D. Approaches to treat immune hot, altered and cold tumours with combination immunotherapies. *Nat. Rev. Drug Discov.* **2019**, *18*, 197–218. [CrossRef]
44. Otsuki, Y.; Saya, H.; Arima, Y. Prospects for new lung cancer treatments that target EMT signaling. *Dev. Dyn.* **2018**, *247*, 462–472. [CrossRef]
45. Byers, L.A.; Diao, L.; Wang, J.; Saintigny, P.; Girard, L.; Peyton, M.; Shen, L.; Fan, Y.; Giri, U.; Tumula, P.K.; et al. An epithelial-mesenchymal transition gene signature predicts resistance to EGFR and PI3K inhibitors and identifies Axl as a therapeutic target for overcoming EGFR inhibitor resistance. *Clin. Cancer Res.* **2013**, *19*, 279–290. [CrossRef] [PubMed]
46. Camidge, D.R.; Pao, W.; Sequist, L.V. Acquired resistance to TKIs in solid tumours: Learning from lung cancer. *Nat. Rev. Clin. Oncol.* **2014**, *11*, 473–481. [CrossRef] [PubMed]
47. Zhang, Z.; Lee, J.C.; Lin, L.; Olivas, V.; Au, V.; Laframboise, T.; Abdel-Rahman, M.; Wang, X.; Levine, A.D.; Rho, J.K.; et al. Activation of the AXL kinase causes resistance to EGFR-targeted therapy in lung cancer. *Nat. Genet.* **2012**, *44*, 852–860. [CrossRef] [PubMed]
48. Dongre, A.; Rashidian, M.; Reinhardt, F.; Bagnato, A.; Keckesova, Z.; Ploegh, H.L.; Weinberg, R.A. Epithelial-to-Mesenchymal Transition Contributes to Immunosuppression in Breast Carcinomas. *Cancer Res.* **2017**, *77*, 3982–3989. [CrossRef] [PubMed]

49. Creighton, C.J.; Li, X.; Landis, M.; Dixon, J.M.; Neumeister, V.M.; Sjolund, A.; Rimm, D.L.; Wong, H.; Rodriguez, A.; Herschkowitz, J.I.; et al. Residual breast cancers after conventional therapy display mesenchymal as well as tumor-initiating features. *Proc. Natl. Acad. Sci. USA* **2009**, *106*, 13820–13825. [CrossRef]
50. Allison Stewart, C.; Tong, P.; Cardnell, R.J.; Sen, T.; Li, L.; Gay, C.M.; Masrorpour, F.; Fan, Y.; Bara, R.O.; Feng, Y.; et al. Dynamic variations in epithelial-to-mesenchymal transition (EMT), ATM, and SLFN11 govern response to PARP inhibitors and cisplatin in small cell lung cancer. *Oncotarget* **2017**, *8*, 28575–28587. [CrossRef]
51. Lou, Y.; Diao, L.; Cuentas, E.R.; Denning, W.L.; Chen, L.; Fan, Y.H.; Byers, L.A.; Wang, J.; Papadimitrakopoulou, V.A.; Behrens, C.; et al. Epithelial-Mesenchymal Transition Is Associated with a Distinct Tumor Microenvironment Including Elevation of Inflammatory Signals and Multiple Immune Checkpoints in Lung Adenocarcinoma. *Clin. Cancer Res.* **2016**, *22*, 3630–3642. [CrossRef] [PubMed]
52. Kim, J.; Bae, J.S. Tumor-Associated Macrophages and Neutrophils in Tumor Microenvironment. *Mediat. Inflamm.* **2016**, *2016*, 6058147. [CrossRef] [PubMed]
53. Carron, E.C.; Homra, S.; Rosenberg, J.; Coffelt, S.B.; Kittrell, F.; Zhang, Y.; Creighton, C.J.; Fuqua, S.A.; Medina, D.; Machado, H.L. Macrophages promote the progression of premalignant mammary lesions to invasive cancer. *Oncotarget* **2017**, *8*, 50731–50746. [CrossRef] [PubMed]
54. Comijn, J.; Berx, G.; Vermassen, P.; Verschueren, K.; van Grunsven, L.; Bruyneel, E.; Mareel, M.; Huylebroeck, D.; van Roy, F. The two-handed E box binding zinc finger protein SIP1 downregulates E-cadherin and induces invasion. *Mol. Cell* **2001**, *7*, 1267–1278. [CrossRef]
55. Huber, M.A.; Kraut, N.; Beug, H. Molecular requirements for epithelial-mesenchymal transition during tumor progression. *Curr. Opin. Cell Biol.* **2005**, *17*, 548–558. [CrossRef]
56. Peinado, H.; Olmeda, D.; Cano, A. Snail, Zeb and bHLH factors in tumour progression: An alliance against the epithelial phenotype? *Nat. Rev. Cancer* **2007**, *7*, 415–428. [CrossRef]
57. Yang, J.; Mani, S.A.; Donaher, J.L.; Ramaswamy, S.; Itzykson, R.A.; Come, C.; Savagner, P.; Gitelman, I.; Richardson, A.; Weinberg, R.A. Twist, a master regulator of morphogenesis, plays an essential role in tumor metastasis. *Cell* **2004**, *117*, 927–939. [CrossRef]
58. Eger, A.; Aigner, K.; Sonderegger, S.; Dampier, B.; Oehler, S.; Schreiber, M.; Berx, G.; Cano, A.; Beug, H.; Foisner, R. DeltaEF1 is a transcriptional repressor of E-cadherin and regulates epithelial plasticity in breast cancer cells. *Oncogene* **2005**, *24*, 2375–2385. [CrossRef]
59. Gregory, P.A.; Bracken, C.P.; Bert, A.G.; Goodall, G.J. MicroRNAs as regulators of epithelial-mesenchymal transition. *Cell Cycle* **2008**, *7*, 3112–3117. [CrossRef]
60. Bracken, C.P.; Gregory, P.A.; Kolesnikoff, N.; Bert, A.G.; Wang, J.; Shannon, M.F.; Goodall, G.J. A double-negative feedback loop between ZEB1-SIP1 and the microRNA-200 family regulates epithelial-mesenchymal transition. *Cancer Res.* **2008**, *68*, 7846–7854. [CrossRef] [PubMed]
61. Burk, U.; Schubert, J.; Wellner, U.; Schmalhofer, O.; Vincan, E.; Spaderna, S.; Brabletz, T. A reciprocal repression between ZEB1 and members of the miR-200 family promotes EMT and invasion in cancer cells. *EMBO Rep.* **2008**, *9*, 582–589. [CrossRef]
62. Gregory, P.A.; Bert, A.G.; Paterson, E.L.; Barry, S.C.; Tsykin, A.; Farshid, G.; Vadas, M.A.; Khew-Goodall, Y.; Goodall, G.J. The miR-200 family and miR-205 regulate epithelial to mesenchymal transition by targeting ZEB1 and SIP1. *Nat. Cell Biol.* **2008**, *10*, 593–601. [CrossRef]
63. Korpal, M.; Lee, E.S.; Hu, G.; Kang, Y. The miR-200 family inhibits epithelial-mesenchymal transition and cancer cell migration by direct targeting of E-cadherin transcriptional repressors ZEB1 and ZEB2. *J. Biol. Chem.* **2008**, *283*, 14910–14914. [CrossRef]
64. Park, S.M.; Gaur, A.B.; Lengyel, E.; Peter, M.E. The miR-200 family determines the epithelial phenotype of cancer cells by targeting the E-cadherin repressors ZEB1 and ZEB2. *Genes Dev.* **2008**, *22*, 894–907. [CrossRef]
65. Shimono, Y.; Zabala, M.; Cho, R.W.; Lobo, N.; Dalerba, P.; Qian, D.; Diehn, M.; Liu, H.; Panula, S.P.; Chiao, E.; et al. Downregulation of miRNA-200c links breast cancer stem cells with normal stem cells. *Cell* **2009**, *138*, 592–603. [CrossRef]
66. Wellner, U.; Schubert, J.; Burk, U.C.; Schmalhofer, O.; Zhu, F.; Sonntag, A.; Waldvogel, B.; Vannier, C.; Darling, D.; zur Hausen, A.; et al. The EMT-activator ZEB1 promotes tumorigenicity by repressing stemness-inhibiting microRNAs. *Nat. Cell Biol.* **2009**, *11*, 1487–1495. [CrossRef] [PubMed]

67. Ceppi, P.; Mudduluru, G.; Kumarswamy, R.; Rapa, I.; Scagliotti, G.V.; Papotti, M.; Allgayer, H. Loss of miR-200c expression induces an aggressive, invasive, and chemoresistant phenotype in non-small cell lung cancer. *Mol. Cancer Res.* **2010**, *8*, 1207–1216. [CrossRef] [PubMed]
68. Hu, X.; Schwarz, J.K.; Lewis, J.S., Jr.; Huettner, P.C.; Rader, J.S.; Deasy, J.O.; Grigsby, P.W.; Wang, X. A microRNA expression signature for cervical cancer prognosis. *Cancer Res.* **2010**, *70*, 1441–1448. [CrossRef] [PubMed]
69. Gibbons, D.L.; Lin, W.; Creighton, C.J.; Rizvi, Z.H.; Gregory, P.A.; Goodall, G.J.; Thilaganathan, N.; Du, L.; Zhang, Y.; Pertsemlidis, A.; et al. Contextual extracellular cues promote tumor cell EMT and metastasis by regulating miR-200 family expression. *Genes Dev.* **2009**, *23*, 2140–2151. [CrossRef]
70. Ahn, Y.H.; Gibbons, D.L.; Chakravarti, D.; Creighton, C.J.; Rizvi, Z.H.; Adams, H.P.; Pertsemlidis, A.; Gregory, P.A.; Wright, J.A.; Goodall, G.J.; et al. ZEB1 drives prometastatic actin cytoskeletal remodeling by downregulating miR-34a expression. *J. Clin. Investig.* **2012**, *122*, 3170–3183. [CrossRef] [PubMed]
71. Yang, Y.; Ahn, Y.H.; Gibbons, D.L.; Zang, Y.; Lin, W.; Thilaganathan, N.; Alvarez, C.A.; Moreira, D.C.; Creighton, C.J.; Gregory, P.A.; et al. The Notch ligand Jagged2 promotes lung adenocarcinoma metastasis through a miR-200-dependent pathway in mice. *J. Clin. Investig.* **2011**, *121*, 1373–1385. [CrossRef] [PubMed]
72. Ungewiss, C.; Rizvi, Z.H.; Roybal, J.D.; Peng, D.H.; Gold, K.A.; Shin, D.H.; Creighton, C.J.; Gibbons, D.L. The microRNA-200/Zeb1 axis regulates ECM-dependent beta1-integrin/FAK signaling, cancer cell invasion and metastasis through CRKL. *Sci. Rep.* **2016**, *6*, 18652. [CrossRef] [PubMed]
73. Schliekelman, M.J.; Gibbons, D.L.; Faca, V.M.; Creighton, C.J.; Rizvi, Z.H.; Zhang, Q.; Wong, C.H.; Wang, H.; Ungewiss, C.; Ahn, Y.H.; et al. Targets of the tumor suppressor miR-200 in regulation of the epithelial-mesenchymal transition in cancer. *Cancer Res.* **2011**, *71*, 7670–7682. [CrossRef]
74. Mahmoud, S.M.; Paish, E.C.; Powe, D.G.; Macmillan, R.D.; Grainge, M.J.; Lee, A.H.; Ellis, I.O.; Green, A.R. Tumor-infiltrating CD8+ lymphocytes predict clinical outcome in breast cancer. *J. Clin. Oncol.* **2011**, *29*, 1949–1955. [CrossRef] [PubMed]
75. Garcia-Martinez, E.; Gil, G.L.; Benito, A.C.; Gonzalez-Billalabeitia, E.; Conesa, M.A.; Garcia Garcia, T.; Garcia-Garre, E.; Vicente, V.; Ayala de la Pena, F. Tumor-infiltrating immune cell profiles and their change after neoadjuvant chemotherapy predict response and prognosis of breast cancer. *Breast Cancer Res.* **2014**, *16*, 488. [CrossRef]
76. Iglesia, M.D.; Vincent, B.G.; Parker, J.S.; Hoadley, K.A.; Carey, L.A.; Perou, C.M.; Serody, J.S. Prognostic B-cell signatures using mRNA-seq in patients with subtype-specific breast and ovarian cancer. *Clin. Cancer Res.* **2014**, *20*, 3818–3829. [CrossRef]
77. Liu, S.; Lachapelle, J.; Leung, S.; Gao, D.; Foulkes, W.D.; Nielsen, T.O. CD8+ lymphocyte infiltration is an independent favorable prognostic indicator in basal-like breast cancer. *Breast Cancer Res.* **2012**, *14*, R48. [CrossRef]
78. Hudis, C.A. Trastuzumab–mechanism of action and use in clinical practice. *N. Engl. J. Med.* **2007**, *357*, 39–51. [CrossRef]
79. Shurin, M.R. Dual role of immunomodulation by anticancer chemotherapy. *Nat. Med.* **2013**, *19*, 20–22. [CrossRef]
80. Zitvogel, L.; Galluzzi, L.; Smyth, M.J.; Kroemer, G. Mechanism of action of conventional and targeted anticancer therapies: Reinstating immunosurveillance. *Immunity* **2013**, *39*, 74–88. [CrossRef]
81. Kim, K.; Skora, A.D.; Li, Z.; Liu, Q.; Tam, A.J.; Blosser, R.L.; Diaz, L.A., Jr.; Papadopoulos, N.; Kinzler, K.W.; Vogelstein, B.; et al. Eradication of metastatic mouse cancers resistant to immune checkpoint blockade by suppression of myeloid-derived cells. *Proc. Natl. Acad. Sci. USA* **2014**, *111*, 11774–11779. [CrossRef]
82. Emens, L.A.; Kok, M.; Ojalvo, L.S. Targeting the programmed cell death-1 pathway in breast and ovarian cancer. *Curr. Opin. Obstet. Gynecol.* **2016**, *28*, 142–147. [CrossRef]
83. Emens, L.A. Breast Cancer Immunotherapy: Facts and Hopes. *Clin. Cancer Res.* **2018**, *24*, 511–520. [CrossRef]
84. Rizvi, N.A.; Hellmann, M.D.; Snyder, A.; Kvistborg, P.; Makarov, V.; Havel, J.J.; Lee, W.; Yuan, J.; Wong, P.; Ho, T.S.; et al. Cancer immunology. Mutational landscape determines sensitivity to PD-1 blockade in non-small cell lung cancer. *Science* **2015**, *348*, 124–128. [CrossRef] [PubMed]
85. Savas, P.; Salgado, R.; Denkert, C.; Sotiriou, C.; Darcy, P.K.; Smyth, M.J.; Loi, S. Clinical relevance of host immunity in breast cancer: From TILs to the clinic. *Nat. Rev. Clin. Oncol.* **2016**, *13*, 228–241. [CrossRef]
86. Greifenberg, V.; Ribechini, E.; Rossner, S.; Lutz, M.B. Myeloid-derived suppressor cell activation by combined LPS and IFN-gamma treatment impairs DC development. *Eur. J. Immunol.* **2009**, *39*, 2865–2876. [CrossRef]

87. Andersen, M.H.; Schrama, D.; Thor Straten, P.; Becker, J.C. Cytotoxic T cells. *J. Investig. Dermatol.* **2006**, *126*, 32–41. [CrossRef] [PubMed]
88. Berg, R.E.; Forman, J. The role of CD8 T cells in innate immunity and in antigen non-specific protection. *Curr. Opin. Immunol.* **2006**, *18*, 338–343. [CrossRef] [PubMed]
89. Joyce, J.A.; Fearon, D.T. T cell exclusion, immune privilege, and the tumor microenvironment. *Science* **2015**, *348*, 74–80. [CrossRef]
90. Dine, J.; Gordon, R.; Shames, Y.; Kasler, M.K.; Barton-Burke, M. Immune Checkpoint Inhibitors: An Innovation in Immunotherapy for the Treatment and Management of Patients with Cancer. *Asia Pac. J. Oncol. Nurs.* **2017**, *4*, 127–135. [CrossRef]
91. Wei, S.C.; Levine, J.H.; Cogdill, A.P.; Zhao, Y.; Anang, N.A.S.; Andrews, M.C.; Sharma, P.; Wang, J.; Wargo, J.A.; Pe'er, D.; et al. Distinct Cellular Mechanisms Underlie Anti-CTLA-4 and Anti-PD-1 Checkpoint Blockade. *Cell* **2017**, *170*, 1120–1133.e17. [CrossRef]
92. Jackson, S.R.; Yuan, J.; Teague, R.M. Targeting CD8+ T-cell tolerance for cancer immunotherapy. *Immunotherapy* **2014**, *6*, 833–852. [CrossRef]
93. Wherry, E.J.; Kurachi, M. Molecular and cellular insights into T cell exhaustion. *Nat. Rev. Immunol.* **2015**, *15*, 486–499. [CrossRef]
94. Knutson, K.L.; Lu, H.; Stone, B.; Reiman, J.M.; Behrens, M.D.; Prosperi, C.M.; Gad, E.A.; Smorlesi, A.; Disis, M.L. Immunoediting of cancers may lead to epithelial to mesenchymal transition. *J. Immunol.* **2006**, *177*, 1526–1533. [CrossRef]
95. Mahic, M.; Henjum, K.; Yaqub, S.; Bjornbeth, B.A.; Torgersen, K.M.; Tasken, K.; Aandahl, E.M. Generation of highly suppressive adaptive CD8(+)CD25(+)FOXP3(+) regulatory T cells by continuous antigen stimulation. *Eur. J. Immunol.* **2008**, *38*, 640–646. [CrossRef]
96. Yang, L.; Pang, Y.; Moses, H.L. TGF-beta and immune cells: An important regulatory axis in the tumor microenvironment and progression. *Trends Immunol.* **2010**, *31*, 220–227. [CrossRef]
97. Caja, F.; Vannucci, L. TGFbeta: A player on multiple fronts in the tumor microenvironment. *J. Immunotoxicol.* **2015**, *12*, 300–307. [CrossRef]
98. Mani, S.A.; Yang, J.; Brooks, M.; Schwaninger, G.; Zhou, A.; Miura, N.; Kutok, J.L.; Hartwell, K.; Richardson, A.L.; Weinberg, R.A. Mesenchyme Forkhead 1 (FOXC2) plays a key role in metastasis and is associated with aggressive basal-like breast cancers. *Proc. Natl. Acad. Sci. USA* **2007**, *104*, 10069–10074. [CrossRef] [PubMed]
99. Dye, E.S. The antimetastatic function of concomitant antitumor immunity. II. Evidence that the generation of Ly-1+2+ effector T cells temporarily causes the destruction of already disseminated tumor cells. *J. Immunol.* **1986**, *136*, 1510–1515. [PubMed]
100. Luo, H.; Zeng, C.; Fang, C.; Seeruttun, S.R.; Lv, L.; Wang, W. A new strategy using ALDHhigh-CD8+T cells to inhibit tumorigenesis. *PLoS ONE* **2014**, *9*, e103193. [CrossRef]
101. Zhang, Z.; Liu, L.; Cao, S.; Zhu, Y.; MEI, Q. Gene delivery of TIPE2 inhibits breast cancer development and metastasis via CD8+ T and NK cell-mediated antitumor responses. *Mol. Immunol.* **2017**, *85*, 230–237. [CrossRef] [PubMed]
102. Li, Y.; Hofmann, M.; Wang, Q.; Teng, L.; Chlewicki, L.K.; Pircher, H.; Mariuzza, R.A. Structure of natural killer cell receptor KLRG1 bound to E-cadherin reveals basis for MHC-independent missing self recognition. *Immunity* **2009**, *31*, 35–46. [CrossRef]
103. Bottino, C.; Castriconi, R.; Pende, D.; Rivera, P.; Nanni, M.; Carnemolla, B.; Cantoni, C.; Grassi, J.; Marcenaro, S.; Reymond, N.; et al. Identification of PVR (CD155) and Nectin-2 (CD112) as cell surface ligands for the human DNAM-1 (CD226) activating molecule. *J. Exp. Med.* **2003**, *198*, 557–567. [CrossRef] [PubMed]
104. Taube, J.H.; Herschkowitz, J.I.; Komurov, K.; Zhou, A.Y.; Gupta, S.; Yang, J.; Hartwell, K.; Onder, T.T.; Gupta, P.B.; Evans, K.W.; et al. Core epithelial-to-mesenchymal transition interactome gene-expression signature is associated with claudin-low and metaplastic breast cancer subtypes. *Proc. Natl. Acad. Sci. USA* **2010**, *107*, 15449–15454. [CrossRef] [PubMed]
105. Chockley, P.J.; Chen, J.; Chen, G.; Beer, D.G.; Standiford, T.J.; Keshamouni, V.G. Epithelial-mesenchymal transition leads to NK cell-mediated metastasis-specific immunosurveillance in lung cancer. *J. Clin. Investig.* **2018**, *128*, 1384–1396. [CrossRef]
106. Stovgaard, E.S.; Nielsen, D.; Hogdall, E.; Balslev, E. Triple negative breast cancer - prognostic role of immune-related factors: A systematic review. *Acta Oncol.* **2017**. [CrossRef]

107. Xu, C.; Fillmore, C.M.; Koyama, S.; Wu, H.; Zhao, Y.; Chen, Z.; Herter-Sprie, G.S.; Akbay, E.A.; Tchaicha, J.H.; Altabef, A.; et al. Loss of Lkb1 and Pten leads to lung squamous cell carcinoma with elevated PD-L1 expression. *Cancer Cell* **2014**, *25*, 590–604. [CrossRef]
108. Condamine, T.; Gabrilovich, D.I. Molecular mechanisms regulating myeloid-derived suppressor cell differentiation and function. *Trends Immunol.* **2011**, *32*, 19–25. [CrossRef]
109. Welte, T.; Kim, I.S.; Tian, L.; Gao, X.; Wang, H.; Li, J.; Holdman, X.B.; Herschkowitz, J.I.; Pond, A.; Xie, G.; et al. Oncogenic mTOR signalling recruits myeloid-derived suppressor cells to promote tumour initiation. *Nat. Cell Biol.* **2016**, *18*, 632–644. [CrossRef]
110. Svoronos, N.; Perales-Puchalt, A.; Allegrezza, M.J.; Rutkowski, M.R.; Payne, K.K.; Tesone, A.J.; Nguyen, J.M.; Curiel, T.J.; Cadungog, M.G.; Singhal, S.; et al. Tumor Cell-Independent Estrogen Signaling Drives Disease Progression through Mobilization of Myeloid-Derived Suppressor Cells. *Cancer Discov.* **2017**, *7*, 72–85. [CrossRef] [PubMed]
111. Welte, T.; Zhang, X.H.; Rosen, J.M. Repurposing Antiestrogens for Tumor Immunotherapy. *Cancer Discov.* **2017**, *7*, 17–19. [CrossRef]
112. Love, M.I.; Huber, W.; Anders, S. Moderated estimation of fold change and dispersion for RNA-seq data with DESeq2. *Genome Biol.* **2014**, *15*, 550. [CrossRef]
113. Robinson, M.D.; McCarthy, D.J.; Smyth, G.K. edgeR: A Bioconductor package for differential expression analysis of digital gene expression data. *Bioinformatics* **2010**, *26*, 139–140. [CrossRef]
114. Chang, J.T.; Gatza, M.L.; Lucas, J.E.; Barry, W.T.; Vaughn, P.; Nevins, J.R. SIGNATURE: A workbench for gene expression signature analysis. *BMC Bioinformatics* **2011**, *12*, 443. [CrossRef]
115. Farmer, P.; Bonnefoi, H.; Anderle, P.; Cameron, D.; Wirapati, P.; Becette, V.; Andre, S.; Piccart, M.; Campone, M.; Brain, E.; et al. A stroma-related gene signature predicts resistance to neoadjuvant chemotherapy in breast cancer. *Nat. Med.* **2009**, *15*, 68–74. [CrossRef]
116. Brand, T.M.; Iida, M.; Wheeler, D.L. Molecular mechanisms of resistance to the EGFR monoclonal antibody cetuximab. *Cancer Biol. Ther.* **2011**, *11*, 777–792. [CrossRef]
117. George, J.T.; Jolly, M.K.; Xu, S.; Somarelli, J.A.; Levine, H. Survival Outcomes in Cancer Patients Predicted by a Partial EMT Gene Expression Scoring Metric. *Cancer Res.* **2017**, *77*, 6415–6428. [CrossRef]
118. Cristescu, R.; Lee, J.; Nebozhyn, M.; Kim, K.M.; Ting, J.C.; Wong, S.S.; Liu, J.; Yue, Y.G.; Wang, J.; Yu, K.; et al. Molecular analysis of gastric cancer identifies subtypes associated with distinct clinical outcomes. *Nat. Med.* **2015**, *21*, 449–456. [CrossRef]
119. Cheng, W.Y.; Kandel, J.J.; Yamashiro, D.J.; Canoll, P.; Anastassiou, D. A multi-cancer mesenchymal transition gene expression signature is associated with prolonged time to recurrence in glioblastoma. *PLoS ONE* **2012**, *7*, e34705. [CrossRef]
120. Sethi, S.; Macoska, J.; Chen, W.; Sarkar, F.H. Molecular signature of epithelial-mesenchymal transition (EMT) in human prostate cancer bone metastasis. *Am. J. Transl. Res.* **2010**, *3*, 90–99.
121. Chae, Y.K.; Chang, S.; Ko, T.; Anker, J.; Agte, S.; Iams, W.; Choi, W.M.; Lee, K.; Cruz, M. Epithelial-mesenchymal transition (EMT) signature is inversely associated with T-cell infiltration in non-small cell lung cancer (NSCLC). *Sci. Rep.* **2018**, *8*, 2918. [CrossRef]
122. Sugio, T.; Miyawaki, K.; Kato, K.; Sasaki, K.; Yamada, K.; Iqbal, J.; Miyamoto, T.; Ohshima, K.; Maeda, T.; Miyoshi, H.; et al. Microenvironmental immune cell signatures dictate clinical outcomes for PTCL-NOS. *Blood Adv.* **2018**, *2*, 2242–2252. [CrossRef] [PubMed]
123. Ali, H.R.; Provenzano, E.; Dawson, S.J.; Blows, F.M.; Liu, B.; Shah, M.; Earl, H.M.; Poole, C.J.; Hiller, L.; Dunn, J.A.; et al. Association between CD8+ T-cell infiltration and breast cancer survival in 12,439 patients. *Ann. Oncol.* **2014**, *25*, 1536–1543. [CrossRef]
124. Teschendorff, A.E.; Miremadi, A.; Pinder, S.E.; Ellis, I.O.; Caldas, C. An immune response gene expression module identifies a good prognosis subtype in estrogen receptor negative breast cancer. *Genome Biol.* **2007**, *8*, R157. [CrossRef]
125. Rody, A.; Holtrich, U.; Pusztai, L.; Liedtke, C.; Gaetje, R.; Ruckhaeberle, E.; Solbach, C.; Hanker, L.; Ahr, A.; Metzler, D.; et al. T-cell metagene predicts a favorable prognosis in estrogen receptor-negative and HER2-positive breast cancers. *Breast Cancer Res.* **2009**, *11*, R15. [CrossRef] [PubMed]
126. Ascierto, M.L.; Kmieciak, M.; Idowu, M.O.; Manjili, R.; Zhao, Y.; Grimes, M.; Dumur, C.; Wang, E.; Ramakrishnan, V.; Wang, X.Y.; et al. A signature of immune function genes associated with recurrence-free survival in breast cancer patients. *Breast Cancer Res. Treat.* **2012**, *131*, 871–880. [CrossRef] [PubMed]

127. Ascierto, M.L.; Idowu, M.O.; Zhao, Y.; Khalak, H.; Payne, K.K.; Wang, X.Y.; Dumur, C.I.; Bedognetti, D.; Tomei, S.; Ascierto, P.A.; et al. Molecular signatures mostly associated with NK cells are predictive of relapse free survival in breast cancer patients. *J. Transl. Med.* **2013**, *11*, 145. [CrossRef]
128. Perez, E.A.; Thompson, E.A.; Ballman, K.V.; Anderson, S.K.; Asmann, Y.W.; Kalari, K.R.; Eckel-Passow, J.E.; Dueck, A.C.; Tenner, K.S.; Jen, J.; et al. Genomic analysis reveals that immune function genes are strongly linked to clinical outcome in the North Central Cancer Treatment Group n9831 Adjuvant Trastuzumab Trial. *J. Clin. Oncol.* **2015**, *33*, 701–708. [CrossRef]
129. Denkert, C.; Loibl, S.; Noske, A.; Roller, M.; Muller, B.M.; Komor, M.; Budczies, J.; Darb-Esfahani, S.; Kronenwett, R.; Hanusch, C.; et al. Tumor-associated lymphocytes as an independent predictor of response to neoadjuvant chemotherapy in breast cancer. *J. Clin. Oncol.* **2010**, *28*, 105–113. [CrossRef]
130. Forero, A.; Li, Y.; Chen, D.; Grizzle, W.E.; Updike, K.L.; Merz, N.D.; Downs-Kelly, E.; Burwell, T.C.; Vaklavas, C.; Buchsbaum, D.J.; et al. Expression of the MHC Class II Pathway in Triple-Negative Breast Cancer Tumor Cells Is Associated with a Good Prognosis and Infiltrating Lymphocytes. *Cancer Immunol. Res.* **2016**, *4*, 390–399. [CrossRef]
131. Newman, A.M.; Liu, C.L.; Green, M.R.; Gentles, A.J.; Feng, W.; Xu, Y.; Hoang, C.D.; Diehn, M.; Alizadeh, A.A. Robust enumeration of cell subsets from tissue expression profiles. *Nat. Methods* **2015**, *12*, 453–457. [CrossRef] [PubMed]
132. Li, T.; Fan, J.; Wang, B.; Traugh, N.; Chen, Q.; Liu, J.S.; Li, B.; Liu, X.S. TIMER: A Web Server for Comprehensive Analysis of Tumor-Infiltrating Immune Cells. *Cancer Res.* **2017**, *77*, e108–e110. [CrossRef] [PubMed]
133. Azizi, E.; Carr, A.J.; Plitas, G.; Cornish, A.E.; Konopacki, C.; Prabhakaran, S.; Nainys, J.; Wu, K.; Kiseliovas, V.; Setty, M.; et al. Single-Cell Map of Diverse Immune Phenotypes in the Breast Tumor Microenvironment. *Cell* **2018**, *174*, 1293–1308.e36. [CrossRef] [PubMed]

7

Circulating Tumor Cell Detection in Lung Cancer: But to What End?

Véronique Hofman [1,2,3,†], **Simon Heeke** [1,2,†], **Charles-Hugo Marquette** [2,4], **Marius Ilié** [1,2,3] **and Paul Hofman** [1,2,3,*]

1 Laboratory of Clinical and Experimental Pathology, CHU Nice, FHU OncoAge, University Côte d'Azur, 06100 Nice, France; hofman.v@chu-nice.fr (V.H.); heeke.s@chu-nice.fr (S.H.); ilie.m@chu-nice.fr (M.I.)
2 Team 4, IRCAN, FHU OncoAge, University Côte d'Azur, CNRS, INSERM, 06107 Nice CEDEX 02, France; marquette.c@chu-nice.fr
3 Hospital-Integrated Biobank (BB-0033-00025), CHU Nice, FHU OncoAge, University Côte d'Azur, 06100 Nice, France
4 Department of Pneumology and Oncology, CHU Nice, FHU OncoAge, University Côte d'Azur, 06100 Nice, France
* Correspondence: hofman.p@chu-nice.fr
† These authors contributed equally to this work.

Abstract: The understanding of the natural history and biology of lung cancer has been enhanced by studies into circulating tumor cells (CTCs). Fundamental and translational research, as well as clinical trials in the characterization and behavior of these cells, have constantly contributed to improving understanding within the domain of thoracic oncology. However, the use of these CTCs as prognostic and predictive biomarkers has not been adopted to the same extent as circulating free DNA (cf-DNA) in plasma, in the daily practice of thoracic oncologists. However, recent technological advances have firmly put the detection and characterization of CTCs in thoracic oncology back on the agenda, and have opened up perspectives for their routine clinical use. This review discusses the major advances of using CTCs in the domain of thoracic oncology, as well as the envisaged short- and long-term prospects.

Keywords: circulating tumor cells; liquid biopsy; lung cancer; personal medicine; techniques; xenograft

---

1. Introduction

Liquid biopsy (LB) plays a major role in thoracic oncology [1,2]. A number of recent publications and developments within this domain testify to the increasing importance of LB. These studies concern not only fundamental translational and clinical research, but also technological advances [3–7]. They have provided a better understanding of the molecular and cellular mechanisms, the progression of lung cancer, and the treatment of patients. Among these studies, research into mutations in *EGFR* using plasma circulating free DNA (cf-DNA) have led to the use of LB in the clinical routine for patients with advanced stage or metastatic non-small cell lung carcinoma (NSCLC) [2,8–10]. This approach is now used in a large number of hospitals.

The number of detectable biological targets in an LB that are potentially accessible to treatment has increased, and future application of different biomarkers can be envisaged in the short-term [11]. The complexity of molecules for detection in the blood of patients with lung cancer has increased with advances in our understanding of the biology of the different components circulating in the blood. These components include free or complexed nucleic acids, microparticles including exosomes, circulating "non-hematological" cells including circulating tumor cells (CTCs), and proteins of serum and plasma [12–16]. The addition to these analyses of different circulating hematological normal cells (neutrophils, lymphocytes, monocytes, platelets), constituting a "liquid microenvironment", has progressively been envisaged [17,18].

While taking into account the increasing complexity, a number of biomarkers have been developed for use, particularly in the clinic, for the interests of patients with advanced or metastatic lung cancer. Thus, the possibility of detecting activating or resistance mutations induced by molecular therapeutics in plasma cf-DNA has been associated with an explosion in the number of exploratory methods and applications in thoracic oncology [2,19–22]. One of the consequences of these rapid developments concerns the progressive decrease in the interest shown in the analysis of CTCs in thoracic oncology, at least for routine daily practice [23]. However, cf-DNA and CTCs are complementary, and can serve to answer different questions [24]. While genetic assessment might be suitable with both cf-DNA and CTCs, only CTCs might be able to give insights into the seeding of metastases and interactions of CTCs with other circulating blood cells, endothelial cells and, subsequently, different parenchyma [25,26]. cf-DNA and CTCs can be successfully simultaneously assessed in the same patient for a broader insight of tumor burden [27–29]. The absence of robust approaches for the detection of CTCs in clinical routine practice, in the context of the healthcare of these patients, probably explains the decline in interest. This is also due to the facts that CTCs are rarely found in blood, for capture, and that the capturing techniques, which are both very sensitive and specific, still require validation to provide optimal results for use in daily practice [30,31]. A selection of key studies on CTC isolation techniques have been summarized in Table 1. In this regard, the fact that different methods of CTC isolation give conflicting results for the same series of patients has certainly slowed the interest shown in this domain by many investigators [32,33]. Fewer groups around the world study CTC detection compared to groups working on detection of cf-DNA in the area of thoracic oncology. A number of review articles have discussed the advantages and limits of using CTCs or plasma cf-DNA in oncology [34–37]. The majority underline the difficulty of using CTCs as prognostic and predictive biomarkers in daily practice. Where, then, lies the interest in—and the role of—projects aimed at detecting and characterizing CTCs in thoracic oncology? Is it possible to envisage, in the future, the routine use of this type of analysis in the clinic?

This review aims to outline how the study of CTCs in an LB can provide unique and indispensable information in thoracic oncology, and to present the future long- and short-term developments in this domain.

Table 1. Technical advancements in circulating tumor cell (CTC) research for lung cancer.

Study	Histology	Approach	Method	Results	Ref
Hofman et al.	NSCLC	Analysis of preoperative CTCs to predict relapse in early stage NSCLC patients.	ISET™ (Rarecells, Paris, France)	Circulating non-hematologic cells were detected in 102/208 patients with patients with >50 cells having worse prognosis	[38]
Hofman et al.	NSCLC	Assessment of CTCs before radical surgery as prognostic factor.	ISET (Rarecells) and CellSearch™ (Menarini Silicon Biosystems, Bologna, Italy)	CTCs were detected in 69% (144/210) of patients but only in 20% (42/210) of patients with both ISET and CellSearch. Patients where CTCs were detected with both methods had worse prognosis	[33]
Carter et al.	SCLC	Assessment of copy number alterations in CTCs to distinguish chemosensitive from chemorefractory patients	CellSearch™ (Menarini Silicon Biosystems)	31 patients tested. 27–20,815 CTCs per 7.5 mL of blood (median, 836). 83.3% correctly classified cases	[39]
Drapkin et al.	SCLC	Generation of CTC-derived Xenografts.	CTC-iChip^{neg} device ‡	CDX could be obtained with an efficiency of 38%	[40]
Tan et al.	NSCLC	Comparison of EML4-ALK FISH in CTCs and tumor tissues	ClearCell FX™ (ClearBridge Biomedics, Singapore, Singapore)	>90% of concordance. More CTCs in EML4-ALK positive patients (3–15/1.88 mL blood) than in negative patients (0–2).	[41]
Ilie et al.	NSCLC	Analysis of PD-L1 expression on CTCs and white blood cells compared to tumor tissue.	ISET™ (Rarecells)	PD-L1 in CTCs can be detected at 93% concordance to tumor tissue and 73% in white blood cells	[42]
Adams et al.	NSCLC	Sequential analysis of PD-L1 and RAD50 expression in patient undergoing radiotherapy.	CellSieve™ (Creatv MicroTech, Rockville, MD, USA)	CTCs and cancer-associated macrophage-like cells (CAMLs) were detected in up to 100% of 41 patients and presence increased during treatment. RAD50 and PD-L1 expression also increased over time	[43]
Chudziak et al.	SCLC	Comparison of Parsortix™ and CellSearch™ devices for clinical evaluation.	Parsortix™ (Angle PLC. Guildford, UK) and CellSearch™ (Menarini Silicon Biosystems)	1–3780 CTCs per 7.5 mL of blood in CellSearch™ (10/12 samples) and 20–1474 using Parsortix™ (12/12 patients)	[44]
Krebs et al.	NSCLC	Comparison of ISET™ with CellSearch™	ISET (Rarecells) and CellSearch™ (Menarini Silicon Biosystems)	80% positive patients using ISET™ (0–1045, mean = 71 cells) compared to 23% in CellSearch™ (0–78, mean = 4 cells)	[45]
Gorges et al.	NSCLC	Comparison of CellSearch™ with GILUPI CellCollector™	GILUPI CellCollector™ (GILUPI, Potsdam, Germany) and CellSearch™ (Menarini Silicon Biosystems)	58% positive patients with GILUPI™ (1–56, median = 5 cells) compared to 27% with CellSearch™ (1–300 cells)	[46]

‡ The CTC-iChip^{neg} is not commercially available. Abbreviations: non-small cell lung carcinoma (NSCLC), small cell lung carcinoma (SCLC).

2. Opportunities Offered by Studying CTCs in Thoracic Oncology

A couple of opportunities can be specifically associated with CTC detection programs only (Table 2).

Table 2. Methodological approaches in CTC research and main issues.

Approaches	Interests	Issues	Ref
CTCs cultured ex vivo	• Drug testing • Genomic/transcriptomic profiling • Assessment of metastatic cells	• Depends on the number of viable isolated cells • Lack of microenvironment	[47–50]
CDX	• Drug testing • Genomic/transcriptomic profiling	• Lack of human immune cells in microenvironment • Long duration to obtain xenograft	[40,51–53]
CTC-derived explant	• Expanding tumor-derived cells • Large potential for drug screening	• Lack of microenvironment • Long duration to establish	[54]
Single-cell analyses	• Genomic/transcriptomic profiling • Tumor heterogeneity studies • Functional studies (secretion)	• Difficult to get isolated viable CTCs • Technologically challenging	[55–58]
Microemboli tumor cells	• Impact on prognosis • Cell–cell contact interaction studies • Heterogeneity studies	• Difficulty to separate the different CTCs from a cluster	[59]
CTCs & circulating immune cells interaction	• Mechanisms of crosstalk between cells	• Different populations of immune cells • Lack of ex vivo models	[17]
Cytomorphological assessment	• Identification and characterization of specific populations of interest • In situ protein and RNA assessment linking to the cell morphology	• Highly dependent on the isolation technique	[42,60–68]
CTCs quantification at baseline and monitoring	• Real time monitoring of systemic anticancer therapies	• No FDA approved test for lung cancer	[69–71]

CDX = CTC-derived xenograft.

2.1. Developing Xenografts from Circulating Tumor Cells and Cells Cultured In Vitro

Different enrichment techniques allow for the isolation of "viable" CTCs from patients with lung cancer (ClearCell® FX System, VTX-1 Liquid Biopsy System, Parsortix™ Cell Separation System) [72–74] (Figure 1). These techniques represent a crucial development in the use of LB in thoracic oncology. By injecting CTCs into mice, CTC-derived xenograft (CDX) models can be obtained, and the biology of these cells can be studied in vivo. This approach allows for analysis of the proliferation and level of "aggressiveness" of CTCs, their behavior once extravasated from blood and, thus, their metastatic potential. CDX can be developed to examine the response of tumors to different therapeutic molecules and protocols. In theory, these studies can anticipate the response of tumors to certain treatments, depending on the patient, and thus allow the most effective treatment to be proposed. Additionally, CDX can also be used to study primary and secondary mechanisms of resistance to therapeutic molecules. However, the setup of the methodology of CDX is difficult, and the systems of cell enrichment for the isolation of CTCs show variable sensitivity (ClearCell® FX System, VTX-1 Liquid Biopsy System, Parsortix™ Cell Separation System) [72–74]. Finally, the rate of successful development of CDX depends on the number of cells isolated and their ability to proliferate.

At present, the development of CDX in thoracic oncology concerns predominantly small cell lung carcinomas (SCLCs), as shown by several publications in this domain on this type of histology [51–53,75]. One reason for this is the high number of CTCs in the blood of patients with SCLC when at a metastatic phase (mean $\pm$ SD = 1589 $\pm$ 5565 in 7.5 mL of blood), and another is due to the capacity of these CTCs to proliferate [59]. Using these model systems, it is possible to envisage treating patients according to the response of the xenografts to different tested molecules [54,76–78]. Complementary analyses can be performed using cells cultured after dissociation of the CDX tumor [54]. This method allows several million tumor cells to be cultured and tested with different therapeutic molecules [54]. By contrast, few studies concern CDX obtained from NSCLC. Fewer cells are isolated in NSCLC, and their ability to proliferate is lower in comparison to SCLC. Methods have been developed to culture, in vitro, the CTCs, and to thus to analyze their potential to proliferate, their biology, and their sensitivity to different molecules [79]. These approaches are not as advanced as CDX for clinical application.

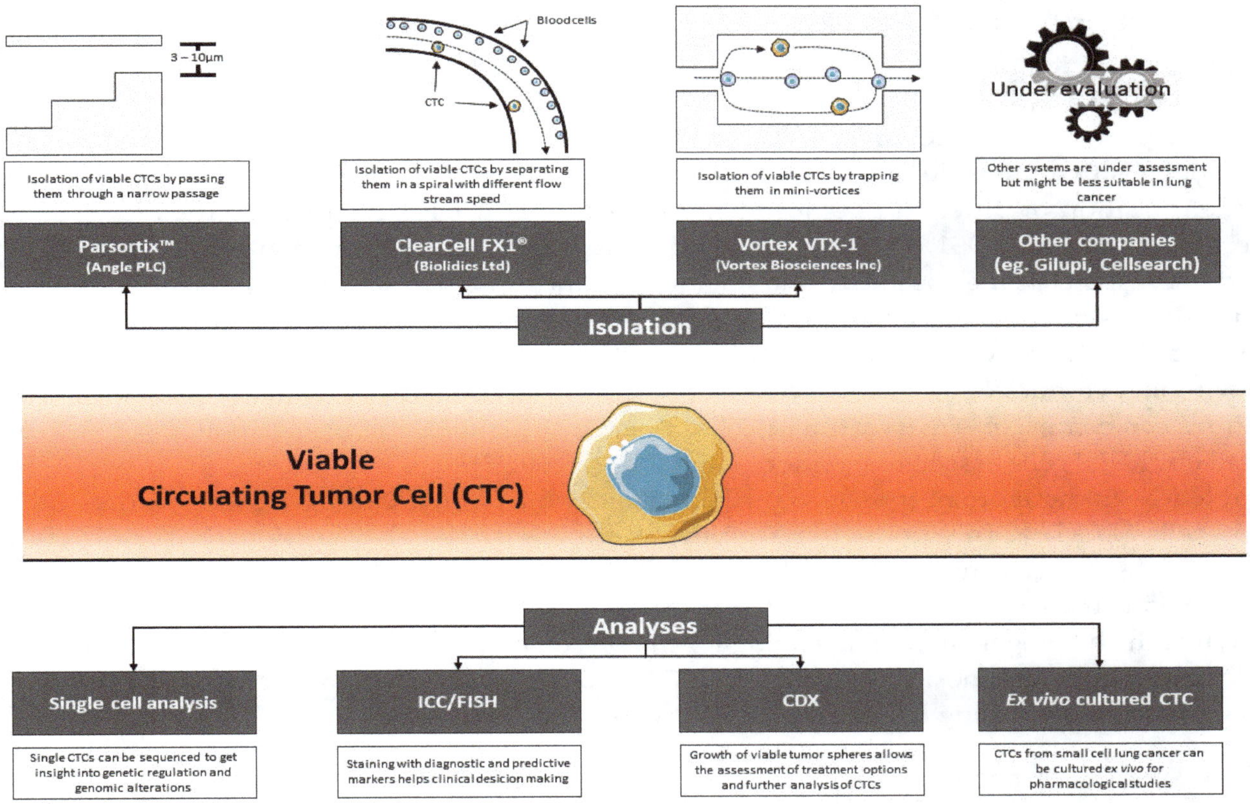

Figure 1. Overview of the different isolation techniques and possibilities in CTC research. Different devices have been developed with Parsortix (Angle PLC, Guildford, UK), ClearCell FX1 (Biolidics, Singapore), and Vortex VTX-1 (Vortex Biosciences, Pleasanton, CA, USA) being the most prominent. However, other CTC isolation systems, like GILUPI (Potsdam, Germany), can also be used for the isolation of viable CTCs. Isolation of viable CTCs then allows for the processing and analysis of cells using numerous approaches.

2.2. *Single-Cell Analysis and Functional Studies*

In contrast to studies on circulating nucleic acids, exosomes, or other blood biomarkers, the analysis of CTCs can define their molecular genetics, epigenetics, transcriptomics, and protein profile [55,56,58]. Thus, a very precise tumor profile and characterization of the phenotype of cells with invasive potential can be studied and can contribute to analyses concerning tumor heterogeneity [30]. Single-cell comparative analyses can be performed with primitive tumors, CTCs, and metastatic tumors from the same patient and thereby provide complementary information concerning the biological mechanisms associated with the progression and dissemination of lung cancers. Using isolated or cultured live cells, these functional studies identify the proteins secreted by CTCs [55]. The EPISPOT technology applied to these live isolated cells is particularly sensitive for the study of the expression and secretion of proteins by CTCs [55]. It has also been demonstrated that CTCs might be directly cultured on microfilters that are used for CTC isolation. This might facilitate CTC culture as it avoids the complicated transfer of CTCs onto cell culture plates, and might strongly increase the time from CTC isolation to plating in a culture medium for growth [80].

Additionally, the development of new technologies, such as the DEPArray^{TM} (Menarini Silicon Biosystems, Bologna, Italy), allows the separation of single cells from a pool of isolated CTCs to get further insight into single-cell dynamics [81,82]. This has been used to determine copy number variations (CNVs) in SCLC patients upon single-cell DNA sequencing [39]. Additionally, NanoArrays have been developed for the single-cell analysis of NSCLC [83].

Finally, single-cell RNAseq approaches from CTCs have been successfully implemented for different solid tumors, like breast and prostatic carcinoma [84,85], and should probably be in use also for lung cancer in the near future [86].

2.3. Correlation between Cytopathological and Molecular Phenotypic Analyses

Some methods of detection of CTCs can visualize and identify the classical cytological criteria of cancer cells that are routinely used in the laboratory for different cytological samples [60,61,87]. The identification of different diagnostic biomarkers (TTF1, p40) or of the predictive response to a therapeutic (ALK, ROS1, PD-L1) can be correlated to these cytomorphological criteria, which considerably increase the specificity and reliability of these methodological approaches [42,62–67,87]. Several studies have reported the extensive morphological heterogeneity of NSCLC CTCs. All the cytological criteria of malignant cells, as well as other criteria and circulating "non-hematological" cells without cytonuclear anomalies were identified. While considering the latter cells, the following questions can be raised: Are they tumor cells? Are they cells with an invasive potential? Or are they normal epithelial cells associated, or not, with CTCs [58,60,87]?

It has been therefore proposed to further categorize CTC in different classes, like disseminated tumor cells (DTC), CTCs undergoing epithelial-to-mesenchymal transition (EMT) (EMTCTCs), and cancer-associated macrophage-like cells (CAMLs), which will further challenge the precise detection and characterization of CTCs [43,88–91].

While the heterogeneity is challenging for the successful identification of CTCs, it also has strong implications on the prognosis, as especially CTCs with a mesenchymal phenotype might have a more severe impact on spreading disease than CTCs with an epithelial phenotype [92–94].

3. What Are the Prospects?

One of the main hurdles facing the analysis of CTCs concerns the large number of methods that have been developed to isolate and characterize CTCs. The number of techniques makes it difficult for an operator to understand and choose a technique, particularly for routine clinical use. The selection by an investigator of a technique is guided by several parameters: (i) the sensitivity and specificity, (ii) the ease of use, (iii) a rapid turnaround time for getting results, (iv) the reproducibility, and (v) the cost. To date, no method answers all these parameters to analyze CTCs in daily practice in the domain of thoracic oncology. Hence, some one concern is improving the methods of detection and characterization of CTCs to make them as competitive as the detection and characterization of cf-DNA, which has been widely adopted in routine clinical practice. Since CTCs in blood are rare occurrences (particularly in NSCLC patients), the optimization of CTC enrichment is essential. Progress in this area will be achieved through a better understanding of the biology of CTCs and the discovery of new specific biomarkers of CTCs, in particular, if they identify "viable" CTCs with aggressive and metastatic potential.

A new avenue of biological investigation has recently emerged with the study of active interactions between circulating hematological cells and CTCs [68,95]. These studies should lead to the discovery of new mechanisms of resistance to cell death by CTCs and, thus, to novel therapeutic targets that induce cell death [68,95].

As for the analyses performed with cf-DNA in plasma (analysis of mutations or of methylation), or other blood biomarkers (plasma microRNA, auto-antibodies, fragments of complement, and plasma proteins), some recent studies suggest that CTCs may be early markers of lung cancer, which may even be detected several months before radiographic emergence of the cancer [69–71,96]. However, these approaches require (i) optimization of the cellular enrichment methods and characterization, (ii) several independent studies, and (iii) inclusion of a large number of patients for validation.

Single-cell genetic and transcriptomic analyses must provide new information on very specific molecular targets for novel therapeutics to be used in the context of personal medicine. Recently developed technological approaches that are being evaluated may contribute to better characterization of CTCs at the single-cell level [58,97]. These complex methodological developments should allow for better understanding of the heterogeneity of CTCs among patients and for the same patient, as well as for identification of CTCs from either primary or metastatic tumors. The molecular characterization of CTCs may compete with or, more likely, provide important complementary information to that obtained from circulating free nucleic acids. One of the obstacles lies in the heterogeneity of CTCs and the variable expression of molecular markers depending on the cell (or cells) isolated [30,39].

Several studies indicate that comparison of the quantity of patient CTCs—at baseline and after treatment—may be a good indicator of prognosis in SCLC [51,98]. Thus, for this pathology, aside from the quantification of cf-DNA in plasma or, as reported more recently, of the tumor mutation load, CTCs may be used, in routine practice as an indicator of the response of tumors to treatment. The possibility of establishing CDX or cells in culture originating from CTCs, and thus of testing therapeutic molecules ex vivo, may benefit the clinical follow-up and care of patients [54,77,78,98]. In a similar manner, cell cultures of millions of cells obtained from CDX should facilitate their molecular analysis [54]. One of the limitations of this approach is the time required to obtain CDX, which is not compatible with care of the majority of patients from whom the CTCs were obtained.

Despite the number of promising studies on NSCLC, the use of CTCs in routine practice remains hypothetical, in particular, for use as a prognostic biomarker. In fact, the quantification of CTCs in this pathology strongly varies according to the techniques used for the same patient, which makes this approach ineffective [33,38,45,99–102]. Moreover, the establishment of CDX is rather challenging for NSCLC [102].

New techniques for detection and characterization of CTCs need to be continually evaluated and examined, which may be difficult for an individual cohort of patients. The standardization of protocols for the isolation, preparation, enrichment, and characterization of CTCs is a prerequisite to presenting international ISO (International Organization for Standardization) norms before their routine clinical use by thoracic oncologists.

4. Conclusions

In thoracic oncology, the use of CTCs is often associated with issues concerning translational research that does not involve immediate use in routine practice. Thus, projects developed with CTCs contrast with applications using plasma cf-DNA that have been employed for a number of years for the care of patients, in particular, in the detection of activating mutations or mutations conferring resistance in *EGFR* [2,8–10]. Until now, a number of technological hurdles prevented the transfer of applications using CTCs into daily practice in thoracic oncology. Transfer to routine practice in real life can only be achieved if solid benefit to the patients is demonstrated, such as choice of therapy according to the number and type of CTCs as well as the expression of certain biomarkers of interest and, more importantly, real benefit in terms of overall survival of patients.

Technological progress on the analysis of CTCs should lead not only to the discovery of novel molecular targets for early diagnosis, but also to new prognostic and predictive biomarkers of the response or resistance to therapeutics. One promising direction concerns the development of CDX, allowing the expansion of tumor cells and their analysis in vivo, as well as the possibility of testing new therapeutic strategies. However, the success of CDX depends on the number of isolated CTCs, which is very low for certain histological types of lung cancer.

The combined and simultaneous study of several elements of LB (CTCs, free circulating nucleic acids, exosomes, proteins, etc.) may permit better assessment of the different phenotypes found using LB, and the associated individual approaches to define reliable diagnostic, prognostic, and predictive parameters [103,104]. Technological progress will permit the combination of different biomarkers at the single-cell level, and will increase our knowledge of CTCs [105,106]. A continual increase in different biomarkers for studying individual patients will evolve from more and more complex studies. In addition, as recently emerging in other areas of medicine, artificial intelligence should rapidly emerge and could integrate the different elements of LB, including CTCs [107,108]. Consequently, CTCs certainly play a key role in this context but, operationally, require further development before coming into daily routine use in thoracic oncology.

Author Contributions: Conceptualization, P.H. and V.H.; methodology, V.H., S.H., C.-H.M., M.I., P.H., writing—original draft preparation, V.H. and P.H.; writing—review and editing, S.H., C.-H.M., M.I.; visualization, S.H. and P.H.

References

1. Bracht, J.W.P.; Mayo-de-Las-Casas, C.; Berenguer, J.; Karachaliou, N.; Rosell, R. The Present and Future of Liquid Biopsies in Non-Small Cell Lung Cancer: Combining Four Biosources for Diagnosis, Prognosis, Prediction, and Disease Monitoring. *Curr. Oncol. Rep.* **2018**, *20*, 70. [CrossRef] [PubMed]
2. Hofman, P. Liquid Biopsy and Therapeutic Targets: Present and Future Issues in Thoracic Oncology. *Cancers* **2017**, *9*, 154. [CrossRef] [PubMed]
3. Alix-Panabières, C.; Mader, S.; Pantel, K. Epithelial-mesenchymal plasticity in circulating tumor cells. *J. Mol. Med.* **2017**, *95*, 133–142. [CrossRef] [PubMed]
4. Bardelli, A.; Pantel, K. Liquid Biopsies, What We Do Not Know (Yet). *Cancer Cell* **2017**, *31*, 172–179. [CrossRef] [PubMed]
5. Li, W.; Wang, H.; Zhao, Z.; Gao, H.; Liu, C.; Zhu, L.; Wang, C.; Yang, Y. Emerging Nanotechnologies for Liquid Biopsy: The Detection of Circulating Tumor Cells and Extracellular Vesicles. *Adv. Mater.* **2018**, e1805344. [CrossRef] [PubMed]
6. Siravegna, G.; Marsoni, S.; Siena, S.; Bardelli, A. Integrating liquid biopsies into the management of cancer. *Nat. Rev. Clin. Oncol.* **2017**, *14*, 531–548. [CrossRef] [PubMed]
7. Sorber, L.; Zwaenepoel, K.; De Winne, K.; Van Casteren, K.; Augustus, E.; Jacobs, J.; Zhang, X.H.; Galdermans, D.; De Droogh, E.; Lefebure, A.; et al. A Multicenter Study to Assess EGFR Mutational Status in Plasma: Focus on an Optimized Workflow for Liquid Biopsy in a Clinical Setting. *Cancers* **2018**, *10*, 290. [CrossRef] [PubMed]
8. Ntzifa, A.; Kroupis, C.; Haliassos, A.; Lianidou, E. A pilot plasma-ctDNA ring trial for the Cobas®EGFR Mutation Test in clinical diagnostic laboratories. *Clin. Chem. Lab. Med.* **2018**. [CrossRef] [PubMed]
9. Rolfo, C.; Mack, P.C.; Scagliotti, G.V.; Baas, P.; Barlesi, F.; Bivona, T.G.; Herbst, R.S.; Mok, T.S.; Peled, N.; Pirker, R.; et al. IASLC Statement Paper: Liquid Biopsy for Advanced Non-Small Cell Lung Cancer (NSCLC). *J. Thorac. Oncol.* **2018**, *13*, 1248–1268. [CrossRef] [PubMed]
10. Sacher, A.G.; Alden, R.S.; Oxnard, G.R. Early Intervention in Lung Cancers With Rapid Plasma Genotyping for EGFR and KRAS Mutations-Reply. *JAMA Oncol.* **2016**, *2*, 1096–1097. [CrossRef] [PubMed]
11. Reimers, N.; Pantel, K. Liquid biopsy: Novel technologies and clinical applications. *Clin. Chem. Lab. Med.* **2018**. [CrossRef] [PubMed]
12. Afrifa, J.; Zhao, T.; Yu, J. Circulating mitochondria DNA, a non-invasive cancer diagnostic biomarker candidate. *Mitochondrion* **2018**. [CrossRef] [PubMed]
13. Anfossi, S.; Babayan, A.; Pantel, K.; Calin, G.A. Clinical utility of circulating non-coding RNAs—An update. *Nat. Rev. Clin. Oncol.* **2018**, *15*, 541–563. [CrossRef] [PubMed]

14. Integrative Analysis of Lung Cancer Etiology and Risk (INTEGRAL) Consortium for Early Detection of Lung Cancer; Guida, F.; Sun, N.; Bantis, L.E.; Muller, D.C.; Li, P.; Taguchi, A.; Dhillon, D.; Kundnani, D.L.; Patel, N.J.; et al. Assessment of Lung Cancer Risk on the Basis of a Biomarker Panel of Circulating Proteins. *JAMA Oncol.* **2018**, *4*, e182078. [CrossRef] [PubMed]
15. Mader, S.; Pantel, K. Liquid Biopsy: Current Status and Future Perspectives. *Oncol. Res. Treat.* **2017**, *40*, 404–408. [CrossRef] [PubMed]
16. Vaidyanathan, R.; Soon, R.H.; Zhang, P.; Jiang, K.; Lim, C.T. Cancer diagnosis: From tumor to liquid biopsy and beyond. *Lab Chip* **2018**, *19*, 11–34. [CrossRef] [PubMed]
17. Leone, K.; Poggiana, C.; Zamarchi, R. The Interplay between Circulating Tumor Cells and the Immune System: From Immune Escape to Cancer Immunotherapy. *Diagnostics* **2018**, *8*, 59. [CrossRef] [PubMed]
18. Zhang, W.-W.; Rong, Y.; Liu, Q.; Luo, C.-L.; Zhang, Y.; Wang, F.-B. Integrative diagnosis of cancer by combining CTCs and associated peripheral blood cells in liquid biopsy. *Clin. Transl. Oncol.* **2018**. [CrossRef] [PubMed]
19. Cabanero, M.; Tsao, M.S. Circulating tumour DNA in EGFR-mutant non-small-cell lung cancer. *Curr. Oncol.* **2018**, *25*, S38–S44. [CrossRef] [PubMed]
20. Kuang, Y.; O'Connell, A.; Sacher, A.G.; Feeney, N.; Alden, R.S.; Oxnard, G.R.; Paweletz, C.P. Monitoring of Response and Resistance in Plasma of EGFR-Mutant Lung Cancer Using Droplet Digital PCR. *Methods Mol. Biol.* **2018**, *1768*, 193–207. [PubMed]
21. Sacher, A.G.; Komatsubara, K.M.; Oxnard, G.R. Application of Plasma Genotyping Technologies in Non-Small Cell Lung Cancer: A Practical Review. *J. Thorac. Oncol.* **2017**, *12*, 1344–1356. [CrossRef] [PubMed]
22. Schrock, A.B.; Welsh, A.; Chung, J.H.; Pavlick, D.; Bernicker, E.H.; Creelan, B.C.; Forcier, B.; Ross, J.S.; Stephens, P.J.; Ali, S.M.; et al. Hybrid Capture-Based Genomic Profiling of Circulating Tumor DNA from Patients with Advanced Non-Small Cell Lung Cancer. *J. Thorac. Oncol.* **2019**, *14*, 255–264. [CrossRef] [PubMed]
23. Duréndez-Sáez, E.; Azkárate, A.; Meri, M.; Calabuig-Fariñas, S.; Aguilar-Gallardo, C.; Blasco, A.; Jantus-Lewintre, E.; Camps, C. New insights in non-small-cell lung cancer: Circulating tumor cells and cell-free DNA. *J. Thorac. Dis.* **2017**, *9*, S1332–S1345. [CrossRef] [PubMed]
24. Wang, L.; Dumenil, C.; Julié, C.; Giraud, V.; Dumoulin, J.; Labrune, S.; Chinet, T.; Emile, J.-F.; He, B.; Leprieur, E.G. Molecular characterization of circulating tumor cells in lung cancer: Moving beyond enumeration. *Oncotarget* **2017**, *8*, 109818–109835. [CrossRef] [PubMed]
25. Pantel, K. Blood-Based Analysis of Circulating Cell-Free DNA and Tumor Cells for Early Cancer Detection. *PLoS Med.* **2016**, *13*, e1002205. [CrossRef] [PubMed]
26. Szczerba, B.M.; Castro-Giner, F.; Vetter, M.; Krol, I.; Gkountela, S.; Landin, J.; Scheidmann, M.C.; Donato, C.; Scherrer, R.; Singer, J.; et al. Neutrophils escort circulating tumour cells to enable cell cycle progression. *Nature* **2019**. [CrossRef] [PubMed]
27. Rossi, G.; Mu, Z.; Rademaker, A.W.; Austin, L.K.; Strickland, K.S.; Costa, R.L.B.; Nagy, R.J.; Zagonel, V.; Taxter, T.J.; Behdad, A.; et al. Cell-Free DNA and Circulating Tumor Cells: Comprehensive Liquid Biopsy Analysis in Advanced Breast Cancer. *Clin. Cancer Res.* **2018**, *24*, 560–568. [CrossRef] [PubMed]
28. Morbelli, S.; Alama, A.; Ferrarazzo, G.; Coco, S.; Genova, C.; Rijavec, E.; Bongioanni, F.; Biello, F.; Dal Bello, M.G.; Barletta, G.; et al. Circulating Tumor DNA Reflects Tumor Metabolism Rather Than Tumor Burden in Chemotherapy-Naive Patients with Advanced Non–Small Cell Lung Cancer: 18 F-FDG PET/CT Study. *J. Nucl. Med.* **2017**, *58*, 1764–1769. [CrossRef] [PubMed]
29. Sundaresan, T.K.; Sequist, L.V.; Heymach, J.V.; Riely, G.J.; Jänne, P.A.; Koch, W.H.; Sullivan, J.P.; Fox, D.B.; Maher, R.; Muzikansky, A.; et al. Detection of T790M, the acquired resistance EGFR mutation, by tumor biopsy versus noninvasive blood-based analyses. *Clin. Cancer Res.* **2016**, *22*, 1103–1110. [CrossRef] [PubMed]
30. Brown, H.K.; Tellez-Gabriel, M.; Cartron, P.-F.; Vallette, F.M.; Heymann, M.-F.; Heymann, D. Characterization of circulating tumor cells as a reflection of the tumor heterogeneity: Myth or reality? *Drug Discov. Today* **2018**. [CrossRef] [PubMed]
31. Hofman, V.; Ilie, M.; Long, E.; Guibert, N.; Selva, E.; Washetine, K.; Mograbi, B.; Mouroux, J.; Vénissac, N.; Reverso-Meinietti, J.; et al. Detection of circulating tumor cells from lung cancer patients in the era of targeted therapy: Promises, drawbacks and pitfalls. *Curr. Mol. Med.* **2014**, *14*, 440–456. [CrossRef] [PubMed]

32. Farace, F.; Massard, C.; Vimond, N.; Drusch, F.; Jacques, N.; Billiot, F.; Laplanche, A.; Chauchereau, A.; Lacroix, L.; Planchard, D.; et al. A direct comparison of CellSearch and ISET for circulating tumour-cell detection in patients with metastatic carcinomas. *Br. J. Cancer* **2011**, *105*, 847–853. [CrossRef] [PubMed]
33. Hofman, V.; Ilie, M.I.; Long, E.; Selva, E.; Bonnetaud, C.; Molina, T.; Vénissac, N.; Mouroux, J.; Vielh, P.; Hofman, P. Detection of circulating tumor cells as a prognostic factor in patients undergoing radical surgery for non-small-cell lung carcinoma: Comparison of the efficacy of the CellSearch Assay^{TM} and the isolation by size of epithelial tumor cell method. *Int. J. Cancer* **2011**, *129*, 1651–1660. [CrossRef] [PubMed]
34. Fici, P. Cell-Free DNA in the Liquid Biopsy Context: Role and Differences Between ctDNA and CTC Marker in Cancer Management. *Methods Mol. Biol.* **2019**, *1909*, 47–73. [PubMed]
35. Ilie, M.; Hofman, V.; Long, E.; Bordone, O.; Selva, E.; Washetine, K.; Marquette, C.H.; Hofman, P. Current challenges for detection of circulating tumor cells and cell-free circulating nucleic acids, and their characterization in non-small cell lung carcinoma patients. What is the best blood substrate for personalized medicine? *Ann. Transl. Med.* **2014**, *2*, 107. [PubMed]
36. Lianidou, E.; Pantel, K. Liquid Biopsies. *Genes Chromosomes Cancer* **2019**, *58*, 219–232. [CrossRef] [PubMed]
37. Lim, M.; Kim, C.-J.; Sunkara, V.; Kim, M.-H.; Cho, Y.-K. Liquid Biopsy in Lung Cancer: Clinical Applications of Circulating Biomarkers (CTCs and ctDNA). *Micromachines* **2018**, *9*, 100. [CrossRef] [PubMed]
38. Hofman, V.; Bonnetaud, C.; Ilie, M.I.; Vielh, P.; Vignaud, J.M.; Fléjou, J.F.; Lantuejoul, S.; Piaton, E.; Mourad, N.; Butori, C.; et al. Preoperative circulating tumor cell detection using the isolation by size of epithelial tumor cell method for patients with lung cancer is a new prognostic biomarker. *Clin. Cancer Res.* **2011**, *17*, 827–835. [CrossRef] [PubMed]
39. Carter, L.; Rothwell, D.G.; Mesquita, B.; Smowton, C.; Leong, H.S.; Fernandez-Gutierrez, F.; Li, Y.; Burt, D.J.; Antonello, J.; Morrow, C.J.; et al. Molecular analysis of circulating tumor cells identifies distinct copy-number profiles in patients with chemosensitive and chemorefractory small-cell lung cancer. *Nat. Med.* **2017**, *23*, 114–119. [CrossRef] [PubMed]
40. Drapkin, B.J.; George, J.; Christensen, C.L.; Mino-Kenudson, M.; Dries, R.; Sundaresan, T.; Phat, S.; Myers, D.T.; Zhong, J.; Igo, P.; et al. Genomic and functional fidelity of small cell lung cancer patient-derived xenografts. *Cancer Discov.* **2018**, *8*, 600–615. [CrossRef] [PubMed]
41. Tan, C.L.; Lim, T.H.; Lim, T.K.; Tan, D.S.-W.; Chua, Y.W.; Ang, M.K.; Pang, B.; Lim, C.T.; Takano, A.; Lim, A.S.-T.; et al. Concordance of anaplastic lymphoma kinase (ALK) gene rearrangements between circulating tumor cells and tumor in non-small cell lung cancer. *Oncotarget* **2016**, *7*, 23251–23262. [CrossRef] [PubMed]
42. Ilié, M.; Szafer-Glusman, E.; Hofman, V.; Chamorey, E.; Lalvée, S.; Selva, E.; Leroy, S.; Marquette, C.-H.; Kowanetz, M.; Hedge, P.; et al. Detection of PD-L1 in circulating tumor cells and white blood cells from patients with advanced non-small-cell lung cancer. *Ann. Oncol. Off. J. Eur. Soc. Med. Oncol.* **2018**, *29*, 193–199. [CrossRef] [PubMed]
43. Adams, D.L.; Adams, D.K.; He, J.; Kalhor, N.; Zhang, M.; Xu, T.; Gao, H.; Reuben, J.M.; Qiao, Y.; Komaki, R.; et al. Sequential Tracking of PD-L1 Expression and RAD50 Induction in Circulating Tumor and Stromal Cells of Lung Cancer Patients Undergoing Radiotherapy. *Clin. Cancer Res.* **2017**, *23*, 5948–5958. [CrossRef] [PubMed]
44. Chudziak, J.; Burt, D.J.; Mohan, S.; Rothwell, D.G.; Mesquita, B.; Antonello, J.; Dalby, S.; Ayub, M.; Priest, L.; Carter, L.; et al. Clinical evaluation of a novel microfluidic device for epitope-independent enrichment of circulating tumour cells in patients with small cell lung cancer. *Analyst* **2016**, *141*, 669–678. [CrossRef] [PubMed]
45. Krebs, M.G.; Hou, J.-M.; Sloane, R.; Lancashire, L.; Priest, L.; Nonaka, D.; Ward, T.H.; Backen, A.; Clack, G.; Hughes, A.; et al. Analysis of circulating tumor cells in patients with non-small cell lung cancer using epithelial marker-dependent and -independent approaches. *J. Thorac. Oncol.* **2012**, *7*, 306–315. [CrossRef] [PubMed]
46. Gorges, T.M.; Penkalla, N.; Schalk, T.; Joosse, S.A.; Riethdorf, S.; Tucholski, J.; Lücke, K.; Wikman, H.; Jackson, S.; Brychta, N.; et al. Enumeration and Molecular Characterization of Tumor Cells in Lung Cancer Patients Using a Novel In Vivo Device for Capturing Circulating Tumor Cells. *Clin. Cancer Res.* **2016**, *22*, 2197–2206. [CrossRef] [PubMed]

47. Yu, M.; Bardia, A.; Aceto, N.; Bersani, F.; Madden, M.W.; Donaldson, M.C.; Desai, R.; Zhu, H.; Comaills, V.; Zheng, Z.; et al. Cancer therapy. Ex vivo culture of circulating breast tumor cells for individualized testing of drug susceptibility. *Science* **2014**, *345*, 216–220. [CrossRef] [PubMed]
48. Wang, R.; Chu, G.C.Y.; Mrdenovic, S.; Annamalai, A.A.; Hendifar, A.E.; Nissen, N.N.; Tomlinson, J.S.; Lewis, M.; Palanisamy, N.; Tseng, H.-R.; et al. Cultured circulating tumor cells and their derived xenografts for personalized oncology. *Asian J. Urol.* **2016**, *3*, 240–253. [CrossRef] [PubMed]
49. Kulasinghe, A.; Perry, C.; Warkiani, M.E.; Blick, T.; Davies, A.; O'Byrne, K.; Thompson, E.W.; Nelson, C.C.; Vela, I.; Punyadeera, C. Short term ex-vivo expansion of circulating head and neck tumour cells. *Oncotarget* **2016**, *7*, 60101–60109. [CrossRef] [PubMed]
50. Grillet, F.; Bayet, E.; Villeronce, O.; Zappia, L.; Lagerqvist, E.L.; Lunke, S.; Charafe-Jauffret, E.; Pham, K.; Molck, C.; Rolland, N.; et al. Circulating tumour cells from patients with colorectal cancer have cancer stem cell hallmarks in ex vivo culture. *Gut* **2017**, *66*, 1802–1810. [CrossRef] [PubMed]
51. Foy, V.; Fernandez-Gutierrez, F.; Faivre-Finn, C.; Dive, C.; Blackhall, F. The clinical utility of circulating tumour cells in patients with small cell lung cancer. *Transl. Lung Cancer Res.* **2017**, *6*, 409–417. [CrossRef] [PubMed]
52. Hodgkinson, C.L.; Morrow, C.J.; Li, Y.; Metcalf, R.L.; Rothwell, D.G.; Trapani, F.; Polanski, R.; Burt, D.J.; Simpson, K.L.; Morris, K.; et al. Tumorigenicity and genetic profiling of circulating tumor cells in small-cell lung cancer. *Nat. Med.* **2014**, *20*, 897–903. [CrossRef] [PubMed]
53. Tellez-Gabriel, M.; Cochonneau, D.; Cadé, M.; Jubellin, C.; Heymann, M.-F.; Heymann, D. Circulating Tumor Cell-Derived Pre-Clinical Models for Personalized Medicine. *Cancers* **2018**, *11*, 19. [CrossRef] [PubMed]
54. Lallo, A.; Gulati, S.; Schenk, M.W.; Khandelwal, G.; Berglund, U.W.; Pateras, I.S.; Chester, C.P.E.; Pham, T.M.; Kalderen, C.; Frese, K.K.; et al. Ex vivo culture of cells derived from circulating tumour cell xenograft to support small cell lung cancer research and experimental therapeutics. *Br. J. Pharmacol.* **2019**, *176*, 436–450. [CrossRef] [PubMed]
55. Alix-Panabières, C.; Pantel, K. Characterization of single circulating tumor cells. *FEBS Lett.* **2017**, *591*, 2241–2250. [CrossRef] [PubMed]
56. Heymann, D.; Téllez-Gabriel, M. Circulating Tumor Cells: The Importance of Single Cell Analysis. *Adv. Exp. Med. Biol.* **2018**, *1068*, 45–58. [PubMed]
57. Miyamoto, D.T.; Ting, D.T.; Toner, M.; Maheswaran, S.; Haber, D.A. Single-Cell Analysis of Circulating Tumor Cells as a Window into Tumor Heterogeneity. *Cold Spring Harb. Symp. Quant. Biol.* **2016**, *81*, 269–274. [CrossRef] [PubMed]
58. Palmirotta, R.; Lovero, D.; Silvestris, E.; Felici, C.; Quaresmini, D.; Cafforio, P.; Silvestris, F. Next-generation Sequencing (NGS) Analysis on Single Circulating Tumor Cells (CTCs) with No Need of Whole-genome Amplification (WGA). *Cancer Genomics Proteomics* **2017**, *14*, 173–179. [CrossRef] [PubMed]
59. Hou, J.-M.; Krebs, M.G.; Lancashire, L.; Sloane, R.; Backen, A.; Swain, R.K.; Priest, L.J.C.; Greystoke, A.; Zhou, C.; Morris, K.; et al. Clinical significance and molecular characteristics of circulating tumor cells and circulating tumor microemboli in patients with small-cell lung cancer. *J. Clin. Oncol.* **2012**, *30*, 525–532. [CrossRef] [PubMed]
60. Lowe, A.C. Circulating Tumor Cells: Applications in Cytopathology. *Surg. Pathol. Clin.* **2018**, *11*, 679–686. [CrossRef] [PubMed]
61. Sundling, K.E.; Lowe, A.C. Circulating Tumor Cells: Overview and Opportunities in Cytology. *Adv. Anat. Pathol.* **2019**, *26*, 56–63. [CrossRef] [PubMed]
62. Catelain, C.; Pailler, E.; Oulhen, M.; Faugeroux, V.; Pommier, A.-L.; Farace, F. Detection of Gene Rearrangements in Circulating Tumor Cells: Examples of ALK-, ROS1-, RET-Rearrangements in Non-Small-Cell Lung Cancer and ERG-Rearrangements in Prostate Cancer. *Adv. Exp. Med. Biol.* **2017**, *994*, 169–179. [PubMed]
63. Ilie, M.; Long, E.; Butori, C.; Hofman, V.; Coelle, C.; Mauro, V.; Zahaf, K.; Marquette, C.H.; Mouroux, J.; Paterlini-Bréchot, P.; et al. ALK-gene rearrangement: A comparative analysis on circulating tumour cells and tumour tissue from patients with lung adenocarcinoma. *Ann. Oncol. Off. J. Eur. Soc. Med. Oncol.* **2012**, *23*, 2907–2913. [CrossRef] [PubMed]
64. Kang, Y.-T.; Kim, Y.J.; Lee, T.H.; Cho, Y.-H.; Chang, H.J.; Lee, H.-M. Cytopathological Study of the Circulating Tumor Cells filtered from the Cancer Patients' Blood using Hydrogel-based Cell Block Formation. *Sci. Rep.* **2018**, *8*, 15218. [CrossRef] [PubMed]

65. Pailler, E.; Adam, J.; Barthélémy, A.; Oulhen, M.; Auger, N.; Valent, A.; Borget, I.; Planchard, D.; Taylor, M.; André, F.; et al. Detection of circulating tumor cells harboring a unique ALK rearrangement in ALK-positive non-small-cell lung cancer. *J. Clin. Oncol.* **2013**, *31*, 2273–2281. [CrossRef] [PubMed]
66. Pailler, E.; Auger, N.; Lindsay, C.R.; Vielh, P.; Islas-Morris-Hernandez, A.; Borget, I.; Ngo-Camus, M.; Planchard, D.; Soria, J.-C.; Besse, B.; et al. High level of chromosomal instability in circulating tumor cells of ROS1-rearranged non-small-cell lung cancer. *Ann. Oncol. Off. J. Eur. Soc. Med. Oncol.* **2015**, *26*, 1408–1415. [CrossRef] [PubMed]
67. Pailler, E.; Faugeroux, V.; Oulhen, M.; Catelain, C.; Farace, F. Routine clinical use of circulating tumor cells for diagnosis of mutations and chromosomal rearrangements in non-small cell lung cancer-ready for prime-time? *Transl. lung cancer Res.* **2017**, *6*, 444–453. [CrossRef] [PubMed]
68. Nicolazzo, C.; Gradilone, A.; Carpino, G.; Gazzaniga, P.; Raimondi, C. Molecular Characterization of Circulating Tumor Cells to Study Cancer Immunoevasion. *Methods Mol. Biol.* **2019**, *1884*, 247–258. [PubMed]
69. Hofman, P. Liquid biopsy for early detection of lung cancer. *Curr. Opin. Oncol.* **2017**, *29*, 73–78. [CrossRef] [PubMed]
70. Ilie, M.; Hofman, V.; Long-Mira, E.; Selva, E.; Vignaud, J.-M.; Padovani, B.; Mouroux, J.; Marquette, C.-H.; Hofman, P. "Sentinel" circulating tumor cells allow early diagnosis of lung cancer in patients with chronic obstructive pulmonary disease. *PLoS ONE* **2014**, *9*, e111597. [CrossRef] [PubMed]
71. Leroy, S.; Benzaquen, J.; Mazzetta, A.; Marchand-Adam, S.; Padovani, B.; Israel-Biet, D.; Pison, C.; Chanez, P.; Cadranel, J.; Mazières, J.; et al. Circulating tumour cells as a potential screening tool for lung cancer (the AIR study): Protocol of a prospective multicentre cohort study in France. *BMJ Open* **2017**, *7*, e018884. [CrossRef] [PubMed]
72. Lee, Y.; Guan, G.; Bhagat, A.A. ClearCell®FX, a label-free microfluidics technology for enrichment of viable circulating tumor cells. *Cytometry A* **2018**, *93*, 1251–1254. [CrossRef] [PubMed]
73. Miller, M.C.; Robinson, P.S.; Wagner, C.; O'Shannessy, D.J. The Parsortix™ Cell Separation System-A versatile liquid biopsy platform. *Cytometry A* **2018**, *93*, 1234–1239. [CrossRef] [PubMed]
74. Sollier-Christen, E.; Renier, C.; Kaplan, T.; Kfir, E.; Crouse, S.C. VTX-1 Liquid Biopsy System for Fully-Automated and Label-Free Isolation of Circulating Tumor Cells with Automated Enumeration by BioView Platform. *Cytometry A* **2018**, *93*, 1240–1245. [CrossRef] [PubMed]
75. Williamson, S.C.; Metcalf, R.L.; Trapani, F.; Mohan, S.; Antonello, J.; Abbott, B.; Leong, H.S.; Chester, C.P.E.; Simms, N.; Polanski, R.; et al. Vasculogenic mimicry in small cell lung cancer. *Nat. Commun.* **2016**, *7*, 13322. [CrossRef] [PubMed]
76. Khandelwal, G.; Miller, C. Improved PDX and CDX Data Processing-Response. *Mol. Cancer Res.* **2018**, *16*, 1814. [CrossRef] [PubMed]
77. Lallo, A.; Schenk, M.W.; Frese, K.K.; Blackhall, F.; Dive, C. Circulating tumor cells and CDX models as a tool for preclinical drug development. *Transl. Lung Cancer Res.* **2017**, *6*, 397–408. [CrossRef] [PubMed]
78. Lallo, A.; Frese, K.K.; Morrow, C.J.; Sloane, R.; Gulati, S.; Schenk, M.W.; Trapani, F.; Simms, N.; Galvin, M.; Brown, S.; et al. The Combination of the PARP Inhibitor Olaparib and the WEE1 Inhibitor AZD1775 as a New Therapeutic Option for Small Cell Lung Cancer. *Clin. Cancer Res.* **2018**, *24*, 5153–5164. [CrossRef] [PubMed]
79. Sharma, S.; Zhuang, R.; Long, M.; Pavlovic, M.; Kang, Y.; Ilyas, A.; Asghar, W. Circulating tumor cell isolation, culture, and downstream molecular analysis. *Biotechnol. Adv.* **2018**, *36*, 1063–1078. [CrossRef] [PubMed]
80. Makarova, O.V.; Adams, D.L.; Divan, R.; Rosenmann, D.; Zhu, P.; Li, S.; Amstutz, P.; Tang, C.-M. Polymer microfilters with nanostructured surfaces for the culture of circulating cancer cells. *Mater. Sci. Eng. C* **2016**, *66*, 193–198. [CrossRef] [PubMed]
81. Fabbri, F.; Carloni, S.; Zoli, W.; Ulivi, P.; Gallerani, G.; Fici, P.; Chiadini, E.; Passardi, A.; Frassineti, G.L.; Ragazzini, A.; et al. Detection and recovery of circulating colon cancer cells using a dielectrophoresis-based device: KRAS mutation status in pure CTCs. *Cancer Lett.* **2013**, *335*, 225–231. [CrossRef] [PubMed]
82. Fernandez, S.V.; Bingham, C.; Fittipaldi, P.; Austin, L.; Palazzo, J.; Palmer, G.; Alpaugh, K.; Cristofanilli, M. TP53 mutations detected in circulating tumor cells present in the blood of metastatic triple negative breast cancer patients. *Breast Cancer Res.* **2014**, *16*, 445. [CrossRef] [PubMed]
83. Park, S.-M.; Wong, D.J.; Ooi, C.C.; Kurtz, D.M.; Vermesh, O.; Aalipour, A.; Suh, S.; Pian, K.L.; Chabon, J.J.; Lee, S.H.; et al. Molecular profiling of single circulating tumor cells from lung cancer patients. *Proc. Natl. Acad. Sci. USA* **2016**, *113*, E8379–E8386. [CrossRef] [PubMed]

84. Ting, D.T.; Wittner, B.S.; Ligorio, M.; Vincent Jordan, N.; Shah, A.M.; Miyamoto, D.T.; Aceto, N.; Bersani, F.; Brannigan, B.W.; Xega, K.; et al. Single-Cell RNA Sequencing Identifies Extracellular Matrix Gene Expression by Pancreatic Circulating Tumor Cells. *Cell Rep.* **2014**, *8*, 1905–1918. [CrossRef] [PubMed]
85. Miyamoto, D.T.; Lee, R.J.; Kalinich, M.; LiCausi, J.; Zheng, Y.; Chen, T.; Milner, J.D.; Emmons, E.; Ho, U.; Broderick, K.; et al. An RNA-based digital circulating tumor cell signature is predictive of drug response and early dissemination in prostate cancer. *Cancer Discov.* **2018**, *8*, 288–303. [CrossRef] [PubMed]
86. Marjanovic, N.D.; Ng, S.R.; Regev, A.; Jacks, T. Abstract A24: Using single-cell RNA-seq approaches to decipher heterogeneity in autochthonous mouse models of small cell lung cancer. In Proceedings of the Fifth AACR-IASLC International Joint Conference: Lung Cancer Translational Science from the Bench to the Clinic, San Diego, CA, USA, 8–11 January 2018; American Association for Cancer Research: Philadelphia, PA, USA, 2018; p. A24.
87. Hofman, V.J.; Ilie, M.; Hofman, P.M. Detection and characterization of circulating tumor cells in lung cancer: Why and how? *Cancer Cytopathol.* **2016**, *124*, 380–387. [CrossRef] [PubMed]
88. Adams, D.L.; Alpaugh, R.K.; Tsai, S.; Tang, C.-M.; Stefansson, S. Multi-Phenotypic subtyping of circulating tumor cells using sequential fluorescent quenching and restaining. *Sci. Rep.* **2016**, *6*, 33488. [CrossRef] [PubMed]
89. Pillai, S.G.; Zhu, P.; Siddappa, C.M.; Adams, D.L.; Li, S.; Makarova, O.V.; Amstutz, P.; Nunley, R.; Tang, C.-M.; Watson, M.A.; et al. Enrichment and Molecular Analysis of Breast Cancer Disseminated Tumor Cells from Bone Marrow Using Microfiltration. *PLoS ONE* **2017**, *12*, e0170761. [CrossRef] [PubMed]
90. Tang, C.-M.; Zhu, P.; Li, S.; Makarova, O.V.; Amstutz, P.T.; Adams, D.L. Filtration and Analysis of Circulating Cancer Associated Cells from the Blood of Cancer Patients. *Methods Mol. Biol.* **2017**, *1572*, 511–524. [PubMed]
91. Tang, C.; Zhu, P.; Li, S.; Makarova, O.V.; Amstutz, P.T.; Adams, D.L. Blood-based biopsies—clinical utility beyond circulating tumor cells. *Cytom. Part A* **2018**, *93*, 1246–1250. [CrossRef] [PubMed]
92. Milano, A.; Mazzetta, F.; Valente, S.; Ranieri, D.; Leone, L.; Botticelli, A.; Onesti, C.E.; Lauro, S.; Raffa, S.; Torrisi, M.R.; et al. Molecular Detection of EMT Markers in Circulating Tumor Cells from Metastatic Non-Small Cell Lung Cancer Patients: Potential Role in Clinical Practice. *Anal. Cell. Pathol.* **2018**, *2018*, 1–12. [CrossRef] [PubMed]
93. Li, S.; Chen, Q.; Li, H.; Wu, Y.; Feng, J.; Yan, Y. Mesenchymal circulating tumor cells (CTCs) and OCT4 mRNA expression in CTCs for prognosis prediction in patients with non-small-cell lung cancer. *Clin. Transl. Oncol.* **2017**, *19*, 1147–1153. [CrossRef] [PubMed]
94. Zhang, X.; Wei, L.; Li, J.; Zheng, J.; Zhang, S.; Zhou, J. Epithelial-mesenchymal transition phenotype of circulating tumor cells is associated with distant metastasis in patients with NSCLC. *Mol. Med. Rep.* **2018**, *19*, 601–608. [CrossRef] [PubMed]
95. Wang, W.-C.; Zhang, X.-F.; Peng, J.; Li, X.-F.; Wang, A.-L.; Bie, Y.-Q.; Shi, L.-H.; Lin, M.-B.; Zhang, X.-F. Survival Mechanisms and Influence Factors of Circulating Tumor Cells. *Biomed. Res. Int.* **2018**, *2018*, 6304701. [CrossRef] [PubMed]
96. Seijo, L.M.; Peled, N.; Ajona, D.; Boeri, M.; Field, J.K.; Sozzi, G.; Pio, R.; Zulueta, J.J.; Spira, A.; Massion, P.P.; et al. Biomarkers in lung cancer screening: Achievements, promises and challenges. *J. Thorac. Oncol.* **2019**, *14*, 343–357. [CrossRef] [PubMed]
97. Di Trapani, M.; Manaresi, N.; Medoro, G. DEPArray^{TM} system: An automatic image-based sorter for isolation of pure circulating tumor cells. *Cytometry A* **2018**, *93*, 1260–1266. [CrossRef] [PubMed]
98. Blackhall, F.; Frese, K.K.; Simpson, K.; Kilgour, E.; Brady, G.; Dive, C. Will liquid biopsies improve outcomes for patients with small-cell lung cancer? *Lancet Oncol.* **2018**, *19*, e470–e481. [CrossRef]
99. Kapeleris, J.; Kulasinghe, A.; Warkiani, M.E.; Vela, I.; Kenny, L.; O'Byrne, K.; Punyadeera, C. The Prognostic Role of Circulating Tumor Cells (CTCs) in Lung Cancer. *Front. Oncol.* **2018**, *8*, 311. [CrossRef] [PubMed]
100. Kulasinghe, A.; Kapeleris, J.; Kimberley, R.; Mattarollo, S.R.; Thompson, E.W.; Thiery, J.-P.; Kenny, L.; O'Byrne, K.; Punyadeera, C. The prognostic significance of circulating tumor cells in head and neck and non-small-cell lung cancer. *Cancer Med.* **2018**, *7*, 5910–5919. [CrossRef] [PubMed]
101. Lindsay, C.R.; Faugeroux, V.; Michiels, S.; Pailler, E.; Facchinetti, F.; Ou, D.; Bluthgen, M.V.; Pannet, C.; Ngo-Camus, M.; Bescher, G.; et al. A prospective examination of circulating tumor cell profiles in non-small-cell lung cancer molecular subgroups. *Ann. Oncol. Off. J. Eur. Soc. Med. Oncol.* **2017**, *28*, 1523–1531. [CrossRef] [PubMed]

102. Morrow, C.J.; Trapani, F.; Metcalf, R.L.; Bertolini, G.; Hodgkinson, C.L.; Khandelwal, G.; Kelly, P.; Galvin, M.; Carter, L.; Simpson, K.L.; et al. Tumourigenic non-small-cell lung cancer mesenchymal circulating tumour cells: A clinical case study. *Ann. Oncol. Off. J. Eur. Soc. Med. Oncol.* **2016**, *27*, 1155–1160. [CrossRef] [PubMed]
103. De Wit, S.; Rossi, E.; Weber, S.; Tamminga, M.; Manicone, M.; Swennenhuis, J.F.; Groothuis-Oudshoorn, C.G.M.; Vidotto, R.; Facchinetti, A.; Zeune, L.L.; et al. Single tube liquid biopsy for advanced non-small cell lung cancer. *Int. J. Cancer* **2018**. [CrossRef]
104. Rothwell, D.G.; Smith, N.; Morris, D.; Leong, H.S.; Li, Y.; Hollebecque, A.; Ayub, M.; Carter, L.; Antonello, J.; Franklin, L.; et al. Genetic profiling of tumours using both circulating free DNA and circulating tumour cells isolated from the same preserved whole blood sample. *Mol. Oncol.* **2016**, *10*, 566–574. [CrossRef] [PubMed]
105. Ortiz, V.; Yu, M. Analyzing Circulating Tumor Cells One at a Time. *Trends Cell Biol.* **2018**, *28*, 764–775. [CrossRef] [PubMed]
106. Salvianti, F.; Pazzagli, M.; Pinzani, P. Single circulating tumor cell sequencing as an advanced tool in cancer management. *Expert Rev. Mol. Diagn.* **2016**, *16*, 51–63. [CrossRef] [PubMed]
107. Ko, J.; Baldassano, S.N.; Loh, P.-L.; Kording, K.; Litt, B.; Issadore, D. Machine learning to detect signatures of disease in liquid biopsies—A user's guide. *Lab Chip* **2018**, *18*, 395–405. [CrossRef] [PubMed]
108. La Porta, C.A.M.; Zapperi, S. Explaining the dynamics of tumor aggressiveness: At the crossroads between biology, artificial intelligence and complex systems. *Semin. Cancer Biol.* **2018**, *53*, 42–47. [CrossRef] [PubMed]

8

New Insights into Long Non-Coding RNA *MALAT1* in Cancer and Metastasis

Yutong Sun [1] **and Li Ma** [2,*]

[1] Department of Molecular and Cellular Oncology, the University of Texas MD Anderson Cancer Center, Houston, TX 77030, USA; ysun2@mdanderson.org

[2] Department of Experimental Radiation Oncology, the University of Texas MD Anderson Cancer Center, Houston, TX 77030, USA

* Correspondence: lma4@mdanderson.org

Abstract: Metastasis-associated lung adenocarcinoma transcript 1 (*MALAT1*) is one of the most abundant, long non-coding RNAs (lncRNAs) in normal tissues. This lncRNA is highly conserved among mammalian species, and based on in vitro results, has been reported to regulate alternative pre-mRNA splicing and gene expression. However, *Malat1* knockout mice develop and grow normally, and do not show alterations in alternative splicing. While *MALAT1* was originally described as a prognostic marker of lung cancer metastasis, emerging evidence has linked this lncRNA to other cancers, such as breast cancer, prostate cancer, pancreatic cancer, glioma, and leukemia. The role described for *MALAT1* is dependent on the cancer types and the experimental model systems. Notably, different or opposite phenotypes resulting from different strategies for inactivating *MALAT1* have been observed, which led to distinct models for *MALAT1*'s functions and mechanisms of action in cancer and metastasis. In this review, we reflect on different experimental strategies used to study *MALAT1*'s functions, and discuss the current mechanistic models of this highly abundant and conserved lncRNA.

Keywords: lncRNA; *MALAT1*; metastasis

---

1. Introduction

Long non-coding RNAs (lncRNAs) are transcripts that are longer than 200 nucleotides (nt) without protein-coding capacity. Despite the exponential growth in lncRNA publications, our understanding of lncRNA functions and mechanisms is still limited, and outstanding caveats and controversies remain in the current lncRNA knowledge [1,2]. The mechanisms of action of some well-known lncRNAs are currently under discussion [3–11]. Questions have also been raised as to whether phenotypes arising from deleting or inactivating a lncRNA gene can be unequivocally attributed to the loss of the lncRNA per se [1]. A recent study revealed opposite effects from the deletion and insertional inactivation of the lncRNA-encoding gene *Haunt*, and remarkably, the gene deletion effect was due to the loss of *Haunt* genomic DNA, which dominated the effect of *Haunt* lncRNA loss [12]. In light of the accumulating evidence for different or opposite phenotypes resulting from different strategies for inactivating the same lncRNA (e.g., *Fendrr*, *Evf2*, and *lincRNA-p21*) in vivo, it has been concluded that genetic rescue experiments, where the lncRNA is re-expressed from an independent transgene, are essential for separating RNA-specific effects from those resulting from the manipulation of the genomic DNA [1]; however, such rescue experiments are generally lacking in the current lncRNA research, especially in cancer studies, making it difficult to interpret many lncRNA results in the cancer field.

Unlike messenger RNAs (mRNAs) and microRNAs (miRNAs), many lncRNAs have poor evolutionary conservation; however, a nuclear lncRNA, metastasis-associated lung adenocarcinoma transcript 1 (*MALAT1*, also known as nuclear enriched abundant transcript 2, *NEAT2*), is exceptionally conserved for lncRNA, and is among the most abundantly expressed lncRNAs in normal tissues [13]. Despite its length (~8 kb in humans and ~7 kb in mice), *MALAT1* is a single-exon gene whose transcript is subject to further processing; for instance, in mice, *Malat1* gives rise to a 7 kb full-length transcript (low expression, nuclear), a 6.7 kb lncRNA (high expression, nuclear), and a 61 nt tRNA-like small RNA (*mascRNA*, exported to the cytoplasm with unknown functions) [14]. At the molecular level, *MALAT1* lncRNA is recruited to nuclear speckles and has been reported to regulate pre-mRNA splicing [13,15]. However, this finding is not supported by *Malat1* knockout mice, which showed normal development and growth and no global difference in alternative splicing [16–18]. In addition, *MALAT1* lncRNA is subject to post-transcriptional modifications, such as N^6-methyladenosine (m6A) [19] and 5-methylcytosine (m5C) [20], but the functional consequences of these modifications remain unknown.

Originally, *MALAT1* was identified as a prognostic marker for poor clinical outcomes (overall survival and metastasis-free survival outcomes) in patients with early-stage non-small cell lung cancer [21]. To date, there are more than 800 publications related to *MALAT1* (the PubMed search word "MALAT1" generated 809 results as of 13 February, 2019) and many of them reported a role of *MALAT1* in cancer, making *MALAT1* one of the most studied lncRNAs. Intriguingly, different studies yielded conflicting results about *MALAT1*'s functions and mechanisms of action. In this review, we discuss the progress and controversies in *MALAT1* research, and reflect on the approaches and experimental design used for lncRNA studies.

2. Does *MALAT1* Regulate Alternative pre-mRNA Splicing and Global Gene Expression?

By performing RNA fluorescent in situ hybridization and protein immunofluorescent staining, Hutchinson et al. found that *MALAT1* lncRNA co-localizes with SC35 nuclear speckles, structures involved in pre-mRNA processing [13]. Subsequently, based on small interfering RNA (siRNA) knockdown results from cultured cell lines, *MALAT1* was identified as a nuclear-retained regulatory RNA that interacts with the serine/arginine-rich family of splicing factors, affects the distribution of splicing factors in nuclear speckle domains, and regulates alternative splicing of pre-mRNAs [15]. Moreover, by using the CHART-seq technology, West at al. identified hundreds of *MALAT1*-binding sites in human cells and most of these sites are on actively transcribed genes, indicating that *MALAT1* might be involved in regulating gene transcription [22]. However, these effects were absent in genetically engineered mouse models lacking *Malat1* expression [16–18].

In 2012, three *Malat1* knockout mouse models, generated by different strategies, were reported by independent groups. Zhang et al. removed a 3 kb genomic region encompassing the 5′ end of *Malat1* and its promoter (Figure 1a) [16]. Eissmann et al. deleted the entire 7 kb mouse *Malat1* gene (Figure 1b) [17]. Nakagawa et al. disrupted the *Malat1* gene by inserting a transcriptional terminator (*lacZ* and the polyadenylation sequences) 69 bp downstream of the transcriptional start site of *Malat1* (Figure 1c); similar to the two gene deletion strategies, this insertional inactivation approach also abrogated *Malat1* RNA expression in mice, as gauged by Northern blot analysis and in situ hybridization [18]. Surprisingly, none of these three models showed phenotypes, and loss of *Malat1* in mice did not affect global gene expression, nuclear speckles, or alternative pre-mRNA splicing [16–18], which argues against the in vitro siRNA knockdown results [13,15,22]. This discrepancy suggests that in vitro findings could be cell line-specific, or rely on specific experimental settings and approaches. Alternatively, *Malat1* may have stress-dependent functions in vivo. It is also possible that additional factors compensate for the effects of *Malat1* loss in mice. These possibilities warrant further investigation.

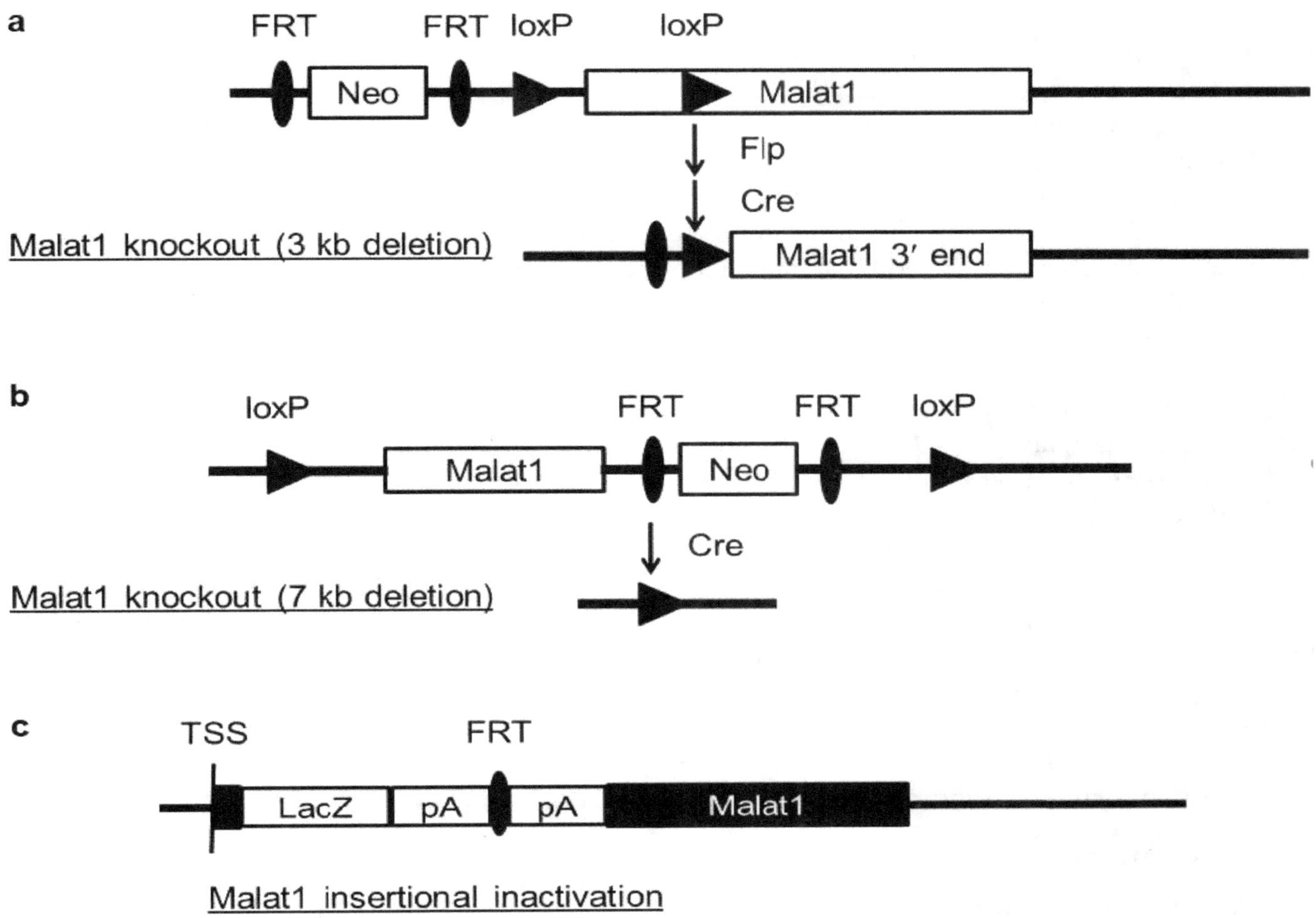

Figure 1. Different strategies used to generate *Malat1* knockout mice. (**a**) A 3 kb genomic region encompassing the 5′ end of *Malat1* and its promoter was deleted. (**b**) The full-length *Malat1*, including 250 bp upstream of the transcriptional start site and 321 bp downstream of the 3′ end of *Malat1*, was deleted. (**c**) The β-galactosidase gene (*lacZ*) with polyadenylation sequences (pA) was inserted 69 bp downstream of the transcriptional start site (TSS) of *Malat1*.

3. Is *MALAT1* a Metastasis Promoter or a Metastasis Suppressor?

MALAT1 expression has been shown to be either upregulated or downregulated in human cancers. On one hand, upregulation of *MALAT1* was reported in lung cancer, hepatocellular carcinoma, breast cancer, and colorectal carcinoma, which has been extensively reviewed previously [23–26]. On the other hand, several studies showed that the expression of *MALAT1* is downregulated in glioma [27], colorectal cancer [28], and breast cancer [29,30]. Previous in vitro and xenograft studies demonstrated that *MALAT1* promotes cell proliferation, migration, tumor growth, metastasis, and chemoresistance [31–37]. In contrast, other studies reported that *MALAT1* inhibits cell proliferation, tumor growth, invasion, and epithelial-mesenchymal transition (EMT) [27,28,30,38–40].

As mentioned above, one of the three *Malat1* knockout mouse models harbors a 3 kb deletion of *Malat1*'s promoter and its 5′ end [16]. After breeding these mice to a metastasis-prone transgenic model of breast cancer, MMTV (mouse mammary tumor virus)-PyMT (polyomavirus middle T antigen) mice [41], Arun et al. observed a reduction of lung metastases [42]. Notably, despite no difference in mammary tumor size, *Malat1* gene-deleted PyMT tumors were liquid-filled and much more differentiated with a drastically increased cystic phenotype [42], which might underlie the metastasis reduction observed in this model. In addition, after treating MMTV-PyMT mice with *Malat1* antisense oligonucleotides (ASOs), Arun et al. also observed increased cystic areas in primary tumors and decreased lung metastases [42]. However, unlike genetic deletion, ASO treatment significantly decreased the tumor volume (by ~50%), suggesting that these ASOs have extra effects other than knocking down *Malat1*. Unfortunately, the molecular mechanisms underlying the *Malat1* gene deletion and ASO effects remain unknown.

In stark contrast, after mice with targeted insertional inactivation of *Malat1* [18] were bred to MMTV-PyMT mice of a C57BL/6 strain, our group found that the transcriptional inactivation of *Malat1* induced a striking increase in the number of visible metastatic nodules and in the number and area of metastatic foci in the lungs [29]. Importantly, the metastatic-promoting effect of *Malat1* insertional inactivation, which contradicted the *Malat1* genomic deletion effect, was completely reversed by the genetic add-back of *Malat1* achieved via breeding to mice with targeted transgenic expression of *Malat1* from the *ROSA26* locus [29]. Consistently, after MMTV-PyMT mice on an FVB background were crossed to the *Malat1* transgenic mice on an FVB background, overexpression of *Malat1* markedly suppressed lung metastasis [29]. In contrast to the gene deletion model [42], our group found that *Malat1* wild-type, *Malat1*-inactivated, and *Malat1*-overexpressing PyMT tumors showed similar degrees of cystic areas and high-grade carcinoma areas [29]. Interestingly, insertional disruption of *Malat1* significantly elevated the percentages of circulating tumor cells (CTCs) in the peripheral blood of MMTV-PyMT mice, which was also reversed by restoration of *Malat1* expression. Furthermore, CRISPR (clustered regularly interspaced short palindromic repeats)-Cas9-mediated knockout of *MALAT1* (~650 bp deletion of the 5′ end) in the MDA-MB-231 breast cancer cell line promoted cell migration and invasion in vitro and lung metastasis in vivo, which could be reversed by ectopic expression of mouse *Malat1*. Conversely, overexpression of *Malat1* in LM2 human breast cancer cells and in 4T1 mouse mammary tumor cells led to a pronounced reduction of their lung metastatic ability in experimental metastasis assays [29]. Taken together, targeted inactivation, restoration (genetic rescue), and overexpression of *MALAT1* in multiple in vivo models suggest that the lncRNA *MALAT1* suppresses breast cancer metastasis.

4. Experimental Dissection of *MALAT1* and Other lncRNAs

What led to inconsistent conclusions about *MALAT1*'s function? While it remains to be determined whether this is dependent on different cell/tissue types, cancer types, and genetic backgrounds, we can carefully examine the experimental settings and approaches that have been used to study *MALAT1* and other lncRNAs; this offers important lessons. In fact, substantially different or opposite phenotypes arising from different strategies (e.g., gene deletion, insertional inactivation, CRISPR-Cas9, and RNAi) for inactivating the same lncRNA are not uncommon.

In mice, genetic deletion of the lncRNA *Fendrr* resulted in lung and gastrointestinal tract defects [43], whereas transcriptional terminator insertion led to heart and body wall defects [44]; the defects caused by insertional inactivation were rescued by a *Fendrr* transgene [44]. Moreover, RNAi experiments showed that the lncRNA *Evf2* is important for activating *Dlx5/6* expression [45], but transcriptional terminator insertion in mice caused the opposite effect on *Dlx5/6* expression [46]; the effect caused by insertional inactivation could be rescued by *Evf2* expression from a separate transgene [47]. Strikingly, a recent study reported opposing effects from the lncRNA *Haunt* gene deletion and insertional inactivation [12]. The *Haunt* genomic locus contains enhancers for *HOXA* genes, while *Haunt* lncRNA inhibits *HOXA* expression by binding to chromatin [12]. Yin et al. showed that CRISPR-Cas9-mediated large deletion of the *Haunt* genomic locus attenuated *HOXA* gene activation during retinoic acid-induced embryonic stem cell differentiation, whereas minimal disruption of genomic sequences, such as insertional inactivation by CRISPR knockin, abrogated *Haunt* transcription and upregulated *HOXA* expression [12]. Notably, *Haunt* cDNA was unable to "rescue" the deletion phenotype [12], suggesting that the *Haunt* genomic deletion effect dominated the effect of *Haunt* lncRNA loss. These and other studies strongly demonstrate the importance of rescue experiments.

Two excellent reviews discussed considerations when investigating lncRNAs in general [1,2]. The vast majority of *MALAT1* reports are based on siRNA or short-hairpin RNA (shRNA) experiments, and a few studies [42,48,49] used ASOs. However, nuclear RNAi is not fully established and the RNAi approach can be problematic for nuclear RNAs. Silencing a nuclear RNA by siRNA or shRNA requires nuclear Ago2 and other RNAi factors [50]. It has been shown that subcellular localization of Ago2 depends on cell/tissue types and genetic backgrounds [51].

If a cell line or tissue does not have nuclear Ago2, the specificity of the *MALAT1* siRNA or shRNA should be questioned. It should be noted that antisense RNAs can have substantial non-specific effects, and that an alarming and growing number of claimed anticancer targets have been invalidated due to recent proof for off-target effects of previously used antisense RNAs and chemical inhibitors [52]. For example, MELK was previously identified as a kinase required for tumor cell survival and proliferation in several cancer types. RNAi and small-molecule inhibitors of MELK demonstrated anticancer efficacies in many studies, and one of the MELK inhibitors, OTS167, entered several clinical trials. Recently, however, multiple independent studies [53–56] demonstrated that these results were caused by off-target effects, thereby invalidating MELK as an anticancer target reported by many groups. For these reasons, it is crucial to rule out off-target effects of antisense RNAs by genetic add-back of RNAi-resistant mutants and by multiple loss-of-function approaches. Unfortunately, so far no publication has demonstrated the specificity of the *MALAT1* siRNA, shRNA, or ASO by rescue experiments or by *MALAT1* knockout cells.

Previous cell culture and xenograft studies showed contradictory effects of *MALAT1* on cancer cell growth, proliferation, and invasion [27,30–32,38–40]. With regard to genetically engineered mouse models, opposite phenotypes were also observed. Whereas genetic deletion of *Malat1* in MMTV-PyMT mice inhibited lung metastasis [42], our group found that targeted insertional inactivation of *Malat1* promoted lung metastasis in the PyMT mouse model [29]. It should be noted that we were able to reverse the insertional inactivation phenotype by genetic add-back of *Malat1* using a targeted *Malat1* transgenic model [29], which suggests that the metastasis-promoting effect of *Malat1* inactivation was due to the loss of *Malat1* lncRNA.

Why did the two different *Malat1* knockout mouse models show different phenotypes? As mentioned above, the *Haunt* lncRNA gene deletion effect has been attributed to the loss of the *Haunt* genomic DNA, which dominated the effect of *Haunt* RNA loss [12]. It is possible that the similar scenario applies to the *Malat1* genomic locus versus *Malat1* lncRNA, although the experimental evidence for this hypothesis is lacking at present. Notably, the *Malat1* genomic deletion model showed significant upregulation of *Malat1*'s 12 adjacent genes [42]; in contrast, the *Malat1* insertional inactivation model showed no changes in expression levels of these neighboring genes both in normal tissues and in mammary tumors [29]. It remains to be determined whether this is the reason for the different phenotypes of the two *Malat1* knockout mouse models. Among the concerns about deletion of lncRNA genomic loci is that large deletions may eliminate regulatory elements for other genes or destroy long-range genomic interactions.

As mentioned above, the *Malat1* gene generates several transcripts with different expression levels and localizations. It should be noted that all three different strategies used to generate *Malat1* knockout mice eliminated all *Malat1* transcripts including the uncharacterized transcripts, and that our group used full-length *Malat1* to restore its expression in *Malat1*-defecient mice and in *MALAT1*-knockout human cells. Among the transcripts derived from the *Malat1* gene locus, the nuclear lncRNA *Malat1* is the predominant form and is expected to be the functional form. Nevertheless, functional dissection of different transcripts warrants future studies.

5. Mechanistic Models of *MALAT1* in Cancer and Metastasis

LncRNAs function through binding to other RNA, genomic DNA, or protein. Specifically, a lncRNA can serve as a scaffold that keeps proteins together, as a guide that helps recruit proteins to specific genomic DNA sequences, or as a molecular decoy (also called "sponge") for proteins and other RNAs. In this section, we discuss several molecular mechanisms by which *MALAT1* regulates tumor progression and metastasis.

5.1. MALAT1 Serves a Competitive Endogenous RNA (ceRNA)

MALAT1 is a long and highly abundant lncRNA that contains many putative binding sites of miRNAs. A number of studies reported that *MALAT1* functions through sponging miRNAs, including miR-145 [57], miR-1 [58], miR-202 [59], miR-200c [60], miR-206 [61], miR-204 [62], and so on. In these studies, the authors typically showed that siRNA-mediated knockdown of *MALAT1* in cancer cell lines resulted in a certain phenotype, such as proliferation, migration, invasion, chemosensitivity, or radiosensitivity, followed by luciferase assays to demonstrate the existence of the miRNA-binding site on *MALAT1*. Then, functional experiments demonstrated that the miRNA and its target gene mediate the effect of *MALAT1*. While the ceRNA model is interesting and *MALAT1* might function as a ceRNA under certain circumstances, more rigorous experiments are needed to prove this model. For instance, the specificity of the siRNAs targeting *MALAT1* or the miRNA targets should be clearly addressed. Moreover, it would be critical to demonstrate that the miRNA-binding site on *MALAT1* is important for its function—key evidence that is generally lacking. In addition, gain-of-function experiments would further strengthen the conclusions. Furthermore, if *MALAT1* functions through sponging multiple miRNAs, it is very challenging to experimentally prove the ceRNA model of *MALAT1* (Figure 2a).

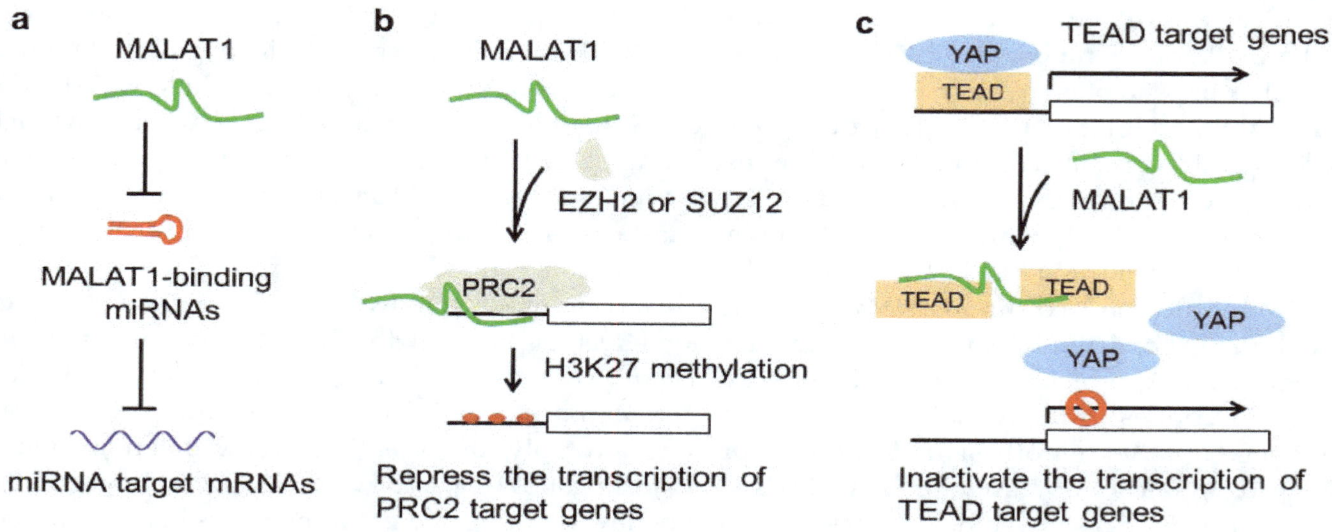

Figure 2. Mechanistic models of *MALAT1* in cancer and metastasis. (**a**) *MALAT1* sponges miRNAs, leading to repression of miRNA target mRNAs. (**b**) *MALAT1* binds PRC2 components and recruits PRC2 to target gene loci. (**c**) *MALAT1* binds, sequesters, and inactivates TEAD.

5.2. MALAT1 Interacts with the PRC2 Complex

Polycomb repressive complex 2 (PRC2) catalyzes histone H3K27 methylation, which plays important roles in transcriptional repression and cancer [63]. *HOTAIR* was the first reported PRC2-binding lncRNA that recruits PRC2 to target gene loci [64]. Subsequently, it has been shown that *HOTAIR* directly interacts with EZH2 [65], and that *HOTAIR* negatively regulates epithelial gene expression through H3K27 trimethylation [66,67]. Recently, additional lncRNAs, including *MALAT1*, have been shown to bind PRC2 components (Figure 2b). Fan et al. reported that *MALAT1* binds SUZ12, a subunit of the PRC2 complex, and that *MALAT1* and SUZ12 mediate TGF-β induced EMT in bladder cancer [68]. Hirata et al. showed that *MALAT1* interacts with EZH2, the catalytic subunit of PRC2, and that both *MALAT1* and EZH2 are required for the EMT in renal cell carcinoma [69]. In addition, several studies showed that the interaction of *MALAT1* with EZH2 is involved in other cancer types, such as prostate cancer [70], gastric cancer [71], and lymphoma [72]. However, it remains unclear whether and how the *MALAT1*-PRC2 interaction specifically regulates the transcription of target genes. Notably, a recent EZH2 RIP-seq assay identified more than 1,000 EZH2-binding lncRNAs [73], while it is unclear whether and how these lncRNAs regulate the activity of EZH2. Similarly, studies from Cech and colleagues revealed promiscuous RNA binding by PRC2 and indicated that mammalian PRC2 binds thousands of RNAs in vivo [74,75]. While the hypothesis that lncRNAs recruit chromatin-modifying complexes to target gene loci is intriguing, questions remain regarding the molecular mechanism by which lncRNAs regulate transcription.

5.3. *MALAT1 Binds and Inactivates TEAD*

Recently, our group performed a chromatin isolation by RNA purification coupled to mass spectrometry (ChIRP-MS) assay to identify *Malat1*'s endogenous binding proteins in mammary tumors from MMTV-PyMT mice. We identified a list of 23 proteins that specifically bind to *Malat1* but not two negative controls (nuclear RNA *U1* and probe-free beads) [29]. Interestingly, all four members of the Tead transcription factor family (Tead1, Tead2, Tead3, and Tead4) were present in this list. Through subsequent validation by ChIRP-Western, RNA pulldown, RIP-qPCR, and UV crosslinking-immunoprecipitation and qPCR (CLIP-qPCR) assays, we found that *MALAT1* binds to the transactivation domain of TEAD proteins, which are unconventional RNA-binding proteins (RBPs), but does not bind to GAPDH, histone H3, or the TEAD co-activator YAP [29]. Moreover, the results from TEAD reporter assays, co-IP, qPCR, ChIP-qPCR, and functional rescue experiments demonstrated that *MALAT1* lncRNA sequesters the transcription factor TEAD, thereby blocking TEAD from associating with its co-activator YAP and target genes, which in turn leads to inhibition of TEAD's transcriptional activity and pro-metastatic function in breast cancer [29] (Figure 2c). It remains to be determined whether *MALAT1* suppresses metastasis by inactivating TEAD in other cancer types. In addition, the functional consequences of the interaction of *Malat1* with its other binding partners warrant further studies.

5.4. *MALAT1 Regulates Multiple Signaling Pathways*

In addition to the Hippo-YAP pathway, *MALAT1* has been reported to regulate other signaling pathways in cancer, including PI3K-AKT, MAPK, WNT, and NF-κB pathways. For instance, by modulating Wnt signaling, *MALAT1* has been shown to regulate cancer cell EMT, migration, invasion, and metastasis [76–78]. *MALAT1* was also found to regulate hepatocellular carcinoma progression through the mTOR pathway [79]. In certain cancer types, a *MALAT1*–NF-κB axis is involved in chemoresistance and EMT [80,81], and PI3K-AKT signaling has been found to mediate the effect of *MALAT1* on metastasis [30,82,83]. Moreover, *MALAT1* may regulate proliferation and metastasis of esophageal squamous cell carcinoma through the ATM-CHK2 pathway [84]. In addition, *MALAT1* has been reported to regulate tumor cell proliferation through the MAPK pathway [27,36]. Unfortunately, validation of these results in genetically engineered mouse models is lacking, and very little is known about the molecular mechanisms by which *MALAT1* regulates these pathways.

6. Conclusions and Future Perspectives

As one of the most abundantly expressed lncRNAs in normal tissues, *MALAT1* has attracted substantial interests from multiple fields including the cancer field. *Malat1* knockout mice are viable and develop normally, suggesting that *MALAT1* is dispensable for development. It remains to be determined whether this lncRNA plays important roles in stress responses or various pathological processes, such as cardiac stress, vascular injury, intestinal injury, immune response, and various oncogenic insults, and whether mice with *Malat1* deficiency show phenotypes in response to external or internal perturbations.

MALAT1 was previously described by many papers as a cancer-promoting and metastasis-promoting lncRNA, while other reports suggested a tumor-suppressing role of *MALAT1*. A major pitfall in these studies was the lack of rescue experiments for loss-of-function approaches. In contrast, our group conducted genetic rescue experiments to demonstrate that the metastasis induction by *Malat1* germline inactivation or somatic knockout (CRISPR-Cas9) was specific to the loss of *MALAT1* lncRNA [29]. This finding underscores the importance of rigorous characterization of lncRNAs, and illustrates how a lncRNA can interact with unconventional RBPs (TEAD proteins) to inhibit metastasis. Non-coding RNA functions should be unambiguously established by rescue experiments in which the RNA expression is restored in knockout cells or knockout mice by means of an independent transgene. Moreover, it is critical to rule out non-specific effects in all types of loss-of-function experiments, including gene deletion, insertional inactivation, CRISPR-Cas9, RNAi, ASO, and chemical inhibition; this is particularly important for the validation of anticancer targets. The current understanding of lncRNAs remains very limited. Moreover, RNA modifications and RBPs can regulate RNA's fate; on the other hand, RBPs, especially unconventional RBPs, could be controlled by RNA, as exemplified by the *MALAT1*-TEAD interaction [29]. We still have a lot to learn about lncRNAs and a lot to expect from the discovery of RNA epigenetics and many new unconventional RBPs. The ongoing and future studies will profoundly advance understanding of the roles of RNA biology in tumor progression and metastasis, and will likely unearth novel anti-metastatic targets for treatment.

Author Contributions: Y.S. and L.M. reviewed and discussed the literature. Y.S. made the outline, wrote a short draft, and made the figures. L.M. wrote the full article based on the short draft. Y.S. and L.M. contributed equally to writing this review.

Acknowledgments: Y.S. and L.M. would like to thank members of the Ma laboratory for their work on *MALAT1* and other non-coding RNAs.

References

1. Bassett, A.R.; Akhtar, A.; Barlow, D.P.; Bird, A.P.; Brockdorff, N.; Duboule, D.; Ephrussi, A.; Ferguson-Smith, A.C.; Gingeras, T.R.; Haerty, W.; et al. Considerations when investigating lncRNA function in vivo. *Elife* **2014**, *3*, e03058. [CrossRef]
2. Kopp, F.; Mendell, J.T. Functional Classification and Experimental Dissection of Long Noncoding RNAs. *Cell* **2018**, *172*, 393–407. [CrossRef]
3. Zhao, J.; Sun, B.K.; Erwin, J.A.; Song, J.J.; Lee, J.T. Polycomb proteins targeted by a short repeat RNA to the mouse X chromosome. *Science* **2008**, *322*, 750–756. [CrossRef]
4. Chen, C.K.; Blanco, M.; Jackson, C.; Aznauryan, E.; Ollikainen, N.; Surka, C.; Chow, A.; Cerase, A.; McDonel, P.; Guttman, M. Xist recruits the X chromosome to the nuclear lamina to enable chromosome-wide silencing. *Science* **2016**, *354*, 468–472. [CrossRef]
5. Wang, C.Y.; Froberg, J.E.; Blum, R.; Jeon, Y.; Lee, J.T. Comment on "Xist recruits the X chromosome to the nuclear lamina to enable chromosome-wide silencing". *Science* **2017**, *356*. [CrossRef]
6. Chen, C.K.; Chow, A.; Lai, M.; Guttman, M. Response to Comment on "Xist recruits the X chromosome to the nuclear lamina to enable chromosome-wide silencing". *Science* **2017**, *356*. [CrossRef]
7. Rinn, J.L.; Kertesz, M.; Wang, J.K.; Squazzo, S.L.; Xu, X.; Brugmann, S.A.; Goodnough, L.H.; Helms, J.A.; Farnham, P.J.; Segal, E.; et al. Functional demarcation of active and silent chromatin domains in human HOX loci by noncoding RNAs. *Cell* **2007**, *129*, 1311–1323. [CrossRef]
8. Li, L.; Liu, B.; Wapinski, O.L.; Tsai, M.C.; Qu, K.; Zhang, J.; Carlson, J.C.; Lin, M.; Fang, F.; Gupta, R.A.; et al. Targeted disruption of Hotair leads to homeotic transformation and gene derepression. *Cell Rep.* **2013**, *5*, 3–12. [CrossRef]
9. Amandio, A.R.; Necsulea, A.; Joye, E.; Mascrez, B.; Duboule, D. Hotair Is Dispensible for Mouse Development. *PLoS Genet.* **2016**, *12*, e1006232. [CrossRef]
10. Li, L.; Helms, J.A.; Chang, H.Y. Comment on "Hotair Is Dispensable for Mouse Development". *PLoS Genet.* **2016**, *12*, e1006406. [CrossRef]
11. Selleri, L.; Bartolomei, M.S.; Bickmore, W.A.; He, L.; Stubbs, L.; Reik, W.; Barsh, G.S. A Hox-Embedded Long Noncoding RNA: Is It All Hot Air? *PLoS Genet.* **2016**, *12*, e1006485. [CrossRef] [PubMed]

12. Yin, Y.; Yan, P.; Lu, J.; Song, G.; Zhu, Y.; Li, Z.; Zhao, Y.; Shen, B.; Huang, X.; Zhu, H.; et al. Opposing Roles for the lncRNA Haunt and Its Genomic Locus in Regulating HOXA Gene Activation during Embryonic Stem Cell Differentiation. *Cell Stem Cell* **2015**, *16*, 504–516. [CrossRef] [PubMed]
13. Hutchinson, J.N.; Ensminger, A.W.; Clemson, C.M.; Lynch, C.R.; Lawrence, J.B.; Chess, A. A screen for nuclear transcripts identifies two linked noncoding RNAs associated with SC35 splicing domains. *BMC Genomics* **2007**, *8*, 39. [CrossRef] [PubMed]
14. Wilusz, J.E.; Freier, S.M.; Spector, D.L. 3'end processing of a long nuclear-retained noncoding RNA yields a tRNA-like cytoplasmic RNA. *Cell* **2008**, *135*, 919–932. [CrossRef] [PubMed]
15. Tripathi, V.; Ellis, J.D.; Shen, Z.; Song, D.Y.; Pan, Q.; Watt, A.T.; Freier, S.M.; Bennett, C.F.; Sharma, A.; Bubulya, P.A.; et al. The nuclear-retained noncoding RNA MALAT1 regulates alternative splicing by modulating SR splicing factor phosphorylation. *Mol. Cell* **2010**, *39*, 925–938. [CrossRef]
16. Zhang, B.; Arun, G.; Mao, Y.S.; Lazar, Z.; Hung, G.; Bhattacharjee, G.; Xiao, X.; Booth, C.J.; Wu, J.; Zhang, C.; et al. The lncRNA Malat1 is dispensable for mouse development but its transcription plays a cis-regulatory role in the adult. *Cell Rep.* **2012**, *2*, 111–123. [CrossRef]
17. Eissmann, M.; Gutschner, T.; Hammerle, M.; Gunther, S.; Caudron-Herger, M.; Gross, M.; Schirmacher, P.; Rippe, K.; Braun, T.; Zornig, M.; et al. Loss of the abundant nuclear non-coding RNA MALAT1 is compatible with life and development. *RNA Biol.* **2012**, *9*, 1076–1087. [CrossRef]
18. Nakagawa, S.; Ip, J.Y.; Shioi, G.; Tripathi, V.; Zong, X.; Hirose, T.; Prasanth, K.V. Malat1 is not an essential component of nuclear speckles in mice. *RNA* **2012**, *18*, 1487–1499. [CrossRef]
19. Liu, N.; Zhou, K.I.; Parisien, M.; Dai, Q.; Diatchenko, L.; Pan, T. N6-methyladenosine alters RNA structure to regulate binding of a low-complexity protein. *Nucleic Acids Res.* **2017**, *45*, 6051–6063. [CrossRef]
20. Amort, T.; Rieder, D.; Wille, A.; Khokhlova-Cubberley, D.; Riml, C.; Trixl, L.; Jia, X.Y.; Micura, R.; Lusser, A. Distinct 5-methylcytosine profiles in poly(A) RNA from mouse embryonic stem cells and brain. *Genome Biol.* **2017**, *18*, 1. [CrossRef]
21. Ji, P.; Diederichs, S.; Wang, W.; Boing, S.; Metzger, R.; Schneider, P.M.; Tidow, N.; Brandt, B.; Buerger, H.; Bulk, E.; et al. MALAT-1, a novel noncoding RNA, and thymosin beta4 predict metastasis and survival in early-stage non-small cell lung cancer. *Oncogene* **2003**, *22*, 8031–8041. [CrossRef]
22. West, J.A.; Davis, C.P.; Sunwoo, H.; Simon, M.D.; Sadreyev, R.I.; Wang, P.I.; Tolstorukov, M.Y.; Kingston, R.E. The long noncoding RNAs NEAT1 and MALAT1 bind active chromatin sites. *Mol. Cell* **2014**, *55*, 791–802. [CrossRef]
23. Gutschner, T.; Hammerle, M.; Diederichs, S. MALAT1—A paradigm for long noncoding RNA function in cancer. *J. Mol. Med. (Berl.)* **2013**, *91*, 791–801. [CrossRef]
24. Yoshimoto, R.; Mayeda, A.; Yoshida, M.; Nakagawa, S. MALAT1 long non-coding RNA in cancer. *Biochim. Biophys. Acta* **2016**, *1859*, 192–199. [CrossRef]
25. Liu, J.; Peng, W.X.; Mo, Y.Y.; Luo, D. MALAT1-mediated tumorigenesis. *Front. Biosci. (Landmark Ed.)* **2017**, *22*, 66–80.
26. Zhao, M.; Wang, S.; Li, Q.; Ji, Q.; Guo, P.; Liu, X. MALAT1: A long non-coding RNA highly associated with human cancers. *Oncol. Lett.* **2018**, *16*, 19–26. [CrossRef]
27. Han, Y.; Wu, Z.; Wu, T.; Huang, Y.; Cheng, Z.; Li, X.; Sun, T.; Xie, X.; Zhou, Y.; Du, Z. Tumor-suppressive function of long noncoding RNA MALAT1 in glioma cells by downregulation of MMP2 and inactivation of ERK/MAPK signaling. *Cell Death Dis.* **2016**, *7*, e2123. [CrossRef]
28. Kwok, Z.H.; Roche, V.; Chew, X.H.; Fadieieva, A.; Tay, Y. A non-canonical tumor suppressive role for the long non-coding RNA MALAT1 in colon and breast cancers. *Int. J. Cancer* **2018**, *143*, 668–678. [CrossRef]
29. Kim, J.; Piao, H.L.; Kim, B.J.; Yao, F.; Han, Z.; Wang, Y.; Xiao, Z.; Siverly, A.N.; Lawhon, S.E.; Ton, B.N.; et al. Long noncoding RNA MALAT1 suppresses breast cancer metastasis. *Nat. Genet.* **2018**, *50*, 1705–1715. [CrossRef]
30. Xu, S.; Sui, S.; Zhang, J.; Bai, N.; Shi, Q.; Zhang, G.; Gao, S.; You, Z.; Zhan, C.; Liu, F.; et al. Downregulation of long noncoding RNA MALAT1 induces epithelial-to-mesenchymal transition via the PI3K-AKT pathway in breast cancer. *Int. J. Clin. Exp. Pathol.* **2015**, *8*, 4881–4891.
31. Li, L.; Feng, T.; Lian, Y.; Zhang, G.; Garen, A.; Song, X. Role of human noncoding RNAs in the control of tumorigenesis. *Proc. Natl. Acad. Sci. USA* **2009**, *106*, 12956–12961. [CrossRef] [PubMed]

32. Ji, Q.; Zhang, L.; Liu, X.; Zhou, L.; Wang, W.; Han, Z.; Sui, H.; Tang, Y.; Wang, Y.; Liu, N.; et al. Long non-coding RNA MALAT1 promotes tumour growth and metastasis in colorectal cancer through binding to SFPQ and releasing oncogene PTBP2 from SFPQ/PTBP2 complex. *Br. J. Cancer* **2014**, *111*, 736–748. [CrossRef] [PubMed]
33. Bi, S.; Wang, C.; Li, Y.; Zhang, W.; Zhang, J.; Lv, Z.; Wang, J. LncRNA-MALAT1-mediated Axl promotes cell invasion and migration in human neuroblastoma. *Tumour Biol.* **2017**, *39*, 1010428317699796. [CrossRef] [PubMed]
34. Li, P.; Zhang, X.; Wang, H.; Wang, L.; Liu, T.; Du, L.; Yang, Y.; Wang, C. MALAT1 Is Associated with Poor Response to Oxaliplatin-Based Chemotherapy in Colorectal Cancer Patients and Promotes Chemoresistance through EZH2. *Mol. Cancer Ther.* **2017**, *16*, 739–751. [CrossRef]
35. Tripathi, V.; Shen, Z.; Chakraborty, A.; Giri, S.; Freier, S.M.; Wu, X.; Zhang, Y.; Gorospe, M.; Prasanth, S.G.; Lal, A.; et al. Long noncoding RNA MALAT1 controls cell cycle progression by regulating the expression of oncogenic transcription factor B-MYB. *PLoS Genet.* **2013**, *9*, e1003368. [CrossRef]
36. Wu, X.S.; Wang, X.A.; Wu, W.G.; Hu, Y.P.; Li, M.L.; Ding, Q.; Weng, H.; Shu, Y.J.; Liu, T.Y.; Jiang, L.; et al. MALAT1 promotes the proliferation and metastasis of gallbladder cancer cells by activating the ERK/MAPK pathway. *Cancer Biol. Ther.* **2014**, *15*, 806–814. [CrossRef] [PubMed]
37. Shen, L.; Chen, L.; Wang, Y.; Jiang, X.; Xia, H.; Zhuang, Z. Long noncoding RNA MALAT1 promotes brain metastasis by inducing epithelial-mesenchymal transition in lung cancer. *J. Neurooncol.* **2015**, *121*, 101–108. [CrossRef] [PubMed]
38. Cao, S.; Wang, Y.; Li, J.; Lv, M.; Niu, H.; Tian, Y. Tumor-suppressive function of long noncoding RNA MALAT1 in glioma cells by suppressing miR-155 expression and activating FBXW7 function. *Am. J. Cancer Res.* **2016**, *6*, 2561–2574. [PubMed]
39. Han, Y.; Zhou, L.; Wu, T.; Huang, Y.; Cheng, Z.; Li, X.; Sun, T.; Zhou, Y.; Du, Z. Downregulation of lncRNA-MALAT1 Affects Proliferation and the Expression of Stemness Markers in Glioma Stem Cell Line SHG139S. *Cell. Mol. Neurobiol.* **2016**, *36*, 1097–1107. [CrossRef]
40. Latorre, E.; Carelli, S.; Raimondi, I.; D'Agostino, V.; Castiglioni, I.; Zucal, C.; Moro, G.; Luciani, A.; Ghilardi, G.; Monti, E.; et al. The Ribonucleic Complex HuR-MALAT1 Represses CD133 Expression and Suppresses Epithelial-Mesenchymal Transition in Breast Cancer. *Cancer Res.* **2016**, *76*, 2626–2636. [CrossRef]
41. Guy, C.T.; Cardiff, R.D.; Muller, W.J. Induction of mammary tumors by expression of polyomavirus middle T oncogene: A transgenic mouse model for metastatic disease. *Mol. Cell. Biol.* **1992**, *12*, 954–961. [CrossRef]
42. Arun, G.; Diermeier, S.; Akerman, M.; Chang, K.C.; Wilkinson, J.E.; Hearn, S.; Kim, Y.; MacLeod, A.R.; Krainer, A.R.; Norton, L.; et al. Differentiation of mammary tumors and reduction in metastasis upon Malat1 lncRNA loss. *Genes Dev.* **2016**, *30*, 34–51. [CrossRef]
43. Sauvageau, M.; Goff, L.A.; Lodato, S.; Bonev, B.; Groff, A.F.; Gerhardinger, C.; Sanchez-Gomez, D.B.; Hacisuleyman, E.; Li, E.; Spence, M.; et al. Multiple knockout mouse models reveal lincRNAs are required for life and brain development. *Elife* **2013**, *2*, e01749. [CrossRef] [PubMed]
44. Grote, P.; Wittler, L.; Hendrix, D.; Koch, F.; Wahrisch, S.; Beisaw, A.; Macura, K.; Blass, G.; Kellis, M.; Werber, M.; et al. The tissue-specific lncRNA Fendrr is an essential regulator of heart and body wall development in the mouse. *Dev. Cell* **2013**, *24*, 206–214. [CrossRef]
45. Feng, J.; Bi, C.; Clark, B.S.; Mady, R.; Shah, P.; Kohtz, J.D. The Evf-2 noncoding RNA is transcribed from the Dlx-5/6 ultraconserved region and functions as a Dlx-2 transcriptional coactivator. *Genes Dev.* **2006**, *20*, 1470–1484. [CrossRef] [PubMed]
46. Bond, A.M.; Vangompel, M.J.; Sametsky, E.A.; Clark, M.F.; Savage, J.C.; Disterhoft, J.F.; Kohtz, J.D. Balanced gene regulation by an embryonic brain ncRNA is critical for adult hippocampal GABA circuitry. *Nat. Neurosci.* **2009**, *12*, 1020–1027. [CrossRef] [PubMed]
47. Berghoff, E.G.; Clark, M.F.; Chen, S.; Cajigas, I.; Leib, D.E.; Kohtz, J.D. Evf2 (Dlx6as) lncRNA regulates ultraconserved enhancer methylation and the differential transcriptional control of adjacent genes. *Development* **2013**, *140*, 4407–4416. [CrossRef] [PubMed]
48. Gutschner, T.; Hammerle, M.; Eissmann, M.; Hsu, J.; Kim, Y.; Hung, G.; Revenko, A.; Arun, G.; Stentrup, M.; Gross, M.; et al. The noncoding RNA MALAT1 is a critical regulator of the metastasis phenotype of lung cancer cells. *Cancer Res.* **2013**, *73*, 1180–1189. [CrossRef] [PubMed]

49. Jadaliha, M.; Zong, X.; Malakar, P.; Ray, T.; Singh, D.K.; Freier, S.M.; Jensen, T.; Prasanth, S.G.; Karni, R.; Ray, P.S.; et al. Functional and prognostic significance of long non-coding RNA MALAT1 as a metastasis driver in ER negative lymph node negative breast cancer. *Oncotarget* **2016**, *7*, 40418–40436. [CrossRef]
50. Gagnon, K.T.; Li, L.; Chu, Y.; Janowski, B.A.; Corey, D.R. RNAi factors are present and active in human cell nuclei. *Cell Rep.* **2014**, *6*, 211–221. [CrossRef]
51. Sharma, N.R.; Wang, X.; Majerciak, V.; Ajiro, M.; Kruhlak, M.; Meyers, C.; Zheng, Z.M. Cell Type- and Tissue Context-dependent Nuclear Distribution of Human Ago2. *J. Biol. Chem.* **2016**, *291*, 2302–2309. [CrossRef] [PubMed]
52. Kaelin, W.G., Jr. Common pitfalls in preclinical cancer target validation. *Nat. Rev. Cancer* **2017**, *17*, 425–440. [CrossRef] [PubMed]
53. Huang, H.T.; Seo, H.S.; Zhang, T.; Wang, Y.; Jiang, B.; Li, Q.; Buckley, D.L.; Nabet, B.; Roberts, J.M.; Paulk, J.; et al. MELK is not necessary for the proliferation of basal-like breast cancer cells. *Elife* **2017**, *6*, e26693. [CrossRef] [PubMed]
54. Lin, A.; Giuliano, C.J.; Sayles, N.M.; Sheltzer, J.M. CRISPR/Cas9 mutagenesis invalidates a putative cancer dependency targeted in on-going clinical trials. *Elife* **2017**, *6*, e24179. [CrossRef] [PubMed]
55. Giuliano, C.J.; Lin, A.; Smith, J.C.; Palladino, A.C.; Sheltzer, J.M. MELK expression correlates with tumor mitotic activity but is not required for cancer growth. *Elife* **2018**, *7*, e32838. [CrossRef] [PubMed]
56. Settleman, J.; Sawyers, C.L.; Hunter, T. Challenges in validating candidate therapeutic targets in cancer. *Elife* **2018**, *7*, e32402. [CrossRef]
57. Lu, H.; He, Y.; Lin, L.; Qi, Z.; Ma, L.; Li, L.; Su, Y. Long non-coding RNA MALAT1 modulates radiosensitivity of HR-HPV+ cervical cancer via sponging miR-145. *Tumour Biol.* **2016**, *37*, 1683–1691. [CrossRef]
58. Jin, C.; Yan, B.; Lu, Q.; Lin, Y.; Ma, L. The role of MALAT1/miR-1/slug axis on radioresistance in nasopharyngeal carcinoma. *Tumour Biol.* **2016**, *37*, 4025–4033. [CrossRef]
59. Zhang, Y.; Chen, Z.; Li, M.J.; Guo, H.Y.; Jing, N.C. Long non-coding RNA metastasis-associated lung adenocarcinoma transcript 1 regulates the expression of Gli2 by miR-202 to strengthen gastric cancer progression. *Biomed. Pharmacother.* **2017**, *85*, 264–271. [CrossRef]
60. Li, Q.; Zhang, C.; Chen, R.; Xiong, H.; Qiu, F.; Liu, S.; Zhang, M.; Wang, F.; Wang, Y.; Zhou, X.; et al. Disrupting MALAT1/miR-200c sponge decreases invasion and migration in endometrioid endometrial carcinoma. *Cancer Lett.* **2016**, *383*, 28–40. [CrossRef]
61. Wang, S.H.; Zhang, W.J.; Wu, X.C.; Zhang, M.D.; Weng, M.Z.; Zhou, D.; Wang, J.D.; Quan, Z.W. Long non-coding RNA Malat1 promotes gallbladder cancer development by acting as a molecular sponge to regulate miR-206. *Oncotarget* **2016**, *7*, 37857–37867. [CrossRef] [PubMed]
62. Hou, Z.; Xu, X.; Zhou, L.; Fu, X.; Tao, S.; Zhou, J.; Tan, D.; Liu, S. The long non-coding RNA MALAT1 promotes the migration and invasion of hepatocellular carcinoma by sponging miR-204 and releasing SIRT1. *Tumour Biol.* **2017**, *39*, 1010428317718135. [CrossRef] [PubMed]
63. Laugesen, A.; Hojfeldt, J.W.; Helin, K. Role of the Polycomb Repressive Complex 2 (PRC2) in Transcriptional Regulation and Cancer. *Cold Spring Harb. Perspect. Med.* **2016**, *6*, a026575. [CrossRef] [PubMed]
64. Gupta, R.A.; Shah, N.; Wang, K.C.; Kim, J.; Horlings, H.M.; Wong, D.J.; Tsai, M.C.; Hung, T.; Argani, P.; Rinn, J.L.; et al. Long non-coding RNA HOTAIR reprograms chromatin state to promote cancer metastasis. *Nature* **2010**, *464*, 1071–1076. [CrossRef] [PubMed]
65. Huang, K.B.; Zhang, S.P.; Zhu, Y.J.; Guo, C.H.; Yang, M.; Liu, J.; Xia, L.G.; Zhang, J.F. Hotair mediates tumorigenesis through recruiting EZH2 in colorectal cancer. *J. Cell. Biochem.* **2018**. [CrossRef] [PubMed]
66. Battistelli, C.; Sabarese, G.; Santangelo, L.; Montaldo, C.; Gonzalez, F.J.; Tripodi, M.; Cicchini, C. The lncRNA HOTAIR transcription is controlled by HNF4alpha-induced chromatin topology modulation. *Cell Death Differ.* **2018**. [CrossRef] [PubMed]
67. Chen, W.M.; Chen, W.D.; Jiang, X.M.; Jia, X.F.; Wang, H.M.; Zhang, Q.J.; Shu, Y.Q.; Zhao, H.B. HOX transcript antisense intergenic RNA represses E-cadherin expression by binding to EZH2 in gastric cancer. *World J. Gastroenterol.* **2017**, *23*, 6100–6110. [CrossRef] [PubMed]
68. Fan, Y.; Shen, B.; Tan, M.; Mu, X.; Qin, Y.; Zhang, F.; Liu, Y. TGF-beta-induced upregulation of malat1 promotes bladder cancer metastasis by associating with suz12. *Clin. Cancer Res.* **2014**, *20*, 1531–1541. [CrossRef]

69. Hirata, H.; Hinoda, Y.; Shahryari, V.; Deng, G.; Nakajima, K.; Tabatabai, Z.L.; Ishii, N.; Dahiya, R. Long Noncoding RNA MALAT1 Promotes Aggressive Renal Cell Carcinoma through Ezh2 and Interacts with miR-205. *Cancer Res.* **2015**, *75*, 1322–1331. [CrossRef]
70. Wang, D.; Ding, L.; Wang, L.; Zhao, Y.; Sun, Z.; Karnes, R.J.; Zhang, J.; Huang, H. LncRNA MALAT1 enhances oncogenic activities of EZH2 in castration-resistant prostate cancer. *Oncotarget* **2015**, *6*, 41045–41055. [CrossRef]
71. Qi, Y.; Ooi, H.S.; Wu, J.; Chen, J.; Zhang, X.; Tan, S.; Yu, Q.; Li, Y.Y.; Kang, Y.; Li, H.; et al. MALAT1 long ncRNA promotes gastric cancer metastasis by suppressing PCDH10. *Oncotarget* **2016**, *7*, 12693–12703. [CrossRef]
72. Kim, S.H.; Kim, S.H.; Yang, W.I.; Kim, S.J.; Yoon, S.O. Association of the long non-coding RNA MALAT1 with the polycomb repressive complex pathway in T and NK cell lymphoma. *Oncotarget* **2017**, *8*, 31305–31317. [CrossRef] [PubMed]
73. Wang, Y.; Xie, Y.; Li, L.; He, Y.; Zheng, D.; Yu, P.; Yu, L.; Tang, L.; Wang, Y.; Wang, Z. EZH2 RIP-seq Identifies Tissue-specific Long Non-coding RNAs. *Curr. Gene Ther.* **2018**, *18*, 275–285. [CrossRef] [PubMed]
74. Wang, X.; Goodrich, K.J.; Gooding, A.R.; Naeem, H.; Archer, S.; Paucek, R.D.; Youmans, D.T.; Cech, T.R.; Davidovich, C. Targeting of Polycomb Repressive Complex 2 to RNA by Short Repeats of Consecutive Guanines. *Mol. Cell* **2017**, *65*, 1056–1067.e5. [CrossRef] [PubMed]
75. Davidovich, C.; Zheng, L.; Goodrich, K.J.; Cech, T.R. Promiscuous RNA binding by Polycomb repressive complex 2. *Nat. Struct. Mol. Biol.* **2013**, *20*, 1250–1257. [CrossRef] [PubMed]
76. Ji, Q.; Liu, X.; Fu, X.; Zhang, L.; Sui, H.; Zhou, L.; Sun, J.; Cai, J.; Qin, J.; Ren, J.; et al. Resveratrol inhibits invasion and metastasis of colorectal cancer cells via MALAT1 mediated Wnt/beta-catenin signal pathway. *PLoS ONE* **2013**, *8*, e78700. [CrossRef] [PubMed]
77. Ying, L.; Chen, Q.; Wang, Y.; Zhou, Z.; Huang, Y.; Qiu, F. Upregulated MALAT-1 contributes to bladder cancer cell migration by inducing epithelial-to-mesenchymal transition. *Mol. Biosyst.* **2012**, *8*, 2289–2294. [CrossRef] [PubMed]
78. Liang, J.; Liang, L.; Ouyang, K.; Li, Z.; Yi, X. MALAT1 induces tongue cancer cells' EMT and inhibits apoptosis through Wnt/beta-catenin signaling pathway. *J. Oral Pathol. Med.* **2017**, *46*, 98–105. [CrossRef]
79. Malakar, P.; Shilo, A.; Mogilevsky, A.; Stein, I.; Pikarsky, E.; Nevo, Y.; Benyamini, H.; Elgavish, S.; Zong, X.; Prasanth, K.V.; et al. Long Noncoding RNA MALAT1 Promotes Hepatocellular Carcinoma Development by SRSF1 Upregulation and mTOR Activation. *Cancer Res.* **2017**, *77*, 1155–1167. [CrossRef] [PubMed]
80. Zhou, X.; Liu, S.; Cai, G.; Kong, L.; Zhang, T.; Ren, Y.; Wu, Y.; Mei, M.; Zhang, L.; Wang, X. Long Non Coding RNA MALAT1 Promotes Tumor Growth and Metastasis by inducing Epithelial-Mesenchymal Transition in Oral Squamous Cell Carcinoma. *Sci. Rep.* **2015**, *5*, 15972. [CrossRef]
81. Ji, D.G.; Guan, L.Y.; Luo, X.; Ma, F.; Yang, B.; Liu, H.Y. Inhibition of MALAT1 sensitizes liver cancer cells to 5-flurouracil by regulating apoptosis through IKKalpha/NF-kappaB pathway. *Biochem. Biophys. Res. Commun.* **2018**, *501*, 33–40. [CrossRef] [PubMed]
82. Jin, Y.; Feng, S.J.; Qiu, S.; Shao, N.; Zheng, J.H. LncRNA MALAT1 promotes proliferation and metastasis in epithelial ovarian cancer via the PI3K-AKT pathway. *Eur. Rev. Med. Pharmacol. Sci.* **2017**, *21*, 3176–3184. [PubMed]
83. Chen, Y.; Huang, W.; Sun, W.; Zheng, B.; Wang, C.; Luo, Z.; Wang, J.; Yan, W. LncRNA MALAT1 Promotes Cancer Metastasis in Osteosarcoma via Activation of the PI3K-Akt Signaling Pathway. *Cell. Physiol. Biochem.* **2018**, *51*, 1313–1326. [CrossRef] [PubMed]
84. Hu, L.; Wu, Y.; Tan, D.; Meng, H.; Wang, K.; Bai, Y.; Yang, K. Up-regulation of long noncoding RNA MALAT1 contributes to proliferation and metastasis in esophageal squamous cell carcinoma. *J. Exp. Clin. Cancer Res.* **2015**, *34*, 7. [CrossRef] [PubMed]

9

Integrated Approaches for the Use of Large Datasets to Identify Rational Therapies for the Treatment of Lung Cancers

Robert J. Cardnell [1], Lauren Averett Byers [1] and Jing Wang [2,*]

1 Department of Thoracic/Head and Neck Medical Oncology, The University of Texas MD Anderson Cancer Center, Houston, TX 77030, USA; rcardnell@mdanderson.org (R.J.C.); lbyers@mdanderson.org (L.A.B.)
2 Department of Bioinformatics and Computational Biology, The University of Texas MD Anderson Cancer Center, Houston, TX 77030, USA
* Correspondence: jingwang@mdanderson.org

Abstract: The benefit and burden of contemporary techniques for the molecular characterization of samples is the vast amount of data generated. In the era of "big data", it has become imperative that we develop multi-disciplinary teams combining scientists, clinicians, and data analysts. In this review, we discuss a number of approaches developed by our University of Texas MD Anderson Lung Cancer Multidisciplinary Program to process and utilize such large datasets with the goal of identifying rational therapeutic options for biomarker-driven patient subsets. Large integrated datasets such as the The Cancer Genome Atlas (TCGA) for patient samples and the Cancer Cell Line Encyclopedia (CCLE) for tumor derived cell lines include genomic, transcriptomic, methylation, miRNA, and proteomic profiling alongside clinical data. To best use these datasets to address urgent questions such as whether we can define molecular subtypes of disease with specific therapeutic vulnerabilities, to quantify states such as epithelial-to-mesenchymal transition that are associated with resistance to treatment, or to identify potential therapeutic agents in models of cancer that are resistant to standard treatments required the development of tools for systematic, unbiased high-throughput analysis. Together, such tools, used in a multi-disciplinary environment, can be leveraged to identify novel treatments for molecularly defined subsets of cancer patients, which can be easily and rapidly translated from benchtop to bedside.

Keywords: bioinformatics; integrated approaches; lung cancer; rational therapy

1. Introduction

While many targeted therapies have been tested in lung cancers, the challenge remains to identify the subset(s) of patients who will respond to these treatments. Integrated approaches are necessary to combine in vitro, in vivo, in silico, and clinical data to identify and validate potential treatments and the cohorts of patients in which these should be used. The University of Texas MD Anderson Lung Cancer Multidisciplinary Program integrates a team of investigators with expertise in biologic, bioinformatics, and clinical studies and has a track record of utilizing high-throughput "-omics" data to identify new therapeutic targets and biomarkers. Here, we discuss three approaches to utilize large datasets with the goal of identifying rational therapeutic options for biomarker-driven patient subsets.

2. Datasets

The approaches described in this manuscript use a combination of publically available clinical datasets accessible through cBioPortal for Cancer Genomics (http://www.cbioportal.org/) or the

National Center for Biotechnology Information (NCBI) (https://www.ncbi.nlm.nih.gov/), and cell line data from the Broad Institute Cancer Cell Line Encyclopedia (CCLE) (https://portals.broadinstitute.org/ccle), the Genomics of Drug Sensitivity in Cancer (GDSC) (https://www.cancerrxgene.org/), and the National Cancer Institute (NCI) Developmental Therapeutics Program (http://sclccelllines.cancer.gov) summarized in Table 1, in additional to data generated at the University of Texas MD Anderson Cancer Center as part of our cell line characterization efforts and clinical trials. The datasets contain a variety of profiling data including genomic, transcriptomic (either array based or RNASeq), methylation, miRNA expression, and protein expression (by reverse phase protein array (RPPA)), as well as drug response for the cell lines and clinical data for patients (e.g., overall survival, progression free survival, smoking history). Compatibility between datasets is crucial and requires taking into account possible batch effects, probe selection in the use of array-based data [1], and fundamental differences in technology (i.e., microarrays versus RNAseq). For example, when comparing cell line drug sensitivity, the manner in which both single agent [2] and combination data [3–6] were generated (e.g., length of experiment, drug dose, and dilution factors) must also be carefully considered, to ensure that the approaches used are compatible, and that the analysis model chosen is adequately supported by the data. Sample source must also be considered, regardless of the type of data available. While cell lines can be used for drug sensitivity assays and candidate biomarker discovery, they do not reflect the role of the tumor stroma and immune microenvironment. Patient derived data, however, do reflect the tumor stroma and immune microenvironment and often include outcome data and other clinical parameters, but do not allow for screening of candidate agents. These considerations highlight some of the underlying reasons behind the assembly of the Multidisciplinary Program, drawing upon a range of expertise from across the institution.

Table 1. Publically available datasets. Summary of publically available datasets used in the approaches presented. * Datasets obtained from the National Center for Biotechnology Information (NCBI) for these analyses include those from George et al., Sato et al. [7,8], BATTLE-1, BATTLE-2, and PROSPECT. # Data types available vary by study. TCGA—The Cancer Genome Atlas; CCLE—Broad Institute Cancer Cell Line Encyclopedia; GDSC—Genomics of Drug Sensitivity in Cancer; SCLC—small cell lung cancer; EMT—epithelial-to-mesenchymal transition.

Resource	Malignancy	Data Types	Pre-Clinical/Clinical	Approach
TCGA [9]	Various	Genomic, transcriptomic, methylation, copy number, proteomic, and clinical #	Clinical	EMT
NCBI * [10]	Various	Genomic, transcriptomic, methylation, copy number and clinical #	Both	EMT, SCLC subgroups
CCLE [11]	Various	Drug sensitivity, genomic, and transcriptomic	Pre-clinical	SCLC subgroups, DISARM
GDSC [12]	Various	Drug sensitivity, genomic, and transcriptomic	Pre-clinical	SCLC subgroups, DISARM
NCI Developmental Therapeutics Program [13]	SCLC	Drug sensitivity, and transcriptomic	Pre-clinical	SCLC subgroups, DISARM
DISARM [14]	Various	Drug sensitivity	Pre-clinical	DISARM

3. Approaches

3.1. Cancer EMT Signature

The concept of epithelial-to-mesenchymal transition (EMT), a process by which epithelial cells lose cellular polarity and cell–cell adhesion and enter a mesenchymal state with enhanced migratory and invasive properties, was first described more than a decade ago in cancer [15,16].

As EMT plays a role in resistance to standard treatments for non-small cell lung cancer (NSCLC) (and other cancers), and no standard method existed to quantify the degree to which a tumor had undergone EMT, we first developed a lung cancer-specific EMT signature, and subsequently a pan-cancer derived signature based on transcriptomic profiling (Figure 1A) [17]. Using gene expression in 54 NSCLC cell lines, the lung cancer EMT signature was first based on those genes whose mRNA expression levels were significantly correlated (either positively or negatively) with at least one of four putative EMT markers—E-cadherin, vimentin, N-cadherin, and/or fibronectin 1. These "seed genes" were selected as they had previously been established as markers of EMT in lung cancers and other epithelial tumor types. Second, the set of genes correlated to the EMT markers was further limited to those with a bimodal expression pattern to facilitate the ability of the signature to dichotomize the cell lines into distinct epithelial and mesenchymal groups. Third, genes correlated to the EMT markers also had to correlate in an independent mRNA microarray dataset to reduce artifacts and identify the most biologically and technically robust genes. We then used the epithelial or mesenchymal status of the cell lines to determine if EMT predicted response to various targeted agents (Figure 1B). As expected, EGFR inhibitors had greater activity in epithelial models. An interesting observation was that the AXL inhibitor SGI7079 was more efficacious in the mesenchymal models. Expression of AXL, a receptor-tyrosine kinase, was higher in the mesenchymal cell lines, suggesting AXL as a novel target in mesenchymal NSCLC. We then tested the efficacy of SGI7079 in an epithelial mouse xenograft model, where we observed single agent activity and a greater than additive effect when combined with erlotinib (Figure 1C). As a clinical validation of our observations, we classified NSCLC patients with prior systemic therapy and subsequent relapse enrolled to the BATTLE-1 (Biomarker-integrated Approaches of Targeted Therapy for Lung Cancer Elimination) [18] clinical trial as either epithelial or mesenchymal. As expected, *EGFR* wild-type patients with an epithelial tumor treated on the erlotinib arm had significantly better eight-week disease control than those with mesenchymal tumors.

To account for the contribution of the tumor microenvironment to EMT, we built on the lung cell line EMT score, to develop a pan-cancer, patient tumor-derived, EMT score [19]. Using an approach similar to the lung-EMT score, we identified mRNAs best correlated with established "seed" markers of EMT (E-cadherin, vimentin, fibronectin, and N-cadherin) across nine distinct, primarily epithelial, solid tumor types from The Cancer Genome Atlas (TCGA) [9]. Using this approach, we identified 77 genes across the nine tumor types tested (breast invasive carcinoma—BRCA, lung squamous cell carcinoma—LUSC, basal-like breast cancer—basal, head and neck squamous cell carcinoma—HNSC, lung adenocarcinoma—LUAD, ovarian carcinoma—OVCA, bladder urothelial cancer—BLCA, uterine corpus endometrial carcinoma—UCEC, and colon adenocarcinoma—COAD). Nineteen genes identified overlapped with the original lung cancer EMT signature, and when applied over 11 tumor types (those used to derive the signature, plus kidney clear cell carcinoma—KIRC, and rectal adenocarcinoma—READ), a wide range of the pan-cancer EMT signature gave a wide range of scores (Figure 1D). As expected, the pan-cancer signatures identify KIRC as highly mesenchymal and both READ and COAD as highly epithelial, in agreement with existing knowledge identifying these cancer types as such.

To better understand tumor gene expression pathways globally dysregulated in the context of EMT, we performed a pathway analysis of all genes correlated with the pan-cancer EMT score in all 11 tumor types. In addition to EMT pathways, among the top hits were pathways related to immune cell signaling. In the context of data generated by our group showing a relationship between EMT and immune escape [20], we investigated the relationship between the EMT score and expression of 20 potentially targetable immune checkpoint genes (Figure 1E). Across all the tumor types tested, we observed a strong positive correlation between EMT score and expression of the targetable immune checkpoint genes. This enrichment of immune target expression in mesenchymal tumors corroborated other work in our group in lung cancer where lung adenocarcinomas with a high lung cell line EMT score had high expression of PD-L1, which is a target of miR-200, which is also a suppressor of EMT and metastasis [20].

As a validation of the association between EMT and immune checkpoint genes, we stained lung adenocarcinoma sections included in a tissue microarray developed from the PROSPECT trial for expression of PD-L1. Automated quantification of immunohistochemistry (IHC) staining (H-score, calculated by multiplying extent and intensity of staining [21]) showed significantly higher expression of PD-L1 in both tumor and non-tumors cells in tumors with a mesenchymal pan-cancer EMT score (Figure 1F). As PD-L1 expression is a biomarker of response to PD-L1 blockade [22], by virtue of mesenchymal tumors expressing higher PD-L1, our analyses indicate that patients with mesenchymal tumors are more likely to be candidates for PD-L1 blockade, and other similar immune checkpoint blockade treatments.

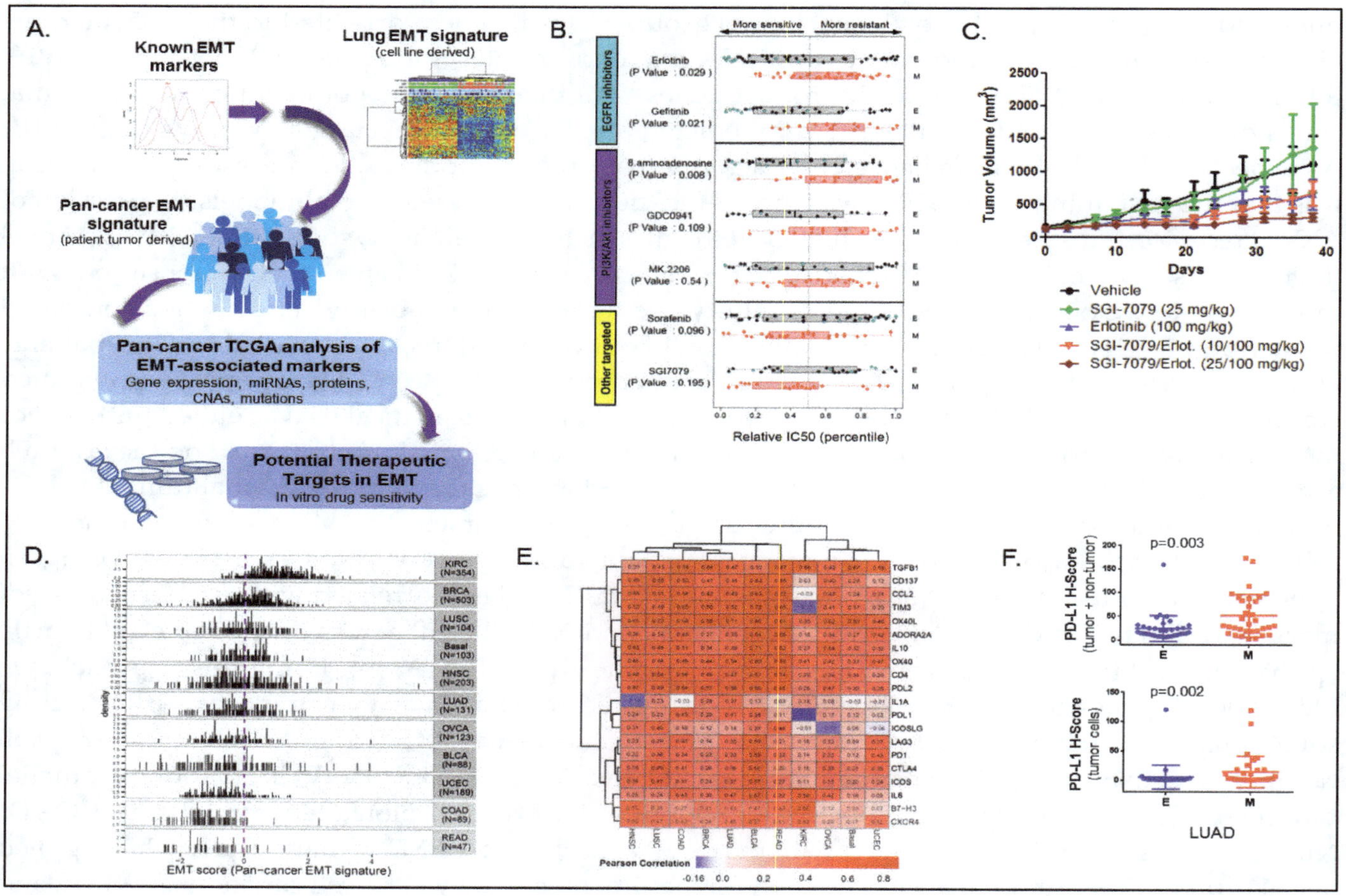

Figure 1. Development of an epithelial-to-mesenchymal transition (EMT) signature. Schematic describing the development of the lung-cancer and pan-cancer EMT scores (**A**). Using the lung-EMT score, mesenchymal cells are less sensitive to EGFR and PI3K inhibition, but are more sensitive to AXL inhibition (**B**). AXL blockade inhibits growth of mesenchymal (A549) non-small cell lung cancer (NSCLC) xenografts (**C**). The Cancer Genome Atlas (TCGA) pan-cancer tumor types display a range of EMT scores (**D**). A mesenchymal pan-cancer EMT score is correlated with higher expression of immune checkpoint genes across multiple cancer types (**E**). Mesenchymal lung adenocarcinoma (LUAD) has higher expression of PD-L1 in both tumor and non-tumor cells by immunohistochemistry (**F**). Adapted from Byers et al. 2013 [17] and Mak et al. 2015 [19].

The approach of using a "seed" to generate cell line and tumor-based signatures to quantify a biological program has been demonstrated in our work both to define alterations in signaling pathways and to identify therapeutic vulnerabilities. This signature generating approach has the potential to be applied to any scenario in which a few known markers describing two distinct morphologies or states have been defined.

3.2. Proteomic Subgrouping of SCLC

Proteomic profiling by RPPA measures a discrete number of targets enriched for druggable and oncologically important pathways (typically around 200 total/phosphorylated proteins) [23,24], and offers significant advantages over other profiling approaches. For example, proteomics, unlike DNA- or RNA-based profiling, directly measures pathway activation and candidate target expression (i.e., the protein "target" itself) [25]. Furthermore, protein biomarkers, particularly those that can be assayed by IHC have the potential for rapid translation into the clinic, as illustrated by the clinical use of PD-L1 IHC in NSCLC [22], and MET IHC in breast cancer [26].

Clinically, SCLC is currently treated as a single disease, with all patients receiving essentially the same standard-of-care (SOC) treatment. The variability in response to SOC seen in the clinic, however, suggested a need to identify subgroups of SCLC with specific vulnerabilities that could be leveraged to develop more personalized approaches. Using proteomic data for 169 targets from a panel of 63 SCLC cell lines [27], we used a model-based clustering method [28,29] to determine the optimal number of clusters. Specifically, the cell lines were categorized into subgroups (range 1–20) using six distinct models, and Bayesian index clustering (BIC) was then applied to determine to optimal number of groups. The optimal model/group combination was then used to segregate the cell lines into two groups. When separated into two groups, we used two sample *t*-tests to compare expression of protein markers between the groups, identifying TTF1 and cMYC as the highest expressed proteins in groups 1 and 2, respectively (Figure 2B). Differences in expression of total protein between the cell line groups were then verified using publically available RNASeq data [30]. As cell culture may impact gene/protein expression, we used two cohorts of human SCLC tumors with gene expression data to validate our observations [7,8]. Using the 38 genes corresponding to total protein differences observed in the cell lines, we clustered the human samples. At the highest level, both patient cohorts separated into two groups, with striking differences in *NKX2-1* (the gene name of TTF1) and *MYC* between the groups.

Having identified two proteomically defined subsets of SCLC, we used a combination of internal [27] and publically available drug sensitivity data [30,32] to determine if these groupings drove differential responses to candidate treatments. Having identified a large number of targeted agents with differential sensitivity between the two subgroups of SCLC, we were intrigued to see if we could use information about the drug targets to identify targets common to multiple drugs. Adapting our clustering data, as expression of TTF1 is bimodal, we segregated the cell lines into two groups (TTF1 high and low) and identified drugs that had a minimum three-fold difference in mean IC_{50} between TTF1 high and low cell lines. We then used an in-house curated drug target database that includes the primary, secondary, and tertiary targets of a given agent to generate a "Drug-TargEt ConsTellation map" (DTECT map—Figure 3). The DTECT map identified multiple common targets including Aurora Kinase and the PI3K/mTOR pathway, similar to the group-based analysis (Figure 2), confirming the validity of the approach. DTECT mapping is an approach that can be used to identify high priority drug targets in any situation where cell lines can be dichotomized on the basis of gene or protein expression, or other statuses such as epithelial versus mesenchymal. The Aurora Kinase inhibitor alisertib has shown pre-clinical and clinical activity in a number of cancer types, including SCLC [33,34]. However, in a phase II study of paclitaxel with alisertib or placebo in an unselected relapsed/refractory SCLC cohort, treatment with alisertib did not improve response rates or survival [35]. As our sub-group comparisons, as well as DTECT mapping using both TTF1 and cMYC expression, had all indicated that Aurora Kinase inhibition was more effective in cMYC high SCLC cell lines, we performed a supervised analysis of candidate proteomic biomarkers of response to single agent alisertib in a panel of 51 SCLC cell lines [31]. Using two approaches (correlating IC_{50} values to protein expression, and comparing protein expression between the most and least sensitive models), high cMYC expression was the top biomarker of sensitivity to alisertib. A retrospective analysis of biopsies from patients enrolled in the phase II trial of alisertib, based on our preliminary data, showed a strong association between cMYC protein expression and improved progression free survival, validating our pre-clinical analyses, despite only being evaluable in a small number of patients [35]. Alisertib is no longer in clinical development for SCLC, in large part because of the lack of efficacy in the unselected phase II trial. An alternative study in an SCLC population selected for patients with tumors that express high levels of cMYC or low TTF1 (for which CLIA certified assays are available) may have yielded a positive outcome and highlights the utility of high-throughput biomarker discovery in the development and subsequent use of novel therapeutics.

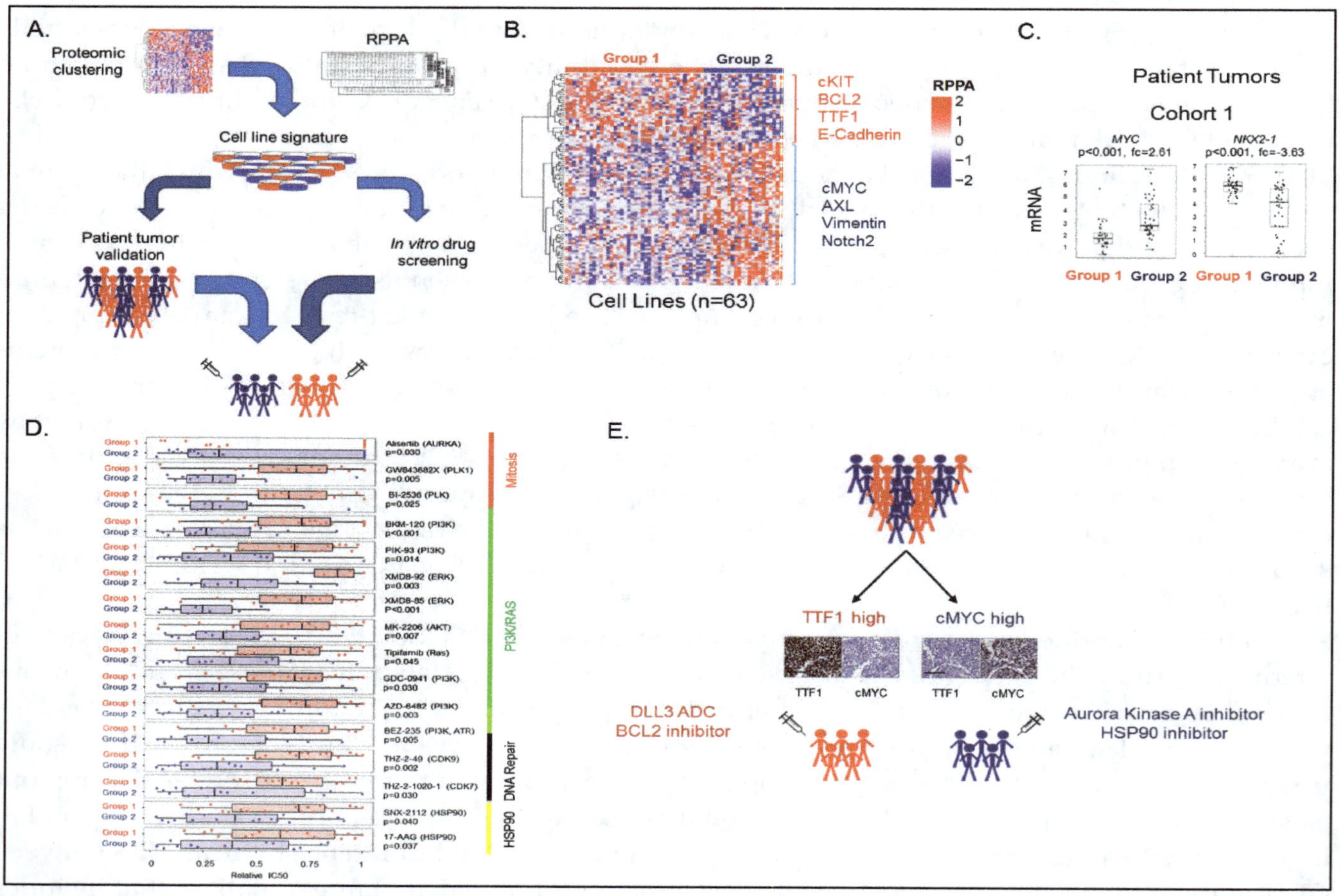

Figure 2. Proteomic subtyping of SCLC. Schematic of how SCLC was divided into two molecular subgroups using proteomic profiling data from 63 cell lines (**A**). Supervised hierarchical analysis shows distant protein expression patterns between the two cell line subgroups (**B**). Comparison of *MYC* and *NKX2-1* expression between the two subsets in patient tumors (**C**). Comparison of relative IC_{50} values between the two subsets shows group 2 (TTF1 low) to be more sensitive to a range of targeted agents (**D**). Working model of how SCLC patients may be divided into two groups (**E**) based on immunohistochemistry (IHC) tests currently in clinical use with different therapeutic vulnerabilities between the groups. Adapted from Cardnell et al 2017 [31]. RPPA—reverse phase protein array.

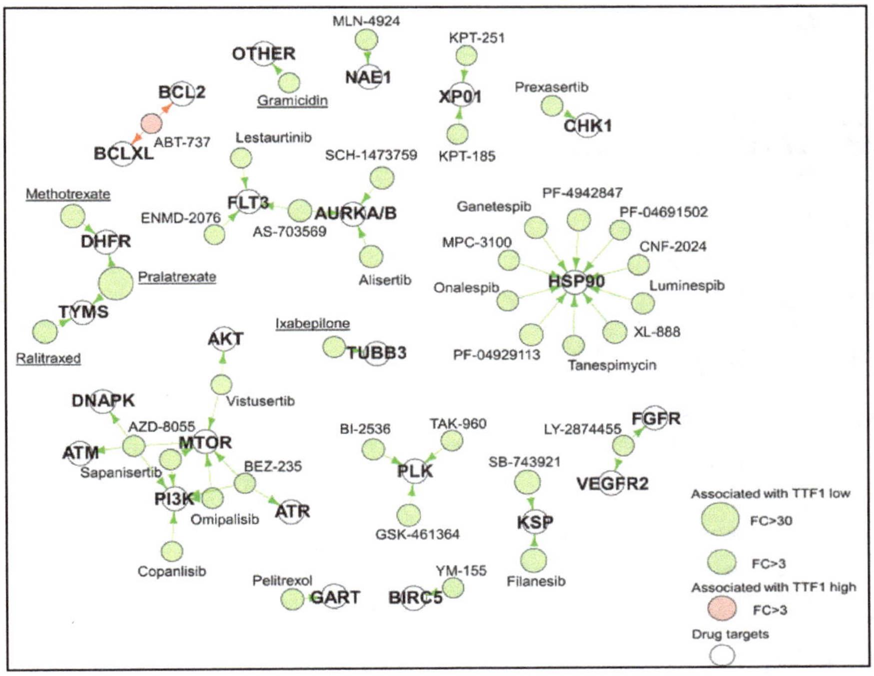

Figure 3. Drug-target constellation (DTECT) mapping. DTECT map of drugs differentially sensitive between TTF1 high and low SCLC cell line (Fold Change (FC) > 3.0, $p < 0.001$). Drugs with differential sensitivity are mapped by their primary, secondary, and tertiary targets. Underlined drugs are either FDA approved or licensed for use in Canada/Europe. Adapted from Cardnell et al. 2017 [31].

3.3. DISARM

Over recent years, a tremendous quantity of publically available drug-sensitivity data has been generated using a plethora of therapeutic agents across multiple cancer types [30,32,36–38]. Our tools and approaches to utilizing this data have, however, not developed at the same rate. Pre-clinical data generated in unselected populations may result in potential therapies being discarded because of their lack of efficacy in the overall population despite their potential efficacy in a targeted population (e.g., Aurora Kinase inhibitors in MYC high SCLC). Similarly, answering the supposedly simple question of, "if a group of tumor models are resistant to a given drug, to what are they sensitive?" is not easily addressed and is often unintentionally biased by the researchers' pre-existing knowledge. To address this, we developed DISARM (Differential Sensitivity Analysis for Resistant Malignancies), a bioinformatics tool designed to identify drugs with efficacy in models that are resistant to a reference drug [39]. DISARM operates by comparing IC_{50} values for two drugs (the reference and candidate drugs), placing them into a 2×2 table to identify instances in which a significant number of models are sensitive to a candidate drug and are resistant to the reference drug (Figure 4A). DISARM calculates a score—the DISARM score—for each drug combination that follows a standard distribution. A higher DISARM score corresponds to a higher significance level, the minimum score is zero and, while there is no theoretical maximum to the score, a score of ≥ 2 is considered to be meaningful. This approach was validated using two clinical paradigms where there is an approved treatment option (candidate drug) for patients with tumors resistant to standard of care (reference drug). One such scenario is the treatment of metastatic NSCLC with exon 19 deletions or *L858R* mutations in *EGFR*. Here, SOC therapy includes the tyrosine kinase (TKI) inhibitor erlotinib (EGFR inhibitor), to which resistance invariably develops, approximately half of which occurs through the acquisition of an additional *T790M* mutation in *EGFR*. A second generation EGFR inhibitor—osimertinib—is, however, effective in patients with *EGFR T970M* erlotinib-resistance mutations. Using response values to both erlotinib and osimertinib from a previous study [40], DISARM successfully identified osimertinib as a candidate for cell lines with *T970M EGFR* mutations (Figure 4A).

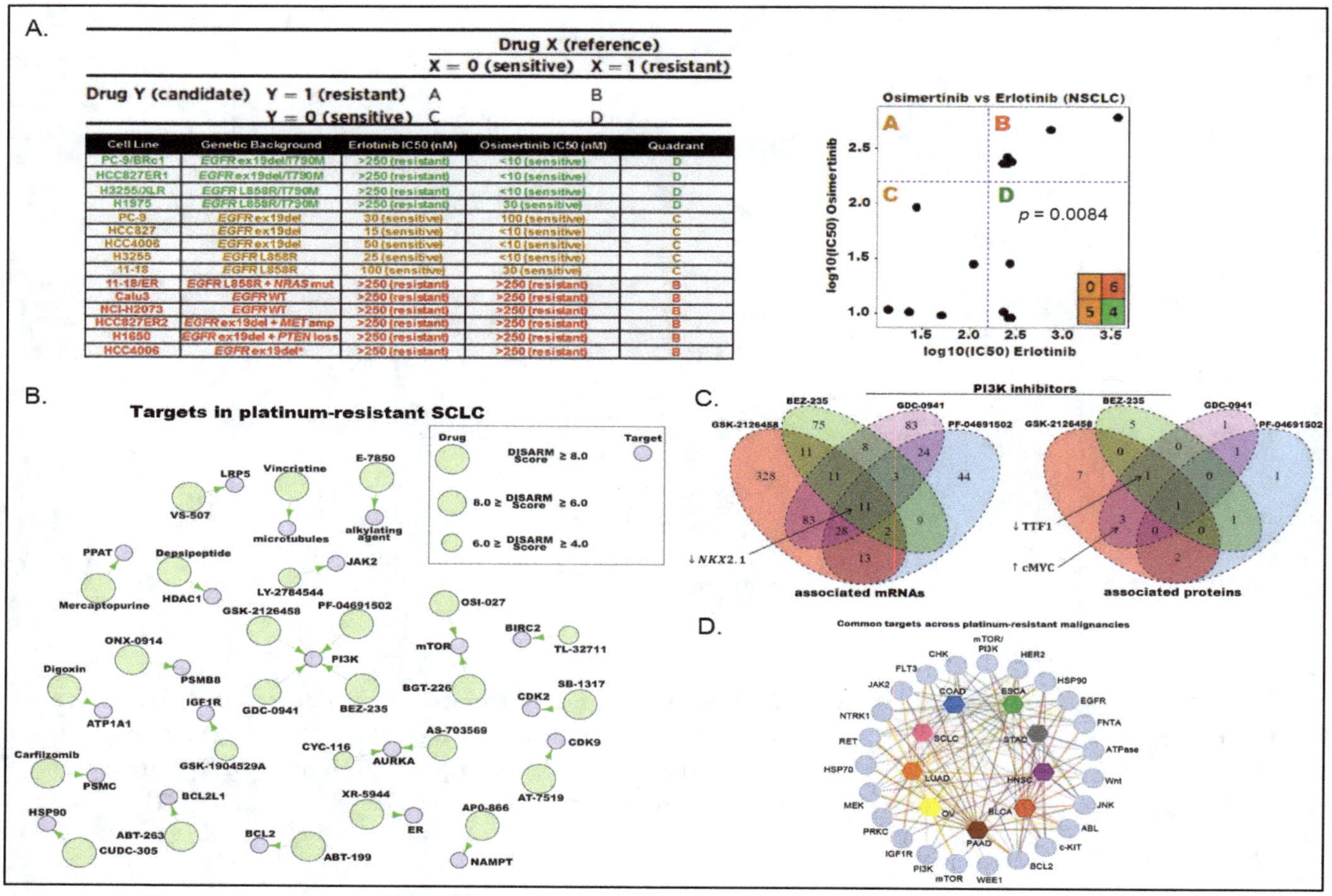

Figure 4. DISARM. DISARM places cell lines, based on IC_{50} data, into a 2 × 2 grid. Using data for erlotinib (reference) and osimertinib (candidate), DISARM correctly identifies osimertinib as a candidate drug in erlotinib-resistant *EGFR T970M* mutant NSCLC (**A**). DTECT mapping of top candidate drugs identified by DISARM in cisplatin-resistant SCLC (**B**). Venn diagrams depicting shared mRNA and protein biomarkers of sensitivity to multiple PI3K inhibitors in platinum-resistant SCLC (**C**). Map demonstrating the interrelatedness of drug targets identified as candidate drugs for cisplatin-resistant disease across multiple cancer types (**D**). Adapted from Gay et al. 2018 [39].

We subsequently used DISARM to interrogate data from a large NCI funded drug screen effort in SCLC [30]. Using sensitivity to platinum, the backbone to all frontline SOC treatments for SCLC [41] to which resistance develops rapidly and almost universally, as the reference drug, we applied DISARM to the problem of platinum-resistance in SCLC. Using cisplatin sensitivity data from our laboratory and data from 526 FDA approved an investigational anti-cancer agent [30], DISARM selected 31 candidate drugs (including 26 with defined molecular targets) for use in platinum-resistant SCLC. The 26 candidate drugs with defined molecular targets, all of which had DISARM scores ≥4.0 were then plotted using a DTECT map of their primary target, which revealed a number of common targets including PI3K, mTOR, and Aurora Kinase A (Figure 4B). We then tested if cell lines identified by DISARM on the basis of their sensitivity to a candidate drugs targeting the same molecule shared common biomarkers of sensitivity. Comparing mRNA [30] and protein expression data [27,42] between cell lines identified as sensitive and resistant by DISARM, we identified low expression of the gene *NKX2-1* and its protein (TTF1) as common markers of sensitivity to PI3K inhibitors (Figure 4C), in agreement with our proteomic subtyping of SCLC (Figure 2D) [31].

As platinum-resistance is not unique to SCLC, we expanded our analysis to include nine solid tumor types for which platinum-based therapy is an established frontline therapy according to National Comprehensive Cancer Network (NCCN) guidelines [43]. These included SCLC, NSCLC, stomach adenocarcinoma (STAD), pancreatic adenocarcinoma (PAAD), ovarian (OV), head and neck squamous cell carcinoma (HSC), esophageal carcinoma (ESCA), colon adenocarcinoma (COAD), and bladder carcinoma (BLCA). Using IC_{50} data for 138 drugs for which there were adequate data across these nine tumor types in the GDSC database [32], we used DISARM to identify common drugs and drug targets across cisplatin-resistant models of different tumor types (Figure 4D). Although sensitivity to many candidate drugs varies between cisplatin-sensitive and -resistant disease for many tumor types, some patterns did emerge. For example, vinblastine and etoposide consistently performed better in cisplatin-resistant models, with DISARM scores of ≥ 2 in 4/7 and 5/7 tumor types tested, respectively. DISARM analyses also revealed a number of common drug targets across multiple platinum-resistant malignancies including PI3K, mTOR, MEK, BCL-2, and HSP-90.

In order to make DISARM available to the broader cancer research community, we also developed a Java-Script based webtool to all investigators to query the available databases with a disease, reference drug, and cut-offs for sensitivity of their choice. The DISARM web-based tool is available at http://ibl.mdanderson.org/DISARM/index. The analyses presented here and in the DISARM manuscript are only the beginning of how this approach can be used to interrogate in vitro data from datasets that are yet to be incorporated, such as the Connectivity Map [44] and from individual investigators. While not yet explored in our analyses, DISARM has the potential to be applied beyond the setting of in vitro drug response data. If properly adapted and validated, DISARM-like approaches could be applied in the analysis of in vivo drug response data using parameters such as tumor volume or $\Delta T/\Delta C$ in lieu of IC_{50} values. Taking the concept further, scenarios in which DISARM could be used in the analysis of clinical data combining together tumor types with shared drug resistance can also be envisioned.

4. Conclusions

The approaches reviewed here represent the work of a large multi-disciplinary team that utilized large datasets to develop approaches for the unbiased classification of models/tumors and identification of novel candidate drugs. These approaches have incorporated both large cell line datasets (proteomic profiling, transcriptomic data, genomic data, and drug sensitivity data) from multiple sources along with patient derived data (transcriptomic, genomic, immunohistochemical, and clinical) from large collaborative efforts (TCGA), publically available data (George et al., Sato et al.; [7,8]), as well as clinical trials (BATTLE-1, BATTLE-2, PROSPECT; [18,21,45]) from multiple cancer types. One example of how these and related approaches have altered our approach to the treatment of lung cancer patients is the discovery of SLFN11 as a biomarker of response to PARP inhibition in SCLC. A proteomic comparison of NSCLC and SCLC led to the initial discovery of PARP1 as a potential therapeutic target in SCLC [42], which was validated in vitro, in vivo, and in SCLC patients [46,47]. Further biomarker analysis using proteomic and transcriptomic profiling data in combination with response data to PARP inhibition in cell lines and PDX models led to the identification of SLFN11 as a biomarker of response [48]. Subsequent retrospective analysis of biopsies from patients enrolled in a Phase II study of temozolomide with or without veliparib (a PARP inhibitor) showed a survival advantage for patients with SLFN11 positive tumors (by IHC) who received veliparib [49].

The tools developed by the University of Texas MD Anderson Lung Cancer Multidisciplinary Program have been highly productive for advancing our understanding of both thoracic and extra-thoracic cancers, particular in expanding our knowledge of the mechanisms of resistance to treatment and identifying new treatment options for patients for whom no treatment options currently exist. These tools, used in the context of multi-disciplinary teams, have the potential to be further leveraged to explore a variety of questions about the biology of lung and other cancers, but most importantly, have the potential to translate into novel, biomarker-driven, personalized treatments for our patients.

Acknowledgments: The authors would like to acknowledge the key members of the Lung Cancer Multidisciplinary Program, without who these studies could not have been conducted, including John V. Heymach, Ignacio I. Wistuba, Jack Roth, Bonnie S. Glisson, Don L. Gibbons, Vali Papadimitrakopoulou, Junya Fujimoto, Lixia Diao, Pan Tong, Lerong Li, C. Allison Stewart, and Carl M. Gay.

References

1. Tong, P.; Diao, L.; Shen, L.; Li, L.; Heymach, J.V.; Girard, L.; Minna, J.D.; Coombes, K.R.; Byers, L.A.; Wang, J. Selecting Reliable mRNA Expression Measurements Across Platforms Improves Downstream Analysis. *Cancer Inform.* **2016**, *15*, 81–89. [CrossRef] [PubMed]
2. Tong, P.; Coombes, K.R.; Johnson, F.M.; Byers, L.A.; Diao, L.; Liu, D.D.; Lee, J.J.; Heymach, J.V.; Wang, J. drexplorer: A tool to explore dose-response relationships and drug-drug interactions. *Bioinformatics* **2015**, *31*, 1692–1694. [CrossRef] [PubMed]
3. University of Alabama School of Medicine. MacSynergy II. Available online: http://www.uab.edu/medicine/peds/macsynergy (accessed on 11 January 2019).
4. Bliss, C. The toxicity of poisons applied jointly. *Ann. Appl. Biol.* **1939**, *26*, 585–615. [CrossRef]
5. Chou, T.C.; Talalay, P. Quantitative analysis of dose-effect relationships: The combined effects of multiple drugs or enzyme inhibitors. *Adv. Enzyme Regul.* **1984**, *22*, 27–55. [CrossRef]
6. Prichard, M.N.; Shipman, C., Jr. A three-dimensional model to analyze drug-drug interactions. *Antivir. Res.* **1990**, *14*, 181–205. [CrossRef]
7. George, J.; Lim, J.S.; Jang, S.J.; Cun, Y.; Ozretic, L.; Kong, G.; Leenders, F.; Lu, X.; Fernandez-Cuesta, L.; Bosco, G.; et al. Comprehensive genomic profiles of small cell lung cancer. *Nature* **2015**, *524*, 47–53. [CrossRef] [PubMed]
8. Sato, T.; Kaneda, A.; Tsuji, S.; Isagawa, T.; Yamamoto, S.; Fujita, T.; Yamanaka, R.; Tanaka, Y.; Nukiwa, T.; Marquez, V.E.; et al. PRC2 overexpression and PRC2-target gene repression relating to poorer prognosis in small cell lung cancer. *Sci. Rep.* **2013**, *3*, 1911. [CrossRef] [PubMed]
9. TCGA. Available online: https://cancergenome.nih.gov/ (accessed on 11 January 2019).
10. NCBI. Available online: https://www.ncbi.nlm.nih.gov/ (accessed on 11 January 2019).
11. CCLE. Available online: https://portals.broadinstitute.org/ccle (accessed on 11 January 2019).
12. GDSC. Available online: https://www.cancerrxgene.org/ (accessed on 11 January 2019).
13. NCI-DTP. Available online: http://sclccelllines.cancer.gov/ (accessed on 11 January 2019).
14. DISARM. Available online: http://ibl.mdanderson.org/DISARM/index.html (accessed on 11 January 2019).
15. Larue, L.; Bellacosa, A. Epithelial–mesenchymal transition in development and cancer: Role of phosphatidylinositol 3′ kinase/AKT pathways. *Oncogene* **2005**, *24*, 7443. [CrossRef]
16. Radisky, D.C. Epithelial-mesenchymal transition. *J. Cell Sci.* **2005**, *118*, 4325–4326. [CrossRef]
17. Byers, L.A.; Diao, L.; Wang, J.; Saintigny, P.; Girard, L.; Peyton, M.; Shen, L.; Fan, Y.; Giri, U.; Tumula, P.K.; et al. An epithelial-mesenchymal transition gene signature predicts resistance to EGFR and PI3K inhibitors and identifies Axl as a therapeutic target for overcoming EGFR inhibitor resistance. *Clin. Cancer Res.* **2013**, *19*, 279–290. [CrossRef]
18. Kim, E.S.; Herbst, R.S.; Wistuba, I.I.; Lee, J.J.; Blumenschein, G.R., Jr.; Tsao, A.; Stewart, D.J.; Hicks, M.E.; Erasmus, J., Jr.; Gupta, S.; et al. The BATTLE trial: Personalizing therapy for lung cancer. *Cancer Discov.* **2011**, *1*, 44–53. [CrossRef] [PubMed]
19. Mak, M.P.; Tong, P.; Diao, L.; Cardnell, R.J.; Gibbons, D.L.; William, W.N.; Skoulidis, F.; Parra, E.R.; Rodriguez-Canales, J.; Wistuba, I.I.; et al. A Patient-Derived, Pan-Cancer EMT Signature Identifies Global Molecular Alterations and Immune Target Enrichment Following Epithelial-to-Mesenchymal Transition. *Clin. Cancer Res.* **2016**, *22*, 609–620. [CrossRef] [PubMed]
20. Chen, L.; Gibbons, D.L.; Goswami, S.; Cortez, M.A.; Ahn, Y.H.; Byers, L.A.; Zhang, X.; Yi, X.; Dwyer, D.; Lin, W.; et al. Metastasis is regulated via microRNA-200/ZEB1 axis control of tumour cell PD-L1 expression and intratumoral immunosuppression. *Nat. Commun.* **2014**, *5*, 5241. [CrossRef] [PubMed]
21. Tang, X.; Kadara, H.; Behrens, C.; Liu, D.D.; Xiao, Y.; Rice, D.; Gazdar, A.F.; Fujimoto, J.; Moran, C.; Varella-Garcia, M.; et al. Abnormalities of the TITF-1 lineage-specific oncogene in NSCLC: Implications in lung cancer pathogenesis and prognosis. *Clin. Cancer Res.* **2011**, *17*, 2434–2443. [CrossRef] [PubMed]

22. Ilie, M.; Hofman, V.; Dietel, M.; Soria, J.C.; Hofman, P. Assessment of the PD-L1 status by immunohistochemistry: Challenges and perspectives for therapeutic strategies in lung cancer patients. *Virchows Arch.* **2016**, *468*, 511–525. [CrossRef] [PubMed]
23. Tabchy, A.; Hennessy, B.T.; Gonzalez-Angulo, A.M.; Bernstam, F.M.; Lu, Y.; Mills, G.B. Quantitative proteomic analysis in breast cancer. *Drugs Today* **2011**, *47*, 169–182. [CrossRef] [PubMed]
24. Tibes, R.; Qiu, Y.; Lu, Y.; Hennessy, B.; Andreeff, M.; Mills, G.B.; Kornblau, S.M. Reverse phase protein array: Validation of a novel proteomic technology and utility for analysis of primary leukemia specimens and hematopoietic stem cells. *Mol. Cancer Ther.* **2006**, *5*, 2512–2521. [CrossRef] [PubMed]
25. Lu, Y.; Ling, S.; Hegde, A.M.; Byers, L.A.; Coombes, K.; Mills, G.B.; Akbani, R. Using reverse-phase protein arrays as pharmacodynamic assays for functional proteomics, biomarker discovery, and drug development in cancer. *Semin. Oncol.* **2016**, *43*, 476–483. [CrossRef] [PubMed]
26. Zagouri, F.; Bago-Horvath, Z.; Rossler, F.; Brandstetter, A.; Bartsch, R.; Papadimitriou, C.A.; Dimitrakakis, C.; Tsigginou, A.; Papaspyrou, I.; Giannos, A.; et al. High MET expression is an adverse prognostic factor in patients with triple-negative breast cancer. *Br. J. Cancer* **2013**, *108*, 1100–1105. [CrossRef]
27. Cardnell, R.J.; Feng, Y.; Mukherjee, S.; Diao, L.; Tong, P.; Stewart, C.A.; Masrorpour, F.; Fan, Y.; Nilsson, M.; Shen, Y.; et al. Activation of the PI3K/mTOR Pathway following PARP Inhibition in Small Cell Lung Cancer. *PLoS ONE* **2016**, *11*, e0152584. [CrossRef]
28. Fraley, C.; Raferty, A. MCLUST: Software for model-based cluster analysis. *J. Classif.* **1999**, *16*, 297–306. [CrossRef]
29. Fraley, C.; Raferty, A. Enhanced model-based clustering, density estimation, and discriminant analysis software: MCLUST. *J. Classif.* **2003**, *20*, 263–286. [CrossRef]
30. Polley, E.; Kunkel, M.; Evans, D.; Silvers, T.; Delosh, R.; Laudeman, J.; Ogle, C.; Reinhart, R.; Selby, M.; Connelly, J.; et al. Small Cell Lung Cancer Screen of Oncology Drugs, Investigational Agents, and Gene and microRNA Expression. *J. Natl. Cancer Inst.* **2016**, *108*. [CrossRef] [PubMed]
31. Cardnell, R.J.; Li, L.; Sen, T.; Bara, R.; Tong, P.; Fujimoto, J.; Ireland, A.S.; Guthrie, M.R.; Bheddah, S.; Banerjee, U.; et al. Protein expression of TTF1 and cMYC define distinct molecular subgroups of small cell lung cancer with unique vulnerabilities to aurora kinase inhibition, DLL3 targeting, and other targeted therapies. *Oncotarget* **2017**, *8*, 73419–73432. [CrossRef] [PubMed]
32. Yang, W.; Soares, J.; Greninger, P.; Edelman, E.J.; Lightfoot, H.; Forbes, S.; Bindal, N.; Beare, D.; Smith, J.A.; Thompson, I.R.; et al. Genomics of Drug Sensitivity in Cancer (GDSC): A resource for therapeutic biomarker discovery in cancer cells. *Nucleic Acids Res.* **2013**, *41*, D955-961. [CrossRef] [PubMed]
33. Niu, H.; Manfredi, M.; Ecsedy, J.A. Scientific Rationale Supporting the Clinical Development Strategy for the Investigational Aurora A Kinase Inhibitor Alisertib in Cancer. *Front. Oncol.* **2015**, *5*, 189. [CrossRef]
34. Melichar, B.; Adenis, A.; Lockhart, A.C.; Bennouna, J.; Dees, E.C.; Kayaleh, O.; Obermannova, R.; DeMichele, A.; Zatloukal, P.; Zhang, B.; et al. Safety and activity of alisertib, an investigational aurora kinase A inhibitor, in patients with breast cancer, small-cell lung cancer, non-small-cell lung cancer, head and neck squamous-cell carcinoma, and gastro-oesophageal adenocarcinoma: A five-arm phase 2 study. *Lancet Oncol.* **2015**, *16*, 395–405. [CrossRef]
35. Owonikoko, T.; Nackaerts, K.; Scoszi, T.; Ostoros, G.; Baik, C.; Mark, Z.; Ullmann, C.D.; Niu, H.; Sheldon-Waniga, E.; Leonard, E.J.; et al. Randomized Phase 2 Study of the Investigational Aurora A Kinase (AAK) Inhibitor Alisertib (MLN8237) + Paclitaxel versus Placebo + Paclitaxel as Second-Line Therapy for Small Cell Lung Cancer (SCLC). *Ann. Oncol.* **2016**, *27*. [CrossRef]
36. Barretina, J.; Caponigro, G.; Stransky, N.; Venkatesan, K.; Margolin, A.A.; Kim, S.; Wilson, C.J.; Lehar, J.; Kryukov, G.V.; Sonkin, D.; et al. The Cancer Cell Line Encyclopedia enables predictive modelling of anticancer drug sensitivity. *Nature* **2012**, *483*, 603–607. [CrossRef]
37. Holbeck, S.L.; Collins, J.M.; Doroshow, J.H. Analysis of Food and Drug Administration-approved anticancer agents in the NCI60 panel of human tumor cell lines. *Mol. Cancer Ther.* **2010**, *9*, 1451–1460. [CrossRef]
38. Teicher, B.A.; Silvers, T.; Selby, M.; Delosh, R.; Laudeman, J.; Ogle, C.; Reinhart, R.; Parchment, R.; Krushkal, J.; Sonkin, D.; et al. Small cell lung carcinoma cell line screen of etoposide/carboplatin plus a third agent. *Cancer Med.* **2017**, *6*, 1952–1964. [CrossRef] [PubMed]
39. Gay, C.M.; Tong, P.; Cardnell, R.J.; Sen, T.; Su, X.; Ma, J.; Bara, R.O.; Johnson, F.M.; Wakefield, C.; Heymach, J.V.; et al. Differential Sensitivity Analysis for Resistant Malignancies (DISARM) Identifies Common Candidate Therapies across Platinum-Resistant Cancers. *Clin. Cancer Res.* **2018**. [CrossRef] [PubMed]

40. Cross, D.A.; Ashton, S.E.; Ghiorghiu, S.; Eberlein, C.; Nebhan, C.A.; Spitzler, P.J.; Orme, J.P.; Finlay, M.R.; Ward, R.A.; Mellor, M.J.; et al. AZD9291, an irreversible EGFR TKI, overcomes T790M-mediated resistance to EGFR inhibitors in lung cancer. *Cancer Discov.* **2014**, *4*, 1046–1061. [CrossRef] [PubMed]
41. NCCN. Available online: http://www.nccn.org/professionals/physician_gls/pdf/sclc.pdf (accessed on 11 January 2019).
42. Byers, L.A.; Wang, J.; Nilsson, M.B.; Fujimoto, J.; Saintigny, P.; Yordy, J.; Giri, U.; Peyton, M.; Fan, Y.H.; Diao, L.; et al. Proteomic Profiling Identifies Dysregulated Pathways in Small Cell Lung Cancer and Novel Therapeutic Targets Including PARP1. *Cancer Discov.* **2012**, *2*, 798–811. [CrossRef] [PubMed]
43. NCCN. Available online: https://www.nccn.org/professionals/physician_gls/default.aspx (accessed on 11 January 2019).
44. Subramanian, A.; Narayan, R.; Corsello, S.M.; Peck, D.D.; Natoli, T.E.; Lu, X.; Gould, J.; Davis, J.F.; Tubelli, A.A.; Asiedu, J.K.; et al. A Next Generation Connectivity Map: L1000 Platform and the First 1,000,000 Profiles. *Cell* **2017**, *171*, 1437–1452. [CrossRef] [PubMed]
45. Papadimitrakopoulou, V.; Lee, J.J.; Wistuba, I.I.; Tsao, A.S.; Fossella, F.V.; Kalhor, N.; Gupta, S.; Byers, L.A.; Izzo, J.G.; Gettinger, S.N.; et al. The BATTLE-2 Study: A Biomarker-Integrated Targeted Therapy Study in Previously Treated Patients With Advanced Non-Small-Cell Lung Cancer. *J. Clin. Oncol.* **2016**, *34*, 3638–3647. [CrossRef] [PubMed]
46. Cardnell, R.J.; Feng, Y.; Diao, L.; Fan, Y.H.; Masrorpour, F.; Wang, J.; Shen, Y.; Mills, G.B.; Minna, J.D.; Heymach, J.V.; et al. Proteomic markers of DNA repair and PI3K pathway activation predict response to the PARP inhibitor BMN 673 in small cell lung cancer. *Clin. Cancer Res.* **2013**, *19*, 6322–6328. [CrossRef] [PubMed]
47. de Bono, J.; Ramanathan, R.K.; Mina, L.; Chugh, R.; Glaspy, J.; Rafii, S.; Kaye, S.; Sachdev, J.; Heymach, J.; Smith, D.C.; et al. Phase I, Dose-Escalation, Two-Part Trial of the PARP Inhibitor Talazoparib in Patients with Advanced Germline BRCA1/2 Mutations and Selected Sporadic Cancers. *Cancer Discov.* **2017**, *7*, 620–629. [CrossRef]
48. Stewart, C.A.; Tong, P.; Cardnell, R.J.; Sen, T.; Li, L.; Gay, C.M.; Masrorpour, F.; Fan, Y.; Bara, R.O.; Feng, Y.; et al. Dynamic variations in epithelial-to-mesenchymal transition (EMT), ATM, and SLFN11 govern response to PARP inhibitors and cisplatin in small cell lung cancer. *Oncotarget* **2017**, *8*, 28575–28587. [CrossRef] [PubMed]
49. Pietanza, M.C.; Waqar, S.N.; Krug, L.M.; Dowlati, A.; Hann, C.L.; Chiappori, A.; Owonikoko, T.K.; Woo, K.M.; Cardnell, R.J.; Fujimoto, J.; et al. Randomized, Double-Blind, Phase II Study of Temozolomide in Combination with Either Veliparib or Placebo in Patients with Relapsed-Sensitive or Refractory Small-Cell Lung Cancer. *J. Clin. Oncol.* **2018**, *36*, 2386–2394. [CrossRef]

The Presence of Concomitant Mutations Affects the Activity of EGFR Tyrosine Kinase Inhibitors in EGFR-Mutant Non-Small Cell Lung Cancer (NSCLC) Patients

Anna Maria Rachiglio [1,†], Francesca Fenizia [1,†], Maria Carmela Piccirillo [2,†], Domenico Galetta [3], Lucio Crinò [4], Bruno Vincenzi [5], Emiddio Barletta [6], Carmine Pinto [7], Francesco Ferraù [8], Matilde Lambiase [1], Agnese Montanino [9], Cristin Roma [1], Vienna Ludovini [10], Elisabetta Sara Montagna [3], Antonella De Luca [1], Gaetano Rocco [11,‡], Gerardo Botti [12], Francesco Perrone [2], Alessandro Morabito [9] and Nicola Normanno [1,*]

1 Cell Biology and Biotherapy Unit, Istituto Nazionale Tumori-IRCCS-Fondazione G. Pascale, 80131 Naples, Italy; anmarachiglio@yahoo.it (A.M.R.); francesca.fenizia@hotmail.it (F.F.); matilde.lambiase@libero.it (M.L.); cristin.roma@gmail.com (C.R.); antoneldel@hotmail.com (A.D.L.)
2 Clinical Trials Unit, Istituto Nazionale Tumori-IRCCS-Fondazione G. Pascale, 80131 Naples, Italy; m.piccirillo@istitutotumori.na.it (M.C.P.); f.perrone@istitutotumori.na.it (F.P.)
3 Medical Oncology, National Cancer Research Center "Giovanni Paolo II", 70126 Bari, Italy; galetta@oncologico.bari.it (D.G.); es.montagna@libero.it (E.S.M.)
4 Istituto Scientifico per lo Studio e la Cura dei Tumori (IRST), 47014 Meldola (FC), Italy; lucio.crino@irst.emr.it
5 Medical Oncology, Campus Bio-Medico University of Rome, 00128 Rome, Italy; b.vincenzi@unicampus.it
6 Medical Oncology, "G. Rummo" Hospital, 82100 Benevento, Italy; emiddiobarletta@libero.it
7 Medical Oncology, AUSL-IRCCS di Reggio Emilia, 42123 Reggio Emilia, Italy; carmine.pinto@asmn.re.it
8 Medical Oncology, "S. Vincenzo" Hospital, 98039 Taormina (ME), Italy; francescoferrau@tin.it
9 Medical Oncology, Thoraco-Pulmonary Department, Istituto Nazionale Tumori-IRCCS-Fondazione G. Pascale, 80131 Naples, Italy; a.montanino@istitutotumori.na.it (A.M.); a.morabito@istitutotumori.na.it (A.M.)
10 Department of Medical Oncology, Santa Maria della Misericordia Hospital, 06129 Perugia, Italy; oncolab@hotmail.com
11 Thoracic Surgery, Thoraco-Pulmonary Department, Istituto Nazionale Tumori-IRCCS-Fondazione G. Pascale, 80131 Naples, Italy; g.rocco@istitutotumori.na.it
12 Surgical Pathology Unit, Istituto Nazionale Tumori-IRCCS-Fondazione G. Pascale, 80131 Naples, Italy; g.botti@istitutotumori.na.it
* Correspondence: n.normanno@istitutotumori.na.it or nicnorm@yahoo.com; Tel./Fax: +39-081-5903826
† These authors equally contributed to the paper.
‡ Thoracic Service, Department of Surgery, Memorial Sloan-Kettering Cancer Center, 1275 York Avenue, New York, NY 10065, USA.

Abstract: Recent findings suggest that a fraction of EGFR-mutant non-small-cell lung cancers (NSCLC) carry additional driver mutations that could potentially affect the activity of EGFR tyrosine kinase inhibitors (TKIs). We investigated the role of concomitant KRAS, NRAS, BRAF, PIK3CA, MET and ERBB2 mutations (other mutations) on the outcome of 133 EGFR mutant patients, who received first-line therapy with EGFR TKIs between June 2008 and December 2014. Analysis of genomic DNA by Next Generation Sequencing (NGS) revealed the presence of hotspot mutations in genes other than the EGFR, including KRAS, NRAS, BRAF, ERBB2, PIK3CA, or MET, in 29/133 cases (21.8%). A p.T790M mutation was found in 9/133 tumour samples (6.8%). The progression free survival (PFS) of patients without other mutations was 11.3 months vs. 7 months in patients with other mutations (log-rank test univariate: $p = 0.047$). In a multivariate Cox regression model including the presence of other mutations, age, performance status, smoking status, and the presence of p.T790M mutations, the presence of other mutations was the only factor significantly associated with PFS (Hazard Ratio

1.63, 95% CI 1.04–2.58; $p = 0.035$). In contrast, no correlation was found between TP53 mutations and patients' outcome. These data suggest that a subgroup of EGFR mutant tumours have concomitant driver mutations that might affect the activity of first-line EGFR TKIs.

Keywords: lung cancer; EGFR mutations; EGFR TKIs

---

1. Introduction

Non-small-cell lung cancer (NSCLC) with epidermal growth factor receptor (EGFR) mutations has long been regarded as a single entity. However, the response rate of EGFR-mutant patients to first-line EGFR tyrosine kinase inhibitors (TKIs) ranged between 56% and 84% in clinical trials [1]. Accordingly, the duration of the response varies significantly among patients, thus suggesting that EGFR-mutant NSCLC is a heterogeneous group of tumours. In this respect, the mechanisms involved in the acquired resistance to EGFR TKIs have much better been identified as compared with factors affecting the intrinsic sensitivity to EGFR inhibition [2].

Evidence suggests that EGFR mutations are an early event in non-smoke related carcinogenesis of the lung [3]. A number of studies have also shown that EGFR mutations are usually mutually exclusive with other driver mutations. In particular, EGFR and KRAS mutations have been rarely found in the same tumours in early studies of genetic alterations in lung cancer and KRAS mutations are regarded as a biomarker of resistance to EGFR TKIs [4]. Nevertheless, recent reports that used more sensitive techniques of analysis have demonstrated that some EGFR-mutant tumours might also carry mutations in genes that have been up to now classified as mutually exclusive with EGFR and that are potentially involved in either primary or acquired resistance to EGFR TKIs. In particular, co-existence of EGFR mutations with KRAS, NRAS, BRAF, MET, and/or PIK3CA variants has been demonstrated in different studies [5–10].

Case reports showed that patients carrying both EGFR and either KRAS or PIK3CA mutations might benefit from treatment with EGFR TKIs [8,11,12]. In contrast, other studies have suggested that the presence of additional coexisting mutations is associated with a reduced response to EGFR TKIs and with a shorter progression free survival (PFS) [7,13]. A significantly higher frequency of additional mutations in different genes including TP53, KRAS, PIK3CA, BRAF, ERBB2, MET, NRAS, and PTEN, was reported in EGFR mutant patients that did not respond to EGFR TKIs as compared with responders [9]. In addition, patients carrying somatic mutations in the PI3K/AKT/mTOR pathway had a shorter PFS and overall survival (OS) when compared to patients without mutations. Finally, different studies have suggested that mutations in TP53 are associated with shorter PFS in EGFR mutant NSCLC patients receiving treatment with EGFR TKIs [7,13–17].

In this study we analysed by next-generation sequencing (NGS), using a targeted sequencing panel, a cohort of 133 EGFR mutant NSCLC patients, who received first-line therapy with EGFR TKIs. In particular, we assessed whether the presence of concomitant somatic mutations in KRAS, NRAS, BRAF, PIK3CA, MET, and ERBB2 might affect the activity of EGFR TKIs in EGFR mutant NSCLC. We focused on these genetic alterations because they can activate signalling pathways that have been demonstrated in previous studies to be involved in the de novo and/or acquired resistance to EGFR TKIs.

2. Results

2.1. Patients' Characteristics

One hundred and thirty-three consecutive patients with advanced or metastatic EGFR mutant NSCLC treated in seven Italian centres between June 2008 and December 2014 were included in the study. Patients' characteristics are shown in Table 1. Median age was 71 years (range 41–92). As expected in a cohort of EGFR mutant NSCLC, the majority of the patients were women (92/133; 69.2%) and never smokers (81/132; 61.4%). According to EGFR mutation analyses carried with routine diagnostic methods including Real Time PCR and pyrosequencing, an EGFR exon 19 deletion was carried by 83/133 patients (62.4%); 39/133 (29.3%) had an EGFR p.L858R point mutation and 11/133 (8.3%) had different EGFR mutations. Most of the patients included in the study received the EGFR TKI gefitinib as first-line treatment (114/133; 85.7%). Eleven out 133 (8.3%) patients received erlotinib and 8/133 (6.0%) afatinib (Table 1). No statistical differences were observed between the two groups (patients with or without other mutations) with respect to the different clinical and pathological variables, including the type of first-line TKI (Table 1).

Table 1. Patients' characteristics.

Characteristics	All (N = 133)	Pts without Other Mutations (N = 104)	Pts with Other Mutations (N = 29)	*p*-Value
Age, median (range)	71 (41–92)	71 (41–92)	69 (42–84)	0.31 *
Gender, n (%)				
Male	41 (31)	32 (31)	9 (31)	0.98 §
Female	92 (69)	72 (69)	20 (69)	
Smoking habits, n (%)				
Never smoker	81 (61)	63 (61)	18 (62)	0.93 §
Ever smoker	51 (38)	40 (39)	11 (38)	
Unknown	1 (1)	1 (<1)	-	
EGFR mutation type, n (%)				
Exon 19 del	83 (62)	66 (63)	17 (59)	0.36 §
p.L858R	39 (29)	28 (27)	11 (38)	
Other	11 (8)	10 (10)	1 (3)	
1st line EGFR TKI				
Gefitinib	114 (86)	91 (87)	23 (79)	0.47 §
Erlotinib	11 (8)	8 (8)	3 (10)	
Afatinib	8 (6)	5 (5)	3 (10)	

* Kruskal-Wallis test. § Chi square test. Abbreviations: Pts: patients.

2.2. *Mutational Landscape of EGFR Mutant Tumours*

All 133 samples were successfully analysed by targeted sequencing. In 11/133 of cases, this analysis did not detect the EGFR mutation identified in diagnostic routine analysis, probably because of the lower sensitivity of the NGS panel. However, we confirmed the presence of the same EGFR variant found by routine diagnostic methods in all cases using a more sensitive technique such as the droplet digital PCR (ddPCR). All EGFR variants not identified by NGS were at allelic frequencies close to or below 2%, which is the limit of detection of the NGS panel.

Hotspot mutations in either KRAS, NRAS, BRAF, ERBB2, PIK3CA or MET genes were detected in 29/133 cases (21.8%) (Figure 1). A total of 36 mutations were identified, with 5 cases showing more than one variant additional to the EGFR mutation. Very surprisingly, 14/133 cases had an alteration in KRAS gene, which accounted for a consistent part of the total number of mutations detected (14/36 mutations) in genes different from EGFR. Nine PIK3CA mutations were also identified, whereas the other gene mutations showed a much lower frequency. In most cases, the allelic frequency of the other mutations was different as compared with the EGFR variant, suggesting intra-tumour heterogeneity. In particular, in 19 cases the allelic frequency of the EGFR variant was higher, whereas in 10 cases the frequency of the mutation in other genes was higher.

KRAS mutations were identified at an allelic frequency between 2% and 38%. In 13/14 cases with available tumour or plasma samples the presence of the KRAS mutation was confirmed using ddPCR (Table 2). In eight cases the allelic frequency of the KRAS variant was lower than the EGFR alteration; in the remaining six cases, the allelic frequency of EGFR mutations was lower than KRAS. Indeed, the EGFR ddPCR test confirmed that the EGFR alterations not detected by targeted sequencing were at an allelic frequency close to the limit of detection of this latter method (Table 2).

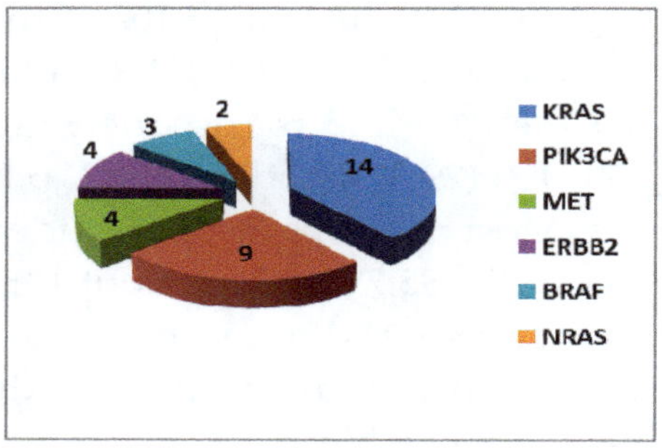

Figure 1. "Other mutations" identified in EGFR-mutant NSCLC cases.

Table 2. KRAS-mutant cases.

PatientID	EGFR		KRAS		PFS	BR
	NGS (VAF)	ddPCR (VAF)	NGS (VAF)	ddPCR (VAF)		
1512#	p.E746_A750del (40%)	-	p.Gly12Cys (3%)	Codon 12/13 mutation (1.93%)	13.19	PR
1616#	p.E746_A750del (58.9%)	-	p.Gly13Asp (11.8%)	Codon 12/13 mutation (10%)	12.3	PR
3426#	mutation not detected	Ex19 del (2.5%)	p.Gly12Asp (38%)	Codon 12/13 mutation (33%)	4.83	SD
3981#	mutation not detected	Ex19 del (1.2%)	p.Gly12Cys (15%)	Codon 12/13 mutation (12%)	2.7	PD
4733#	p.E746_A750 > DP (2.6%)	-	p.Gly12Ala (10.7%)	Codon 12/13 mutation (9.3%)	0.43	PD
4840#	mutation not detected	Ex19 del (0,5%) [1]	p.Gly13Cys (10.1%)	Codon 12/13 mutation (0.4%) [1]	2.14	PD
4990#	mutation not detected	Ex19 del (0.7%)	p.Gly13Cys (28%)	Codon 12/13 mutation (24%)	1.18	PD
5074#	p.E746_A750del (12.8%); p.L858R (16.9%)	-	p.Gly12Cys (3.3%)	Codon 12/13 mutation (0.13%)	3.26	PD
5374#	mutation not detected	Ex19 del (1.8%)	p.Gly12Cys (13.4%)	Codon 12/13 mutation (11%)	4.64	PR
6541#	p.E746_A750del (47.2%)	-	p.Gly13Asp (12.7%)	Codon 12/13 mutation (11.3%)	0.06	NE
6545#	p.L858R (75%)	-	p.Ala59Thr (6.2%)	Tissue and plasma not available	9.87	SD
6548#	p.L858R (55.9%)	-	p.Gln61His (3.3%)	p.Gln61His (0.43%)	6.48	PD
7567#	p.L858R (35.4%); p.T790M (0.9%)	-	p.Gly12Cys (9.2%)	Codon 12/13 mutation (8.7%)	12.43	PR
7964#	p.E746_A750del (56.4%)	-	p.Ala146Thr (2%)	p.Ala146Thr (0.4%)	51.58	CR

[1] test performed on plasma sample. Abbreviations: NGS: next-generation sequencing; VAF: variant allelic frequency; ddPCR: droplet digital PCR, PFS: progression-free survival, in months; BR: best response; PD: progressive disease; SD: stable disease; PR: partial response; CR: complete response; NE: not evaluable.

NGS analysis also revealed the presence of a p.T790M mutation of the EGFR in 9/133 tumour samples (6.8%). In most cases, the frequency of the p.T790M variant was significantly lower as compared with the sensitizing EGFR mutation. The sensitizing and resistance mutations had a similar allelic frequency only in two cases. The p.T790M mutation was detected in 6/9 cases in the initial EGFR analysis performed with diagnostic methods. In the other three cases this variant was not detected because not screened (two cases) or below of the limit of detection (one case). Nevertheless, all patients received treatment with first- or second-generation EGFR TKIs because third-generation EGFR TKIs with activity against the T790M variant was not available at the time of the treatment.

No significant correlation was found between the presence of other mutations and either sex (male vs. female, $p = 0.98$), smoking habit (never-smokers vs. ever-smokers, $p = 0.93$), p.T790M status (p.T790M present vs. absent, $p = 0.39$), or type of EGFR mutation (exon 19 deletions vs. p.L858R vs. other mutations, $p = 0.36$).

Since we used for NGS analysis, a panel that targets 22 genes potentially involved in lung carcinoma, 52 additional variants in genes not included in the primary analysis of this study were also identified (Table S1). In particular, 23 EGFR mutant cases were found to carry mutations in TP53 (17.3%).

2.3. Correlation with Patients' Outcome

At a median follow-up of 36.1 months, 114 PFS events (101 progressions and 13 deaths without documented progression) were recorded. With respect to the mutational status, 88 PFS events were registered among patients without other mutations and 26 in the cohort of patients carrying other mutations. The median PFS of patients without other mutations was 11.3 months vs. seven months in patients with other mutations (Log-rank test univariate: $p = 0.047$) (Figure 2A). Overall, 80 deaths were reported. Median OS was 23.7 months in the group of patients without other mutations and 15.5 months in those with other mutations (Log-rank test univariate: $p = 0.216$) (Figure 2B).

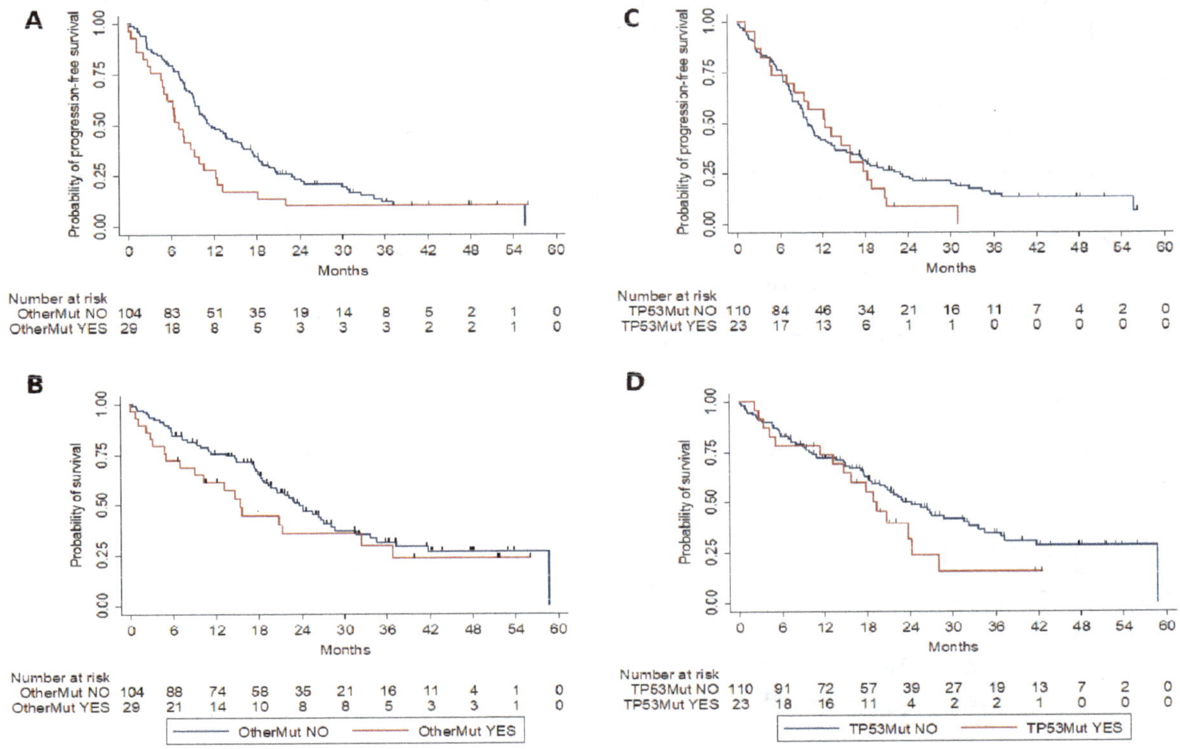

Figure 2. PFS (**A**) and OS (**B**) of EGFR-mutant patients with and without "other mutations"; PFS (**C**) and OS (**D**) of EGFR mutant patients with and without TP53 mutations.

The presence of other mutations did not preclude the possibility of response to EGFR TKIs (Table 3). The median PFS of the different subgroups of patients with specific mutations was generally lower as compared with patients without other mutations (Table 3). However, the small number of patients in these subgroups prevents the possibility of any conclusion.

Table 3. Outcome of patients with and without other mutations.

	No Other Mutation (n = 104)	Any Other Mutation (n = 29)	KRAS MUT (n = 14)	NRAS MUT (n = 2)	BRAF MUT (n = 3)	PIK3CA MUT (n = 9)	ERBB2 MUT (n = 4)	MET MUT (n = 4)
Objective Response Responder, N (%)	71 (68.3%)	17 (58.6%)	6 (42.9%)	2 (100%)	0	7 (77.8%)	1 (25.0%)	4 (100.0%)
Non responder, n (%)	33 (31.7%)	12 (41.4%)	8 (57.1%)	0	3 (100.0%)	2 (22.2%)	3 (75.0%)	0
PFS, months (95% CI)	11.3 (9.4–15.9)	7.0 (4.8–9.9)	4.6 (1.2–12.3)	NA *	3.3 (0.4–NR)	8.7 (5.5–NR)	3.3 (1.2–NR)	6.4 (6.2–NR)
OS, months (95% CI)	23.7 (19.4–28. 1)	15.5 (7.0–32.4)	5.1 (1.2–20.8)	NA *	3.3 (0.8–NR)	36.8 (9.1–NR)	3.3 (2.2–NR)	32.4 (10.3–NR)

NA *: not assessed due to the low number.

Among the KRAS mutant cases, the PFS was significantly shorter in patients with VAF of KRAS mutations higher than EGFR mutations (2.42 months vs. 11.09 months; $p = 0.0081$) as well as the response rate was inferior (16.7% vs. 57.1%). The five patients with more than one variant additional to the EGFR mutation showed a 40% response rate, a median PFS of 5.0 months (95%CI 0.4-NR) and a median OS of 7.0 months (95%CI 0.8–NR), thus confirming the negative predictive value of additional mutations.

In a multivariate Cox regression model including the presence of other mutations, age, performance status, smoking status and the presence of T790M mutations, the presence of other mutations was the only factor significantly associated with PFS (Hazard Ratio -HR 1.63, 95% CI 1.04–2.58; $p = 0.035$) (Table 4). At the same multivariate analysis, the correlation between the presence of other mutations and OS was not statistically significant (HR 1.64, 95% CI 0.96–2.80; $p = 0.072$) (data not shown).

Table 4. Multivariate Cox regression model for PFS.

Variable	HR	95% CI	P
Other mutations	1.63	1.04–2.58	0.03
Sex	0.98	0.6–1.63	0.97
Age	1	0.98–1.02	0.70
Ever smoker	1.22	0.76–1.95	0.41
T790M	1.06	0.53–2.13	0.86

Abbreviations: HR: Hazard ratio.

Since different studies have hypothesized that TP53 mutations might affect the activity of EGFR TKIs, we evaluated the correlation between TP53 variants and survival in our cohort of patients. The median PFS of patients without TP53 mutations was 9.9 months vs. 12.3 months in patients with TP53 mutations (Figure 2C). This difference was not statistically significant at both univariate (HR = 1.25, 95% CI 0.78–1.99; $p = 0.36$) and multivariate (HR = 1.29, 95% CI 0.80–2.08; $p = 0.29$) analysis. Similarly, no significant difference in median OS was observed between patients without (23 months) or with TP53 mutations (18.9 months) (unadjusted HR = 1.45, 95% CI 0.83–2.51, $p = 0.19$; adjusted HR = 1.46 (95% CI 0.83–2.57); $p = 0.19$) (Figure 2D).

3. Discussion

Our results confirm that EGFR-mutant NSCLC is a heterogeneous group of tumours and, in particular, that a fraction of EGFR-mutant tumours carry additional driver mutations. These findings are not surprising because additional driver alterations can be accumulated during tumour progression thus giving rise to tumour heterogeneity [18]. Indeed, driver mutations are almost always clonal, although sub-clonal driver alterations can occur in different tumour types including lung cancer [19,20]. In this respect, it has been recently demonstrated that lung adenocarcinoma contains, on average, 4–7 different clones, with tumours showing >15 clones [21]. We expect that the number of clones and therefore the extent of tumour heterogeneity is higher in tumours with a higher tumour mutation burden. EGFR mutant NSCLC was reported to carry a mean of 4.5 mutations/megabase (Mb) as compared with 9.1 in NSCLC adenocarcinoma [22]. However, the nuclear genome is 3200 Mb and, therefore, EGFR mutant NSCLC do carry a number of somatic variants. A recent study elegantly depicted the intra-tumour heterogeneity of NSCLC [3]. Unfortunately, this study included only 13 EGFR mutant lung carcinoma, thus, providing limited information on the heterogeneity of this subtype of NSCLC. Nevertheless, EGFR mutant tumours with concomitant genetic alterations in PIK3CA, ERBB2, and TP53 were described. In this respect, it must be emphasized that NGS analysis cannot rule out whether the same tumour cell is carrying EGFR mutations and other variants or rather these mutations are present in different sub-clones.

The relative frequency of KRAS mutation in our cohort of EGFR mutant NSCLC was surprisingly high. This might be due to different factors. In contrast with most of European centres, the majority of Italian laboratories do not run the KRAS test before EGFR testing in NSCLC. Therefore, in other countries but not in Italy the EGFR mutation positive population is deprived of KRAS mutations. In addition, the use of targeted sequencing allows to detect mutations at low allelic frequency that are not identified by standard sequencing methods or by whole genome or whole exome sequencing that have a relatively low sensitivity. In this regard, we might expect that the use of high sensitive techniques will reveal an ever increasing level of clonal complexity of human tumours. Importantly, all the KRAS mutations identified with NGS were confirmed by additional analysis thus excluding sequencing artifacts. Interestingly, Hong et al. found KRAS mutations in 6.9% of EGFR mutant lung cancer patients using a liquid biopsy approach [23].

Given that some level of heterogeneity will be present in almost every tumour, the question that needs to be addressed is at what extent this phenomenon might affect the response to target-based agents. Our study confirmed recent reports suggesting that EGFR-mutant tumours carrying additional driver alterations have a reduced sensitivity to EGFR TKIs [23,24]. However, this study is the first to focus on driver alterations that might interfere with EGFR blockade by activating alternative pathways or downstream signalling proteins. Nevertheless, we acknowledge that our study has several limits. First, this was a retrospective collection of cases that might suffer of selection biases. More importantly, we grouped together mutations in different genes that might play a different role in de novo and acquired resistance to EGFR TKIs. For example, KRAS mutations have been reported in different studies as a mechanism of de novo resistance to EGFR TKIs in NSCLC [4]. In contrast, KRAS and NRAS mutations have not been detected in tumour biopsy from patients that progressed following treatment with first-generation TKIs [25]. However, recent reports showed that the levels of KRAS and/or NRAS mutations increase in the liquid biopsy from patients that progressed following treatment with first-, second-, or third-generation EGFR TKIs, thus suggesting that these variants might also play a role in the acquired resistance to these agents [26,27]. While the choice to group different mutations was due to the low frequency of the single variant that would prevent from an analysis with a feasible number of cases, we do recognize that prospective studies in each specific subgroup of mutant patients are necessary to confirm our findings.

Our data confirm that patients with clonal KRAS mutation and sub-clonal EGFR mutation do not benefit from treatment with EGFR TKIs. However, the 8/14 patients with apparent clonal EGFR mutation and sub-clonal KRAS mutation had a median PFS of 11.09 months and a response rate of 57.1%. Therefore, our data suggest that quantitative assessment of both EGFR and KRAS mutations might better identify patients benefiting from EGFR TKI treatment.

We found an EGFR p.T790M mutation in 6.8% of the cases. The p.T790M mutation has been previously reported in approximately 2% of TKI-naive EGFR-mutant tumours when routine diagnostic methods are used for testing [28]. The relatively higher sensitivity of the NGS panel that we employed as compared with routine testing techniques might account for such difference. Previous studies that used highly sensitive methods (sensitivity ~0.1%) found the p.T790M variant in 25%–65% of untreated EGFR mutant NSCLC [29–31]. In these studies, the presence of the p.T790M was correlated with a shorter PFS in patients treated with EGFR TKIs. In our cohort of patients, the p.T790M variant was not an independent factor of shorter PFS. This difference might be due to the relative low number of p.T790M-positive cases. In addition, in 7/9 cases the allelic frequency of the p.T790M was lower as compared with the sensitizing mutations. In this respect, responses to first generation EGFR TKIs have been observed in patients carrying both an EGFR sensitizing and the p.T790M mutation when the resistance mutation is expressed in a minor clone of tumour cells [32].

We could not confirm the correlation between TP53 mutation and shorter PFS that has been reported by different preliminary studies [10,16–19,33]. The frequency of TP53 mutations was only 17.3% in our cohort whereas it ranged between 30.1% and 62% in the above mentioned reports. TP53 mutations have been previously described to occur in 10% to 26% of never smokers with NSCLC [34–36]. Whereas the above highlighted differences in TP53 mutation frequency might be due to either selection of the cases or significant differences in the sensitivity of the testing methods, a population of EGFR mutant NSCLC that is enriched of never-smokers is not expected to carry TP53 mutations at a high frequency. In addition, the correlation of TP53 mutations with PFS was found in the above studies at univariate analysis but it was not confirmed at multivariate analysis. These findings suggest that the predictive role of TP53 mutations should be addressed in much larger cohorts of patients.

4. Materials and Methods

4.1. Study Design

This is a retrospective, observational clinical study that was approved by the Ethic Committee of the Istituto Nazionale Tumouri "Fondazione G. Pascale" (16/14 OSS). The primary objective of the study was to assess whether a correlation exists between detection of mutations in genes potentially associated with resistance to EGFR targeting agents (KRAS, NRAS, BRAF, ERBB2, PIK3CA, and MET, "other mutations") and PFS in EGFR-mutant, advanced or metastatic NSCLC patients that received EGFR TKI treatment as first-line therapy. The study was conducted by using archival material residual from the diagnostic activity and available at the bio-bank of the INT-Fondazione Pascale. The tissue specimens were obtained from 133 patients with advanced or metastatic EGFR mutant NSCLC prior to EGFR TKI treatment. The inclusion criteria were: diagnosis of NSCLC, any histology; EGFR mutation detected with routine diagnostic methods; stage IIIB or IV; no previous systemic treatment for advanced disease; first-line treatment with EGFR TKIs as monotherapy; availability of data on response and PFS; availability of tumour tissue or DNA for NGS analysis. For sample size calculation, we estimated that, with a presumed prevalence of other mutations in 20% of the cases, the registration of 103 events for PFS (i.e., either disease progressions or deaths without progression) could allow an 80% statistical power to identify a HR of progression equal to 0.50 between the two groups (cases without "other mutations" vs. cases with "other mutations"), with alpha level of 0.05.

4.2. Mutational Analysis

The same specimen was used for the initial EGFR mutational analysis and for NGS for all cases included in this study. Tumour samples were analysed with the Ion AmpliSeq Colon and Lung Cancer Panel (Thermofisher, Monza, Italy) using the Ion Torrent semiconductor sequencing. The panel allows to analyse hotspot and targeted regions of the following cancer related genes: EGFR, ALK, ERBB2, ERBB4, FGFR1, FGFR2, FGFR3, MET, DDR2, KRAS, PIK3CA, BRAF, AKT1, PTEN, NRAS, MAP2K1, STK11, NOTCH1, CTNNB1, SMAD4, FBXW7, TP53. Libraries were prepared starting from 10 ng of genomic DNA and analysed on the Agilent® 2100 Bioanalyzer (Agilent Technologies, Milan, Italy). One hundred picomoles of each library were multiplexed and clonally amplified on Ion sphere particles (ISPs) by emulsion PCR performed on the Ion One Touch 2 instrument (Thermo Fisher Scientific, Waltham, MA, USA) with the Ion PGM template OT2 200 kit (Thermo Fisher Scientific, Waltham, MA, USA). The ISPs were enriched, loaded on an Ion 316 chip and sequenced on a PGM sequencer with the Ion PGM™ sequencing 200 kit v2 (Thermo Fisher Scientific, Waltham, MA, USA). The raw data were analyzed using Torrent Suite software v4.6(Thermo Fisher Scientific, Waltham, MA, USA) and variants were detected using Ion Reporter Software v4.6 (Thermo Fisher Scientific, Waltham, MA, USA). Each mutation was verified in the Integrative genome viewer (IGV) from the Broad Institute (http://www.broadinstitute.org/igv/).

We have previously demonstrated that this panel can detect hotspot mutations at allelic frequency ≥2% [33]. 13 KRAS variants were confirmed by droplet digital PCR (ddPCR) using the QX200 Droplet Digital PCR System (Bio-Rad, Milan, Italy) and either the KRAS Screening Multiplex Kit (Bio-Rad, Milan, Italy), a primer-probe mix able to detect seven mutations (G12A, G12C, G12D, G12R, G12S, G12V, G13D) in codon 12 and 13 of the KRAS gene, or specific assays for KRAS mutations in codons 61 and 146, and by the Oncomine Lung cfDNA Assay (Thermo Fisher Scientific, Waltham, MA, USA) for the analysis of plasma-derived circulating cell-free DNA. Similarly, EGFR mutations were analysed by ddPCR by using specific assays for the mutations reported by routine diagnostic assays.

4.3. Study Treatment and Assessments

Patients received gefitinib, erlotinib, or afatinib as first-line therapy in clinical practice, according to availability of drugs and investigator's choice. Drugs were administered orally at standard doses (250 mg for gefitinib; 150 mg for erlotinib; 40 mg for afatinib) once daily until disease progression according to RECIST criteria, intolerable toxicity, or patient refusal. The medical history, concomitant medications, and smoking status of patients included in the study were recorded. The objective tumour response was assessed every eight weeks as for standard clinical practice. Additional assessment could be performed at any time if symptoms or signs appeared that might suggest disease progression.

4.4. Statistical Analyses

PFS was the primary endpoint. It was defined as the time from EGFR TKI treatment start to progression or death, whichever occurred first, or last follow-up date for patients alive and free from progression at the time of the analysis. OS was a secondary endpoint and was defined as the time from EGFR TKI treatment start to death or last follow-up date for alive patients. Median follow-up (mFU) was calculated according to the reverse Kaplan-Meier technique. PFS and OS curves were estimated by Kaplan-Meier product limit method and compared between the two groups (cases without "other mutations" vs. cases with "other mutations") by log-rank test. Hazard ratios were estimated by a Cox proportional hazard model adjusted by gender, age (as a continuous variable), smoking habits (current or previous smoker vs. never smoker), and presence of the T790M mutation. Explorative analyses were done to assess the prognostic value of TP53 mutation in this cohort of patients. Statistical analyses were performed using STATA MP 14.1 (StataCorp LP, College Station, TX, USA).

5. Conclusions

In conclusion, our study suggests that the presence of concurrent mutations in signalling pathways potentially leading to resistance to EGFR blockade might be associated with shorter PFS in patients treated with EGFR TKIs. While these data need confirmation in prospective clinical trials, they suggest that EGFR-mutant NSCLC is a heterogeneous disease and that molecular profiling with NGS panels might help to further select patients who will better benefit treatment with anti-EGFR agents.

Author Contributions: Conceptualization: N.N.; methodology: A.M.R., F.F. (Francesca Fenizia), and M.C.P.; formal analysis: A.M.R., F.F. (Francesca Fenizia), M.C.P., and C.R.; investigation: D.G., L.C., B.V., E.B., C.P., F.F. (Francesco Ferraù), A.M. (Agnese Montanino), V.L., E.S.M., G.R., G.B., F.P., and A.M. (Alessandro Morabito); resources: N.N.; data curation: A.M.R., F.F. (Francesca Fenizia), M.C.P., M.L., and A.D.L.; writing-original draft preparation: A.M.R. and F.F. (Francesca Fenizia); writing-review and editing: N.N.

Acknowledgments: The authors also thank Alessia Iannaccone and Nicoletta Chicchinelli for their technical support.

References

1. Rossi, A.; Pasquale, R.; Esposito, C.; Normanno, N. Should epidermal growth factor receptor tyrosine kinase inhibitors be considered ideal drugs for the treatment of selected advanced non-small cell lung cancer patients. *Cancer Treat. Rev.* **2013**, *39*, 489–497. [CrossRef] [PubMed]
2. Camidge, D.R.; Pao, W.; Sequist, L.V. Acquired resistance to TKIs in solid tumours: Learning from lung cancer. *Nat. Rev. Clin. Oncol.* **2014**, *11*, 473–481. [CrossRef] [PubMed]

3. Jamal-Hanjani, M.; Wilson, G.A.; McGranahan, N.; Birkbak, N.J.; Watkins, T.B.K.; Veeriah, S.; Shafi, S.; Jhonson, H.D.; Mitter, R.; Rosenthal, R.; et al. Tracking the evolution of non-small-cell lung cancer. *N. Engl. J. Med.* **2017**, *376*, 2109–2121. [CrossRef] [PubMed]
4. De Luca, A.; Normanno, N. Predictive biomarkers to tyrosine kinase inhibitors for the epidermal growth factor receptor in non-small-cell lung cancer. *Curr. Drug. Targets* **2010**, *11*, 851–864. [CrossRef] [PubMed]
5. Li, S.; Li, L.; Zhu, Y.; Huang, C.; Qin, Y.; Liu, H.; Ren-Heidenreich, L.; Shi, B.; Ren, H.; Chu, X.; et al. Coexistence of EGFR with KRAS, or BRAF, or PIK3CA somatic mutations in lung cancer: A comprehensive mutation profiling from 5125 Chinese cohorts. *Br. J. Cancer* **2014**, *110*, 2812–2820. [CrossRef] [PubMed]
6. Scheffler, M.; Bos, M.; Gardizi, M.; Konig, K.; Michels, S.; Fassunke, J.; Heydt, C.; Kunstlinger, H.; Ihle, M.; Veckeroth, F.; et al. PIK3CA mutations in non-small cell lung cancer (NSCLC): Genetic heterogeneity, prognostic impact and incidence of prior malignancies. *Oncotarget* **2015**, *6*, 1315–1326. [CrossRef] [PubMed]
7. Bria, E.; Pilotto, S.; Amato, E.; Fassan, M.; Novello, S.; Peretti, U.; Vavala, T.; Kingspergher, S.; Righi, L.; Santo, A.; et al. Molecular heterogeneity assessment by next-generation sequencing and response to gefitinib of EGFR mutant advanced lung adenocarcinoma. *Oncotarget* **2015**, *6*, 12783–12795. [CrossRef] [PubMed]
8. Ju, L.; Han, M.; Zhao, C.; Li, X. EGFR, KRAS and ROS1 variants coexist in a lung adenocarcinoma patient. *Lung Cancer* **2016**, *95*, 94–97. [CrossRef] [PubMed]
9. Lim, S.M.; Kim, H.R.; Cho, E.K.; Min, Y.J.; Ahn, J.S.; Ahn, M.J.; Park, K.; Cho, B.C.; Lee, J.H.; Jeong, H.C.; et al. Targeted sequencing identifies genetic alterations that confer primary resistance to EGFR tyrosine kinase inhibitor (Korean Lung Cancer Consortium). *Oncotarget* **2016**, *7*, 36311–36320. [CrossRef] [PubMed]
10. Lee, T.; Lee, B.; Choi, Y.L.; Han, J.; Ahn, M.J.; Um, S.W. Non-small cell lung cancer with concomitant EGFR, KRAS, and ALK mutation: Clinicopathologic features of 12 cases. *J. Pathol. Transl. Med.* **2016**, *50*, 197–203. [CrossRef] [PubMed]
11. Choughule, A.; Sharma, R.; Trivedi, V.; Thavamani, A.; Noronha, V.; Joshi, A.; Desai, S.; Chandrani, P.; Sundaram, P.; Utture, S.; et al. Coexistence of KRAS mutation with mutant but not wild-type EGFR predicts response to tyrosine-kinase inhibitors in human lung cancer. *Br. J. Cancer* **2014**, *111*, 2203–2204. [CrossRef] [PubMed]
12. Tiseo, M.; Bersanelli, M.; Perrone, F.; Tamborini, E.; Settanni, G.; Busico, A.; Rossi, G.; Ardizzoni, A.; Pelosi, G. Different clinical effects upon separate inhibition of coexisting EGFR and PI3KCA mutations in a lung adenocarcinoma patient. *Lung Cancer* **2015**, *87*, 204–206. [CrossRef] [PubMed]
13. Yu, H.A.; Jordan, E.; Ni, A.; Feldman, D.; Rodriguez, C.; Kim, H.R.; Kris, G.M.; Solit, B.D.; Berger, F.M.; Ladanyi, M.; et al. Concurrent genetic alterations identified by next-generation sequencing in pre-treatment, metastatic EGFR-mutant lung cancers. *J. Clin. Oncol.* **2016**, *34*, 9053. [CrossRef]
14. Canale, M.; Petracci, E.; Delmonte, A.; Chiadini, E.; Dazzi, C.; Papi, M.; Cappeli, L.; Casanova, C.; De Luigi, N.; Mariotti, N.; et al. Impact of TP53 mutations on outcome in EGFR-mutated patients treated with first-line tyrosine kinase inhibitors. *Clin. Cancer Res.* **2017**, *23*, 2195–2202. [CrossRef] [PubMed]
15. Labbe, C.; Korpanty, G.; Tomasini, P.; Doherty, M.; Mascaux, C.; Jao, K.; Pitcher, B.; Pintilie, M.; Leighle, B.N.; Feld, R.; et al. Prognostic and predictive effects of TP53 mutation in patients with EGFR-mutated non-small cell lung cancer (NSCLC). *J. Clin. Oncol.* **2016**, *34*, 11585. [CrossRef]
16. Roeper, J.; Netchaeva, M.; Lueers, A.C.; Regina, P.; Sriba, D.; Willborn, K.; Stropiep, U.; Hallas, C.; Falk, M.; Tiemann, M.; et al. P53 Non-disruptive mutation is a negative Predictive factor for OS and PFS in EGFR M+ NSCLC treated with TKI. In Proceedings of the World Conference on Lung Cancer, Vienna, Austria, 11 October 2016; p. ID5879.
17. Elamin, Y.Y.; Rinsurongkawong, W.; Tran, H.T.; Gold, K.A.; Lewis, J.; Roarty, E.; Futreal, A.; Zhang, J.; Heymach, J. The impact of genomic landscape of EGFR Mutant NSCLC on response to targeted and immune therapy. *J. Thorac. Oncol.* **2016**, *12*, S423–S424. [CrossRef]
18. Alizadeh, A.A.; Aranda, V.; Bardelli, A.; Blanpain, C.; Bock, C.; Borowski, C.; Caldas, C.; Califano, A.; Doherty, M.; Elsner, M.; et al. Toward understanding and exploiting tumor heterogeneity. *Nat. Med.* **2015**, *21*, 846–853. [CrossRef] [PubMed]
19. McGranahan, N.; Favero, F.; De Bruin, E.C.; Birkbak, N.J.; Szallasi, Z.; Swanton, C. Clonal status of actionable driver events and the timing of mutational processes in cancer evolution. *Sci. Transl. Med.* **2015**, *7*, 283ra54. [CrossRef] [PubMed]

20. Normanno, N.; Rachiglio, A.M.; Lambiase, M.; Martinelli, E.; Fenizia, F.; Esposito, C.; Roma, C.; Troiani, T.; Rizzi, D.; Tatangelo, F.; et al. Heterogeneity of KRAS, NRAS, BRAF and PIK3CA mutations in metastatic colorectal cancer and potential effects on therapy in the CAPRI GOIM trial. *Ann. Oncol.* **2015**, *26*, 1710–1714. [CrossRef] [PubMed]
21. Andor, N.; Graham, T.A.; Jansen, M.; Xia, L.C.; Aktipis, C.A.; Petritsch, C.; Ji, P.H.; Maley, C.C. Pan-cancer analysis of the extent and consequences of intratumor heterogeneity. *Nat Med.* **2016**, *22*, 105–113. [CrossRef] [PubMed]
22. Spigel, D.R.; Schrock, A.B.; Fabrizio, D.; Frampton, G.M.; Sun, J.; He, J.; Johnson, L.M.; Bauer, M.T.; Kalemkerian, P.G.; Raez, E.L.; et al. Total mutation burden (TMB) in lung cancer (LC) and relationship with response to PD-1/PD-L1 targeted therapies. *J.Clin. Oncol.* **2016**, *34*, 9017. [CrossRef]
23. Hong, S.; Gao, F.; Fu, S.; Wang, Y.; Fang, W.; Huang, Y.; Zhang, L. Concomitant genetic alterations with response to treatment and epidermal growth factor receptor tyrosine Kinase inhibitors in patients with EGFR-Mutant advanced non-small cell lung cancer. *JAMA Oncol.* **2018**, *4*, 739–742. [CrossRef] [PubMed]
24. Jakobsen, J.N.; Santoni-Rugiu, E.; Grauslund, M.; Melchior, L.; Sorensen, J.B. Concomitant driver mutations in advanced EGFR-mutated non-small-cell lung cancer and their impact on erlotinib treatment. *Oncotarget* **2018**, *9*, 26195–26208. [CrossRef] [PubMed]
25. Ohashi, K.; Sequist, L.V.; Arcila, M.E.; Moran, T.; Chmielecki, J.; Lin, Y.L.; Pan, Y.; Wang, L.; de Stanchina, E.; Shein, K.; et al. Lung cancers with acquired resistance to EGFR inhibitors occasionally harbor BRAF gene mutations but lack mutations in KRAS, NRAS, or MEK1. *Proc. Natl. Acad. Sci. USA* **2012**, *109*, E2127–E2133. [CrossRef] [PubMed]
26. Del Re, M.; Tiseo, M.; Bordi, P.; D'Incecco, A.; Camerini, A.; Petrini, I.; Lucchesi, M.; Inno, A.; Spada, D.; Vasile, E.; et al. Contribution of KRAS mutations and c.2369C > T (p.T790M) EGFR to acquired resistance to EGFR-TKIs in EGFR mutant NSCLC: A study on circulating tumor DNA. *Oncotarget* **2017**, *8*, 13611–13619. [CrossRef] [PubMed]
27. Chabon, J.J.; Simmons, A.D.; Lovejoy, A.F.; Esfahani, M.S.; Newman, A.M.; Haringsma, H.J.; Kurtz, M.D.; Stehr, H.; Schere, F.; Karlovich, A.C.; et al. Circulating tumour DNA profiling reveals heterogeneity of EGFR inhibitor resistance mechanisms in lung cancer patients. *Nat Commun.* **2016**, *7*, 11815. [CrossRef] [PubMed]
28. Yu, H.A.; Arcila, M.E.; Hellmann, M.D.; Kris, M.G.; Ladanyi, M.; Riely, G.J. Poor response to erlotinib in patients with tumors containing baseline EGFR T790M mutations found by routine clinical molecular testing. *Ann. Oncol.* **2014**, *25*, 423–428. [CrossRef] [PubMed]
29. Maheswaran, S.; Sequist, L.V.; Nagrath, S.; Ulkus, L.; Brannigan, B.; Collura, C.V.; Inserra, E.; Diederich, S.; Iafrate, J.; Bell, W.D.; et al. Detection of mutations in EGFR in circulating lung-cancer cells. *N. Engl. J. Med.* **2008**, *359*, 366–377. [CrossRef] [PubMed]
30. Su, K.Y.; Chen, H.Y.; Li, K.C.; Kuo, M.L.; Yang, J.C.H.; Chan, W.K.; Ho, B.C.; Chang, G.C.; Shih, J.Y.; Yu, S.L.; et al. Pretreatment epidermal growth factor receptor (EGFR) T790M mutation predicts shorter EGFR tyrosine kinase inhibitor response duration in patients with non-small-cell lung cancer. *J. Clin. Oncol.* **2012**, *30*, 433–440. [CrossRef] [PubMed]
31. Costa, C.; Molina, M.A.; Drozdowskyj, A.; Gimenez-Capitan, A.; Bertran-Alamillo, J.; Karachaliou, N.; Geravis, R.; Massuti, B.; Wei, J.; Moran, T.; et al. The impact of EGFR T790M mutations and BIM mRNA expression on outcome in patients with EGFR-mutant NSCLC treated with erlotinib or chemotherapy in the randomized phase III EURTAC trial. *Clin. Cancer Res.* **2014**, *20*, 2001–2010. [CrossRef] [PubMed]
32. Morabito, A.; Costanzo, R.; Rachiglio, A.M.; Pasquale, R.; Sandomenico, C.; Franco, R.; Montanino, A.; De Lutio, E.; Rocco, G.; Normanno, N. Activity of gefitinib in a non–small-cell lung cancer patient with both activating and resistance EGFR mutations. *J. Thorac. Oncol.* **2013**, *8*, e59–e60. [CrossRef] [PubMed]
33. Tops, B.B.; Normanno, N.; Kurth, H.; Amato, E.; Mafficini, A.; Rieber, N.; Le Corre, D.; Rachinglio, A.M.; Reiman, A.; Sheli, O.; et al. Development of a semi-conductor sequencing-based panel for genotyping of colon and lung cancer by the Onconetwork consortium. *BMC Cancer.* **2015**, *15*, 26. [CrossRef] [PubMed]
34. Takagi, Y.; Osada, H.; Kuroishi, T.; Mitsudomi, T.; Kondo, M.; Niimi, T.; Saji, S.; Gazdar, A.F.; Takahashi, T.; Minna, J.D.; et al. p53 mutations in non-small-cell lung cancers occurring in individuals without a past history of active smoking. *Br. J. Cancer* **1998**, *77*, 1568–1572. [CrossRef] [PubMed]

35. Husgafvel-Pursiainen, K.; Boffetta, P.; Kannio, A.; Nyberg, F.; Pershagen, G.; Mukeria, A.; Constantinescu, V.; Fortes, C.; Benhamou, S. p53 Mutations and exposure to environmental tobacco smoke in a multicenter study on lung cancer. *Cancer Res.* **2000**, *60*, 2906–2911. [PubMed]
36. Vahakangas, K.H.; Bennett, W.P.; Castren, K.; Welsh, J.A.; Khan, M.A.; Blomeke, B.; Alavanja, C.R.M.; Harris, C.C. p53 and K-ras mutations in lung cancers from former and never-smoking women. *Cancer Res.* **2001**, *61*, 4350–4356. [PubMed]

11

Multiplexed Immunohistochemistry for Molecular and Immune Profiling in Lung Cancer—Just About Ready for Prime-Time

Paul Hofman [1,2], Cécile Badoual [3,4], Fiona Henderson [5], Léa Berland [1], Marame Hamila [1], Elodie Long-Mira [1,2], Sandra Lassalle [1,2], Hélène Roussel [3,4], Véronique Hofman [1,2], Eric Tartour [4,6] and Marius Ilié [1,2,*]

1 Laboratory of Clinical and Experimental Pathology, Hospital-Integrated Biobank (BB-0033-00025), Nice Hospital University, FHU OncoAge, Université Côte d'Azur, Nice 06000, France; hofman.p@chu-nice.fr (P.H.); leaberland370@gmail.com (L.B.); hamila.m@chu-nice.fr (M.H.); long-mira.e@chu-nice.fr (E.L.-M.); lassalle.s@chu-nice.fr (S.L.); hofman.v@chu-nice.fr; ilie.m@chu-nice.fr (V.H.)

2 Team 4, Institute for Research on Cancer and Aging, Nice (IRCAN), INSERM U1081/UMR CNRS 7284, FHU OncoAge, Université Côte d'Azur, Nice 06107, France

3 Department of Pathology, Hôpital Européen Georges Pompidou, APHP, Paris 75015, France; cecile.badoual@aphp.fr (C.B.); helene.roussel@aphp.fr (H.R.)

4 INSERM U970, Université Paris Descartes Sorbonne Paris-Cité, Paris 75015, France; eric.tartour@aphp.fr

5 Department EMEA, Indica Labs, 2469 Corrales Rd Bldg. A-3 Corrales, NM 87048, USA; fhenderson@indicalab.com

6 Department of Immunology, Hôpital Européen Georges Pompidou, Paris 75015, France

* Correspondence: ilie.m@chu-nice.fr

Abstract: As targeted molecular therapies and immuno-oncology have become pivotal in the management of patients with lung cancer, the essential requirement for high throughput analyses and clinical validation of biomarkers has become even more intense, with response rates maintained in the 20%–30% range. Moreover, the list of treatment alternatives, including combination therapies, is rapidly evolving. The molecular profiling and specific tumor-associated immune contexture may be predictive of response or resistance to these therapeutic strategies. Multiplexed immunohistochemistry is an effective and proficient approach to simultaneously identify specific proteins or molecular abnormalities, to determine the spatial distribution and activation state of immune cells, as well as the presence of immunoactive molecular expression. This method is highly advantageous for investigating immune evasion mechanisms and discovering potential biomarkers to assess mechanisms of action and to predict response to a given treatment. This review provides views on the current technological status and evidence for clinical applications of multiplexing and how it could be applied to optimize clinical management of patients with lung cancer.

Keywords: multiplexed; brightfield; chromogenic; fluorescence; molecular; immune profiling; immune-oncology; digital; lung cancer

1. Introduction

Lung cancer is the leading cause of cancer death among males, and the second most common among females worldwide [1]. Approximately 80% of newly diagnosed patients with non-small cell lung cancer (NSCLC) have unresectable locally advanced or metastatic disease [2]. In these patients, current treatment strategies, across all lines of therapy, include chemotherapy regimens based on histology, targeted drugs for patients carrying specific genomic alterations and immunotherapy using immune checkpoint inhibitors (ICIs), in particular monoclonal antibodies targeting programmed cell death-1 (PD-1) and programmed cell death ligand-1 (PD-L1) [3–7]. The development of molecularly targeted therapies, as well as ICIs, has improved outcomes in the metastatic setting for NSCLC patients who harbor somatically activated oncogenes such as *EGFR* and *BRAFV600*, rearranged *ALK* or *ROS1*, or PD-L1 expression ≥50% of tumor cells [3–5]. However, even with these molecular strategies, a large proportion of patients do not attain prolonged disease control, and the 5-year survival rate does not exceed 5% [8–10].

Patients with suspected stage IIIB/IV NSCLC require tissue or cytology sampling to confirm the diagnosis (e.g., adenocarcinoma vs. squamous cell carcinoma vs. other lung histological subtypes), as this determines eligibility for biomarker testing and further therapeutic strategies [11]. Several immunohistochemical (IHC) markers (e.g., TTF1, p40, INSM1) may be needed to confirm and subtype lung carcinoma [12,13]. Additional tumor material is required for interrogating predictive biomarkers, using IHC (e.g., ALK, ROS1, PD-L1), in situ hybridization (ISH; e.g., ALK, ROS1) or sequencing techniques (e.g., *EGFR*, *BRAF* V600E, etc.). Moreover, in the context of precision oncology, lung cancer patients may be enrolled in ongoing clinical trials (https://clinicaltrials.gov/) and tumor samples may be used for basic and clinical research studies [14].

For these procedures, sufficient material of high quality is mandatory. In a large number of cases, the tumor material on which all diagnostic and predictive test must be theoretically be performed might be sparse, containing only a small number of tumor cells [15]. Small biopsy samples with few tumor cells might often only allow diagnosis and classification of tumor subtype, and additional tests may be compromised [11,15].

In the current boost to improve the tailored approach to the clinical management of patients with NSCLC, pathologists and researchers deal continuously with an unresolved dilemma for exploring a growing number of protein biomarkers on small-sized tumor samples. In this context, multiplexed immunohistochemistry (mIHC) has recently emerged as a potent tool for the simultaneous detection of multiple protein biomarkers on the same tissue section to expand the molecular and immune profiling of NSCLC, while preserving tumor material. Over the last years, the role of IHC has been constantly extended to improve diagnosis, and to guide prognosis and treatment of NSCLC patients, while requiring assessment of an increasing number of protein targets. In addition, multiplying serial tissue sections to stain for a single marker per slide, can waste small biopsy specimens, entangle the correlation of section-to-section protein expression, and leave insufficient tumor material for additional analyses [16]. Multiplexing can be carried out using chromogenic or fluorescent staining methods. Complex fluorescent multiplexing systems are currently being developed (reviewed in this Special Focus by Parra et al.) [17]. New approaches compatible with high levels of target multiplexing and suitable for use on formalin-fixed paraffin-embedded (FFPE) samples have recently demonstrated the potential to be transferred to the clinical setting [18–22]. For instance, direct simultaneous assessment by mIHC of both immune and tumor-related pathways and their spatial relationships, in a single tissue sample, may empower more accurate patient stratification for immunotherapy [23].

Finally, in recent years, mIHC technology has seen rapid advancements in image acquisition throughput, image resolution and data accuracy, allowing improvements in pathologist performance by automatically measuring parameters that are hard to achieve reliably by microscope, to extract comprehensive information on biomarker expression levels, co-localization, and compartmentalization. The present manuscript reports on mIHC approaches for molecular and immune profiling in lung cancer.

2. Principles of Multiplexing Staining Methods

2.1. Chromogenic Multiplexed IHC

Technical approaches of brightfield chromogenic mIHC include direct detection of antigens by primary antibodies from the same or different species that are directly labeled with different chromogens. Alternatively, an indirect mIHC detection method can be used with two or more layers of antibodies, allowing for increased amplification of signal [24]. The direct detection approach has several disadvantages, such as lower sensitivity for low abundance targets, the need for sizeable quantities of conjugated antibodies, which are usually more expensive, and the risk that antibody activity could be adversely affected by direct labeling [24]. The indirect approach can be limited by the number of available host species and the use of same species antibodies, which would thus require inactivation between successive cycles of immunolabeling [24].

The unwanted cross-reactivity between primary antibodies from different staining cycles is regarded as the main technical challenge in mIHC. The most frequent solution used to avoid such reactions is manual microwaving or heating of tissue slides to deactivate the preceding antibody [25,26]. Whereas microwaving is often used in research facilities when dealing with antibodies from the same host-species, it may not be an optimal method to be adopted in a routine clinical setting. Variable and heterogeneous results could be obtained by manual processing. Furthermore, microwaving can increase the damage of the tumor tissue and may remove small biopsies from the slides, especially if they have already been antigen retrieved by a previous heat-mediated procedure [27].

Another strategy for preventing cross-reactivity is the use of stripping buffers to elute the primary/secondary antibody complex [27,28]. A number of buffers with different pH, osmolality, detergent content and denaturing features were evaluated to strip the bound antibody complex from previous IHC staining cycles, however this produced variable results across studies. Certain buffers were found to be hazardous, to decolorize H&E stain and/or to reduce nuclear protein staining [27,28].

An alternative, more recent approach named "multiplexed immunohistochemical consecutive staining on single slide" (MICSSS), was developed for use on FFPE samples by applying repetitive cycles of immunoperoxidase labeling, image scanning, then chemical stripping of the chromogenic substrate [20,21]. However, this process can result in a labor-intensive protocol and a prolonged turnaround time to yield results that are not suitable for a routine clinical setting. Moreover, multiplexing may be limited due to tissue degradation after successive serial mIHC cycles [24,29].

More recently, a fully automated mIHC technology using a thermochemical process (heat deactivation; HD) to deactivate an antibody complex between staining cycles on an automated slide stainer was first developed for fluorescent detection, and further applied to brightfield chromogenic detection (Figure 1) [30,31].

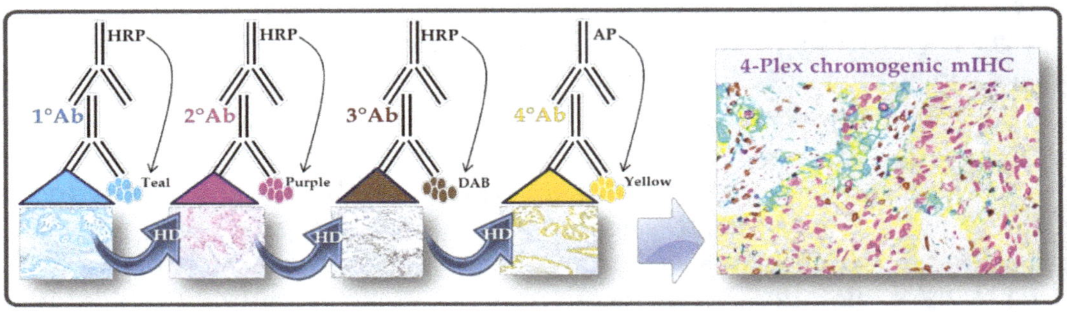

Figure 1. Chromogenic multiplexed immunohistochemistry assay scheme. The assay is using the sequential application of four unmodified primary antibodies with a specific heat deactivation (HD) step between staining cycles.

This technology allows the use of the first antibody from the same host species, detected by the anti-species secondary antibody conjugated to horseradish peroxidase (HRP). In the presence of its substrate, the active HRP, generates in-situ deposition of tyramide within the medium containing the chromogens. The bound primary antibody/secondary antibody complex is then eluted with a citrate/acetate buffer. Thus, the deposited chromogen-conjugated tyramide bounds covalently to the tissue near the first detected antigen. The same procedure is repeated to detect the following antigens [30,31]. Indeed, the sequential stripping may lead to wastage of the conjugated secondary antibodies, whereas the chromogen-conjugated tyramine remains stable by binding covalently to the electron-rich amino acids of detected proteins and by resisting to the elution with the stripping buffer [30,31]. Importantly, the automation allows for standardization of all critical mIHC steps, such as HD, reagent application, washing steps, control of temperatures, evaporation and humidity, while maintaining the integrity of the tissue architecture and the subsequent epitopes [32,33].

To setup a brightfield mIHC assay using sequential detection with unmodified primary antibodies and chromogenic detection, it is essential to optimize assay conditions on the tissue types of interest before testing clinical samples [34]. Thus, an optimal mIHC assay needs to assure several staining performances: (i) equivalent positive/negative signal to single "gold standard" IHC staining, (ii) robust dynamic proportion of low and high protein quantity, (iii) expected cellular staining topology (e.g., whole membrane, cytoplasmic, nuclear localization), and (iv) minimal overlap of chromogenic spectra for co-localized targets [34]. Recent developments have enabled optimal configurations suitable for testing on clinical samples. For instance, the order of chromogen deposition is determined by the effect of HD on each epitope, that is, the most HD-affected epitope is incubated first, with the least affected epitope incubated last.

To offer the best detection sensitivity, other assay parameters must be taken into account such as the optimal epitope retrieval time to balance the signal/background ratio, and to protect the tissue architecture by optimizing the incubation time for each primary antibody [30]. Moreover, the number of antibodies for simultaneous immunolabeling on the same tissue slide has been extended up to six with the availability of additional chromogens [24,33]. In addition, a major technical challenge is the risk of insufficient deactivation of the primary antibody complexes, which could determine cross-reactions and may give false-positive signals. Besides efforts to optimize HD steps during assay validation, the imaging tools can help to anticipate or to detect potential cross-reactions [35].

2.2. *Immunofluorescent Multiplexing*

Many newly identified or discovered biomarkers, especially for cancer immunotherapy, are linked to the tumor microenvironment and need to be analyzed with new methodological tools. For years, it has become increasingly essential to develop staining and interpretation techniques for the different cell populations infiltrating or composing a tissue. This is particularly true in oncology. To date, as previously described, the use of immunohistochemistry can help the visualization of an antibody-antigen conjugation. It has been showed in the last subsection, that an antibody is conjugated to an enzyme, like a peroxidase, can catalyze a color-producing reaction. Alternatively, the antibody can also be tagged with a fluorophore. Nowadays the use of immunofluorescence is far easier due to technical improvement, like the use of stable fluorophores or the possibility to perform staining in paraffin embedded slides. Since years, research teams proposed immunoscoring, using single staining per slide, to identify prognostic factors [36]. However, the tumor microenvironment is too complex to be summarized by the exploration of a single marker. Chromogenic mIHC is one of the alternatives, and even if this technique is much easier to be used routinely, it is limited by the use of 4 antibodies on the same slide. In addition, fluorescence reveals membrane co-localizations (in the membrane or the nucleus), which is more difficult to obtain with the latter technique. Nevertheless, the use of multiple antibodies (mixed or used step by step) was restricted to the specificity of the primary and the risk of false positivity due to cross reactivity between them. Until recently, the single-parametric or even multiparametric (double or triple) staining, revealed by chromomeric or fluorescent staining, were most often read and interpreted directly by the researchers [37], with a lot of technical constraints.

The microenvironment can now be studied using the multiplex fluorescence technique based on tyramide coupled to a fluorophore (e.g., Opal®, PerkinElmer, Waltham, MA, USA). This allows the simultaneous detection of several markers of interest on FFPE tissues. The concept of the technique is very close the one described above, the chromogenic mIHC assay using sequential application of four unmodified primary antibodies with a specific HD step between staining cycles. The main advantage of this technique is the multiplicity of the staining. The technique is based on a conventional fixation on the epitope of interest. The secondary antibody then binds to the primary antibody followed by Opal® HRP polymer and one of the Opal®fluorophore adjunction. After deposition of Opal® reagents, antibodies are stripped after use of a specific microwave to allow subsequent staining of other antigens. These cycles can be repeated at least seven to nine times. This seven to nine color multiplex staining technique makes it possible to more precisely characterize different cells and their interactions with their environment, on the same paraffin slide [38,39]. However, the use of these new techniques requires the acquisition of specific expertise for in situ multiple staining. Automation of this different process is now efficient and several autostainers are able to execute most of the steps previously described.

For the validation of the different panels of multiparametric IHC markers, in particular for the exploration of the immune system, staining can be performed on tonsil tissue sections as this contains lympho-epithelial structures (Figure 2). Before any application on a cohort, especially when it concerns lung sections, the validation of staining on pulmonary tissue sections as a positive control is highly recommended. In addition, the same positive tissue control could be run on the same slide tested with mIHC, such as is currently performed for clinical diagnostic IHC.

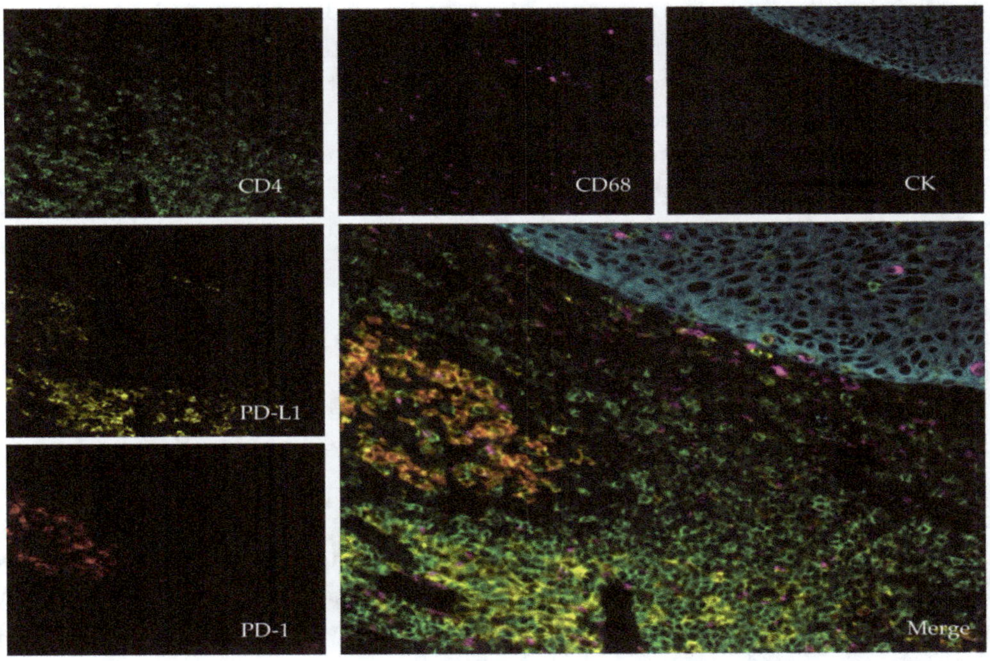

Figure 2. Immunofluorescent multiplexing, image scanned with a spectral scanner (Polaris®; PerkinElmer, Waltham, MA, USA) using 20× magnification. The tissue is a paraffin embedded tonsil. The stains are as follows: pan-Cytokeratin (CK, teal), CD4 (green), CD68 (purple), PD-1 (red), PD-L1 (yellow) and dapi (blue). The central picture compiles the entire staining (merge).

The principle of a multiplex analysis of the tumor microenvironment is the automatic acquisition of a large surface, or the entire slide, quickly and sustainably. Having a fast acquisition time (milliseconds for each illuminated spot) is fundamental for fluorescence techniques because it prevents the "bleaching" which is the progressive extinction of the fluorescent signal after excitation.

3. Clinical and Translational Research Applications: Brief Literature Review and Own Results

Despite the impressive recent achievements in therapeutic strategies for NSCLC treatment, clinical responses have remained limited to subsets of patients, relapse has occurred in the vast majority of patients, and only few effective predictive biomarkers have been defined [40]. The development of more effective predictive biomarkers is needed to optimize patient benefits, minimize the risk of toxicities, and guide combinatorial approaches. In particular, the emerging picture in immune-oncology requires a comprehensive understanding of the tumor microenvironment that is the immune landscape of NSCLC, which results from a complex dynamic cross-talk between the tumor and the immune system [23,40]. Current efforts on novel biomarker candidates include research on identification and quantification of different immune cell subsets, their spatial localization and relationships within tumor areas, the expression of different immune checkpoint markers, tumor mutational burden, and immune gene signatures [23,40]. Thus, the complete picture will be generated by the integrative high-dimensional analysis of the tumor and immune profile based on multiple technological approaches, including mIHC [23].

3.1. *Chromogenic Multiplexed Immunohistochemistry*

The MICSS technology has demonstrated that high-dimensional characterization of the immune contexture before and after treatment with ICIs correlates with response to treatment in cancer patients [20,21]. The immune contexture describes the density, localization, and organization of the immune cells within solid tumors [41]. By analyzing the composition of complex immune cell populations, the neutrophil/dendritic cell density score refined the prognostic value of tumors rich in T-cells and was an independent marker of outcome in NSCLC patients [21].

Another MICSS mIHC platform with computational image processing workflows, including image cytometry, enabled simultaneous evaluation of three 12-antibody biomarker panels in one FFPE tissue section, highlighting the impact of in situ monitoring of immune complexity for patient stratification to improve biomarker discovery and development [20]. The diverse immune complexity within lymphoid- or myeloid-inflamed tumors as detected by this platform, correlates with clinical outcomes and tumor sub-classification in head and neck squamous cell carcinoma. In addition, myeloid-inflamed and T cell exhaustion status correlated with shorter overall survival and the therapeutic response to vaccination therapy in patients with pancreatic ductal adenocarcinoma [20].

Recently, a chromogenic mIHC method revealed that a high density of tumor-associated neutrophils (TANs), but not stromal TANs, may have a divergent prognostic effect in NSCLC, negative in adenocarcinomas, while in squamous cell carcinoma it is a good prognostic factor [42]. Overall, the in situ high-dimensional assessment of immune cells reveals the potential of mIHC to expand the immunoscore in NSCLC patients in a clinically relevant manner [43–45].

Interestingly, a recent clinical trial has supported the role for neoadjuvant immunotherapy in surgically resectable NSCLC, suggesting that the neoadjuvant regimen may lead to early induction of an adaptive anti-tumor immunity, which could be responsible for preventing distant metastases [6]. While this treatment strategy is still in an early stage of clinical development, there are several pending questions that are yet to be answered, including whether the major pathologic response could represent a surrogate end-point for survival and determining the best way to identify upfront patients who may benefit in this setting [46]. With regard to this, the assessment of candidate biomarkers by mIHC on tumor biopsies prior to initiation of neoadjuvant treatment as well as on post-treatment surgical resection samples may be helpful while preserving tumor architecture to assess complete tumor response. Thus, the mIHC approach could be used to standardize the recently described "Immune-Related Pathologic Response Criteria" in a clinical setting [47].

Moreover, another open question that remains to be solved is the use of immunotherapy in special subpopulations, such as elderly patients [48]. Aging is characterized by rebuilding the immune functions, involving both innate and adaptive immunity [49]. By using a brightfield mIHC platform, we recently shown that elderly ≥75 years NSCLC patients have less effective anti-tumor immunoreactivity [33]. While further validation in a larger population is required, our findings suggest that distinct immune pathways may lead to poor outcome in elderly patients with lung adenocarcinoma [33]. Several previous studies demonstrated that the $CD4^+/CD8^+$ ratio may give more prognostic information than either marker alone in solid tumors [50–52].

As outlined above, mIHC provides a unique sample-sparing analytical tool to characterize limited clinical tissue samples by multiplexing targets of interest. This method also has the potential to improve clinical diagnostic accuracy and facilitate histopathological interpretation.

We recently developed in our laboratory (Laboratory of Clinical and Experimental Pathology, Nice, France) two automated brightfield 4-Plex mIHC assays to comprehensively characterize NSCLC major histotypes by multiplexing three conventional IHC markers (e.g., TTF1, p40, AE1/AE3) and three predictive biomarkers (*ALK, ROS1, BRAFV600E*) cleared by the US Food and Drug Administration/European Conformity-*In Vitro* Diagnostic (FDA/CE-IVD) [22]. Some pathology laboratories use chromogenic mIHC on FFPE samples but stain for no more than two markers per tissue slide [45]. The two assays demonstrated no antigenicity loss, steric interference or increased cross-reactivity, providing an analytical tool that can be integrated in a routine clinical workflow [22]. In addition, there are some concerns on the extent to which a multi-color background with color overlap on whole-slide samples could influence the visual interpretation of critical biomarkers. In particular, the PD-L1 expression can be heterogeneous and variably expressed in either tumor or immune cells [53]. By excluding the PD-L1 expressing cells that are unstained with keratin and TTF1 as per tumor-infiltrating immune cells expressing PD-L1, the chromogenic mIHC assay made the visual interpretation straightforward and less ambiguous (Figure 3).

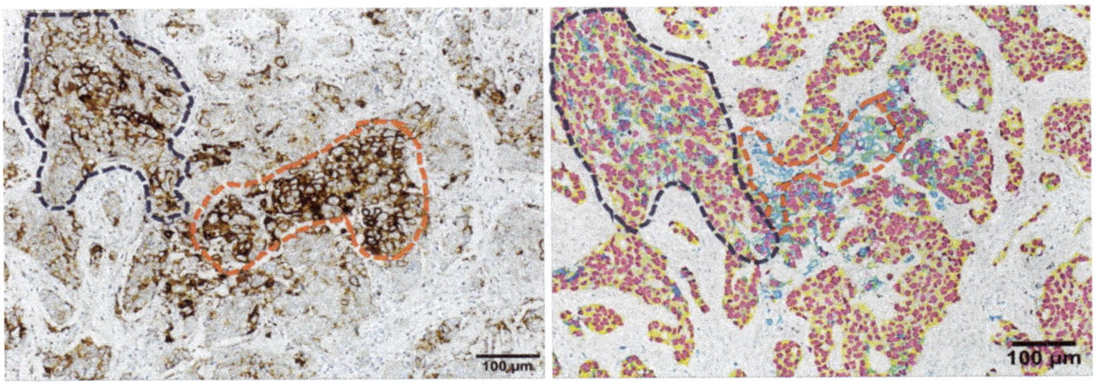

(a) (b)

Figure 3. Interpretation of the programmed death-ligand 1 (PD-L1) staining in serial whole-tissue formalin-fixed paraffin embedded samples from a lung adenocarcinoma case. (**a**) PD-L1 expression revealed by conventional immunoperoxidase staining; (**b**) PD-L1 expression revealed by chromogenic multiplexed immunohistochemistry, with the anti-TTF1 antibody colored in purple, anti-AE1/AE3 in yellow and anti-PD-L1 SP263 in teal. Blue dotted line: tumor area; red dotted line, immune cells.

As the restricted tissue size is a major issue for the management of the vast majority of solid tumors, and individual antibodies rarely demonstrate 100% specificity in the determination of malignancy or cell lineage, a chromogenic mIHC approach with specific multiple protein markers can provide valuable diagnostic information and has the potential to enhance the clinical significance of histological subtyping by delivering substantial prognostic information with therapeutic consequences [54,55].

3.2. Immunofluorescent Multiplexing

3.2.1. Localization of Immune Cells and Their Relationships with Immunosuppressive Markers in the Tumor Microenvironment

The multiplex immunofluorescence techniques better distinguish the stromal and the tumor compartment and thus have allowed for a more detailed description of the topography of immune cells in cancer. Cruz et al. found that T lymphocytes were predominantly concentered in stromal compartment instead of the epithelial compartment in NSCLC [56]. Based on a quantitative immunofluorescence study, a comparative analysis of the expression of immunosuppressive molecules (e.g., PD-L1, IDO-1, B7H4) with the infiltration of intratumoral cells in lung cancer showed that PD-L1 and IDO-1 were consistently associated with prominent B- and T-cell infiltrates, but B7-H4 was not [57]. This could be explained by the role of IFNγ produced by immune cells in regulating PD-L1 and IDO-1 in the tumor microenvironment [58].

3.2.2. Novel Prognostic Composite Biomarker based on Fluorescence in Situ Multiplexing

One of the first clinical studies based on fluorescent digital pathology was the work of Schalper et al., who reported that the infiltration of intratumoral $CD3^+$ and $CD8^+$T cells was associated with a better overall survival in lung cancer patients [59]. For the $CD8^+$T cell infiltration, this prognostic impact was independent from age, tumor size, histology and stage in multivariate analyses [59]. This technology also allows us to better define the prognostic value of immune cells depending on their localization in the tumor microenvironment. For example, after neoadjuvant chemotherapy, high levels of epithelial but not stromal $CD4^+CD3^+$T lymphocytes correlated with better survival in patients with NSCLC [60].

A more complex cell phenotype could also be better characterized with this multiparametric analysis. A novel subpopulation of $CD8^+$T cells called resident memory T cells appear to play a major role in immunosurveillance, as they localize in close contact with epithelial tumor cells [61]. They are defined by a composite phenotype including various biomarkers such as CD103, CD49a, CD69 (Figure 4).

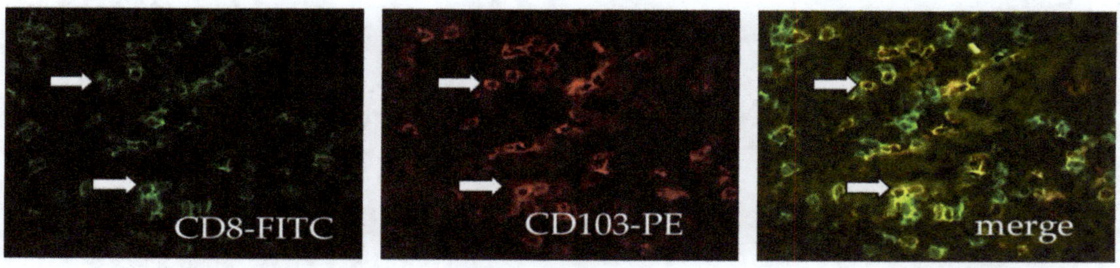

(a) (b) (c)

Figure 4. Infiltration of resident memory T cells ($CD103^+CD8^+$T cells) in human lung cancer. Frozen tissue sections derived from lung adenocarcinoma patients were stained by immunofluorescence with antibodies directed against human (**a**) CD8 (green), and (**b**) CD103 (red). (**c**) The co-localization of CD8 and CD103 markers can be detected by merging the mono-stained pictures. The arrows indicate double positive cells. Staining with isotype controls was included for each experiment (20$\times$ magnification).

We previously demonstrated that high levels of intratumoral infiltration with a resident memory $CD8^+$T cells are associated with a better clinical outcome of NSCLC patients, both in univariate and multivariate analyses [62]. These were a more powerful prognostic marker than the infiltration of total $CD8^+$T cells. These data were then confirmed by various clinical studies [63,64].

This technique also allows us to focus beyond just one cell type, and to integrate the relationships that exist between immune cells in the various compartments of tumors and the relative impact of these cellular relationships on the future of patients. For example, a high effector $CD8^+$T cell/regulatory T cell ratio in the tumor nest is correlated with a better overall survival than when each cell measured independently [65].

3.2.3. Fluorescence Multiplexing Technique to Predict Clinical Response to Immunotherapy

Various parameters such as PD-L1, the expression of PD-1 and the intratumoral infiltration of $CD8^{+}$T cells are considered, especially when combined together, as potential predictive biomarkers of clinical response to immunotherapy [66]. Parra et al., observed higher levels of PD-L1 expression on tumor cells and an increase in the infiltration of T cells and PD-1^{+}T cells in the tumor microenvironment of NSCLC after neoadjuvant chemotherapy [60]. These findings confirm studies in other cancers reporting that neoadjuvant chemotherapy, whatever the regimen, makes the tumor microenvironment more permissive to immunotherapy [67,68]. These results suggest that it would be worthwhile to combine chemotherapy and immunotherapy before surgical resection of locally advanced lung cancer.

Using a quantitative multiplex immunofluorescence technique, we reported that *EGFR*-mutated NSCLC weakly expressed PD-L1 and was not infiltrated by $CD8^{+}$T cells suggesting that it would not be prone to respond to immunotherapy [69]. This hypothesis was then clinically confirmed in various clinical trials [70]. Interestingly, we found that a subpopulation of NSCLC displaying chromosomal rearrangement of the *ALK* gene expressed significant levels of PD-L1 on their tumor cells and were infiltrated by PD-$1^{+}$$CD8^{+}$T cells [69]. However, other studies showed that concurrent $CD8^{+}$T cells and high PD-L1 expression on tumor cells tend to be rare in *ALK* positive NSCLCs [71,72]. Clinical trials did not confirm the sensitivity of this cancer subtype to the blockade of PD-1/PD-L1 axis [71]. This may suggest that other resistance mechanisms occur in this population such as the possible co-expression of inhibitory receptors on T cells or the infiltration of immunosuppressive cells [73,74]. Finally, an increase of T cells with a quiescent phenotype defined by a low proliferation and activation status (Ki67 and Granzyme negative) correlated with better overall survival in NSCLC patients treated by anti-PD-1/PD-L1 [75]. Interestingly, in NSCLC patients not treated by immunotherapy, this population of "dormant" T cells did not correlate with a better clinical outcome, supporting the fact that these cells could represent a true predictive biomarker of response to immunotherapy and not a prognostic marker [75].

4. Image Analysis of Multiplexed Staining

Until recently, pathologic analysis of the IHC signal remained a subjective and time-consuming procedure, wherein the staining intensity, localization and amount had to be manually assessed. Therefore, despite development of practical scoring systems, such as the H-score, the scoring decision is still directly influenced by visual bias [76,77]. Nowadays, with the advent of precision digital immune-oncology, pathologists face a technological transition phase. The convergence of tissue-based mIHC along with automated computer-aided imaging technologies has the potential to make complex information more accessible in routine clinical workflows, improving prognostic and predictive patient stratification [78]. Image analysis and artificial intelligence tools and fields of application in immune-oncology have been outlined in a recent review by Koelzer et al. [78].

The improvement in digital imaging processing systems has opened new doors towards an unbiased, unsupervised, and automatic IHC image analysis by measurement of optical density, which is proportional to the expression extent of specific antigens [77]. Furthermore, application of an automated scoring method for mIHC signals might help pathologists in quantitative comparisons and produce a more accurate characterization of the tumor microenvironment. The mIHC digital image must have the correct stains unmixed into their constituent chromogens for each individual biomarker. Moreover, in order to obtain accurate identification, segmentation and profiling of tumor and immune cells, the mIHC image analysis has to assure the same quantity of chromogen in the color mixture [35]. Several technologies have been developed to decompose each pixel into a collection of constituent signals and the fractions from each of them, in order to convert the whole image into analyte-specific image channels [79]. However, the maximum number of stains that can be unmixed was limited to three, as the linear system had insufficient equations for cases of more than three stains [35]. Alternatively, a novel multi-spectral image deconvolution algorithm has been developed to handle more than three colors and to maintain the biological properties of the protein markers [35].

An increasing number of automated digital pathology systems are being used to analyze information from mIHC technology, such as HALO (Indica Labs, London, UK) [80] for up to five colors, Vectra/inForm (PerkinElmer, Waltham, MA, USA) for up to three colors [81], the "Aperio Color Deconvolution Algorithm" or SlidePath (Leica Biosystems, Wetzlar, Germany) for up to three colors [82], BLISS workstation (Bacus Laboratories, Lombard, IL, USA) for up to four colors but restricted to one region-of-interest (ROI), Tissue Studio® 4.0 (Definiens, Munich, Germany) for up to two colors [83], the "Automated Cellular Imaging System" (ACIS III, Dako, Glostrup, Denmark), and Mirax HistoQuant (3DHistech, Budapest, Hungary) [84].

In our own experience we have used HALO, which is an automated quantitative digital pathology platform, compatible with all major microscope/slide scanners and non-proprietary tiff/jpeg formats and allowing for whole-slide and field-of-view analyses. Modules used for mIHC analysis include mIHC (brightfield mIHC), a tissue classifier module for tissue differentiation (e.g., tumor vs. stroma), and a spatial analysis module for interrogating spatial distributions of cell populations within the same, or serial tissue sections. Occasionally, it is critical to separate out the tumor and stroma into two classes, in order to determine the percentage of tumor cells positive for x, versus the percentage of stromal cells positive for x. Manually annotating these regions is extremely laborious and therefore automatic detection of these two regions is required for high-throughput analysis. HALO uses two different machine learning classifiers for automatic tissue detection: the random forest classifier and HALO-AI. The random forest classifier uses the random forest algorithm to assign pixels to a certain class based on color and texture. A random forest classifier is very quick to create and is effective in applications such as differentiating between tumor and stroma as shown in Figure 5. The Serial Section module also allows one to create a classifier on one stain (e.g., an H&E image), and then superimpose the classification onto a registered serial section. Therefore, there is no need to have a tumor marker on each serial section to achieve tumor/stroma separation.

The random forest classifier is quick and easy to set-up but will often suffer when presented with multiple variable tissue staining; such is often true for large clinical cohorts. In such situations HALO-AI, a deep learning classifier can be used. HALO-AI is a convolutional neural network for pattern recognition within a tissue section. Whilst a pathologist's input is increased relative to random forest, the training results in a highly robust classifier that can be used across large cohorts. HALO-AI can even be trained to recognize different tissue classes across different stains. The probability map and conversion to annotation features can also be used in HALO-AI.

Once the selected classifier has been created and saved, it can then be used in the mIHC analysis in HALO. In brightfield, the mIHC module allows the pathologist to detect up to 5 stains, including an exclusion stain, in any cell compartment (nucleus, cytoplasm, membrane). The exclusion stain option can be used to exclude tar within lung tissue. An example of a mIHC analysis in HALO is shown in Figure 6.

Prior to running the mIHC analysis, pathologists can define specific phenotypes such as active T cells (e.g., dual-positive cells for brown and purple stains will be identified as dual positive for CD8 and Ki67; Figure 6).

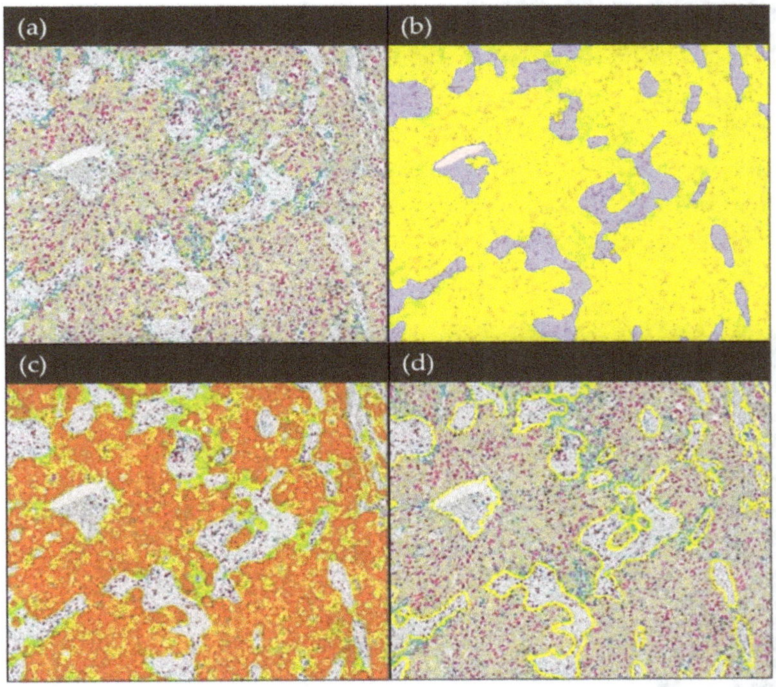

Figure 5. Tissue classification using the random forest classifier in non-small cell lung cancer tissue (20× magnification). (**a**) The multiplexed immunohistochemistry (mIHC) image was scanned with a Nanozoomer 2.0-HT Scanner (Hamamatsu photonics, Hamamatsu, Japan). The stains are as follows: Pan-cytokeratin (yellow), CD8 (brown), Ki67 (purple), PD-L1 (teal) and hematoxylin (dark purple). (**b**) The random forest classifier in HALO was used to separate the image into three classes: tumor, stroma and microscope glass slide. The classifier mask is shown overlaying the mIHC image where classified tumor regions are shown in yellow, stroma regions in purple, and the microscope glass slide in pale pink. (**c**) The probability threshold used by the random forest to detect tumor regions was increased to 70%. A heatmap is displayed where the red regions represent areas most likely to be tumor regions, and the green regions that are less likely. No mask will appear in areas where pixels have below 70% probability of being in the tumor class. (**d**) The classifier to annotations option was used whereby regions can automatically be annotated from the classification mask; only the tumor has been annotated (shown in yellow).

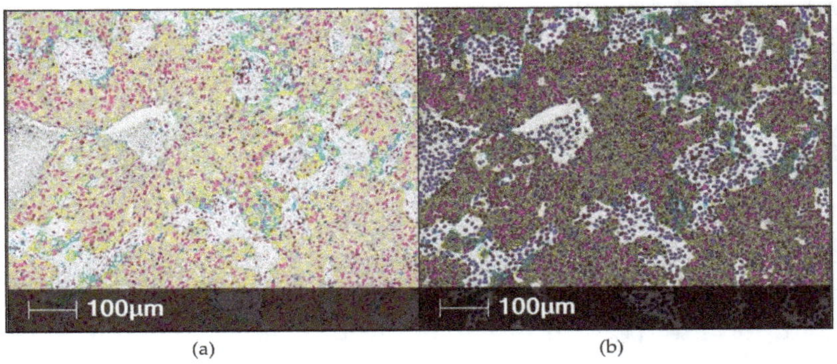

Figure 6. Automated digital analysis of multiplexed immunohistochemistry (mIHC) using the HALO software in non-small cell lung cancer tissue. (**a**) The mIHC image was scanned with a Nanozoomer 2.0-HT Scanner (Hamamatsu photonics, Hamamatsu, Japan) using 20x magnification. The stains are as follows: Pan-cytokeratin (yellow), CD8 (brown), Ki67 (purple), PD-L1 (teal) and hematoxylin (dark purple). (**b**) The HALO mark-up image shows colors similar to the original stain color and in the same cell compartment (nucleus/cytoplasm/membrane as the stain is found. The user can select different colors to be used in the mark-up image if they wish.

When this is run in conjunction with the pre-made classifier, information about the number of cells with a specific phenotype in both the tumor and the stroma can be obtained. Additionally, HALO's interactive cell-by-cell data table allows easy localization of the phenotyped cells on the image. In the example analysis in Figure 7, outputs will include those for the entire image, those specific to the tumor and those specific to the stroma. Other outputs include the number of cells positive for each stain in each compartment, number of cells with different stain co-localizations, the average optical density values for each stain in each compartment, cell/nucleus/cytoplasm/membrane area, and tissue areas in square microns.

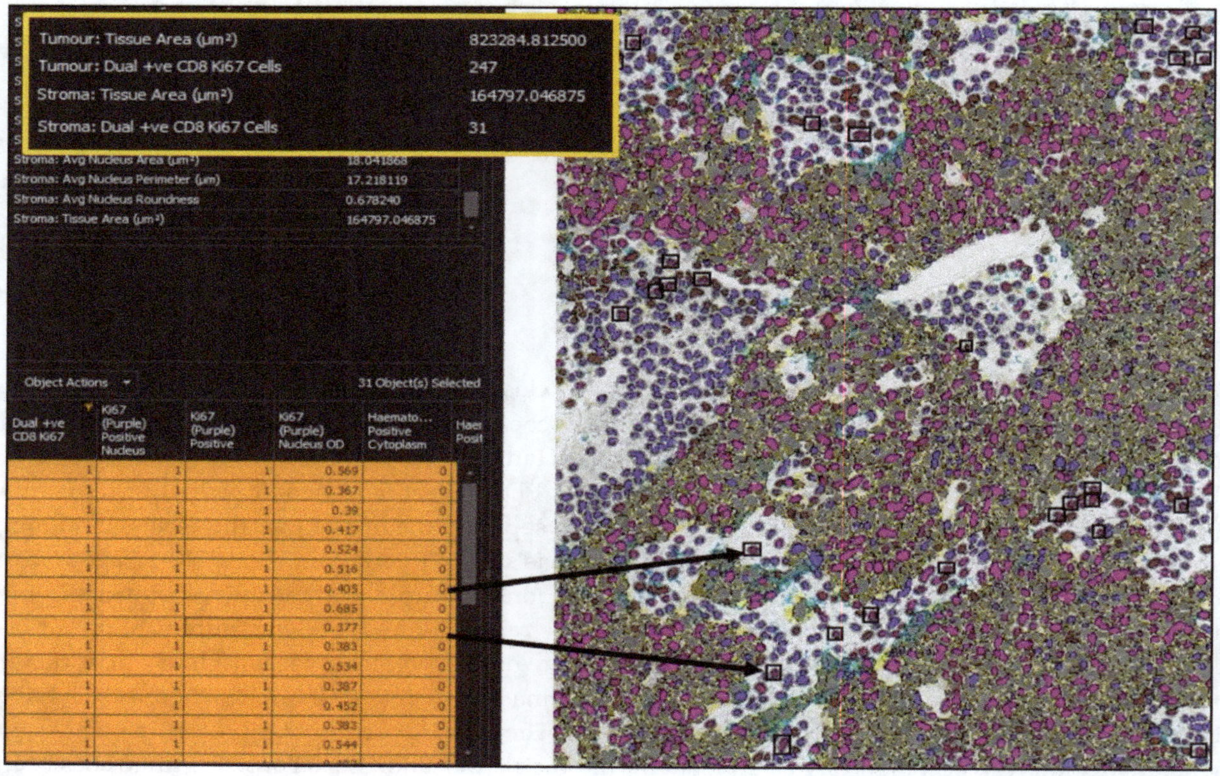

Figure 7. Results of a multiplexed immunohistochemistry (mIHC) analysis in HALO. The top left table provides the summary results from the analysis; important outputs in this analysis are the density of cells co-expressing both CD8 and Ki67 in the tumor and stroma, and so the data relating to this has been highlighted. The bottom left table is HALO's interactive cell-by-cell data table, which can be mined to find specific cell types. Here, only cells that are positive for CD8 and Ki67 and are in the stroma have been selected. HALO will find the cells selected in the image viewer (right, 20× magnification) by putting a black box around each cell.

After running a mIHC analysis in HALO, the pathologist then has the option to generate spatial information using the spatial analysis module. As outlined above, spatial information is becoming increasingly important in cancer research, prominently in the immune-oncology field [36,85]. Three different types of spatial analysis can be performed in HALO: nearest neighbor, proximity analysis and invasive margin analysis. Nearest neighbor outputs will calculate the average distance of two cell populations based on their nearest neighbors. Proximity analysis allows you to calculate the number of cells of one phenotype (e.g., CD8+ cytotoxic T lymphocytes) within a defined distance of another cell type. Lastly, the invasive margin analysis allows you to count the number of cells within a user defined distance of the invasive margin.

Similarly, the HALO image analysis software was recently used to demonstrate the divergent state of exhaustion of the PD-1 receptor in T cells with impaired effector cytokine production, while producing CXCL13, which mediates immune cell recruitment to tertiary lymphoid structures [80].

Importantly, the presence of PD-1^{high} cells was strongly predictive for both response and survival in a cohort of NSCLC patients treated with a PD-1 blocking agent [80].

In the immunofluorescence multiplexing field, the use of scanners (fluorescent or spectral) represents a major technological advance by enabling the utilization of multiple and sometimes unstable fluorochromes (e.g., phycoerythrins) and thus more than 7 different antibodies on the same slide. For example, Vectra® systems or Polaris®(PerkinElmer) allow the capture of information by spectral resolution in the visible and in the near infrared band (bandwidth between 420 and 900 nm). Vectra® or Polaris® allows extremely precise quantitative (cell-by-cell) management of the markings of different tissue samples, in brightfield or fluorescence detection. Detection and phenotypic characterization of cells in tissues, combined with bioinformatic image analysis is possible thanks to the InForm® software (PerkinElmer). This software allows automatic analysis of parameters that cannot be accurately discerned by the human eye (cell forms, multiple molecule networks, vascular network).

Franchising of autofluorescence by the "Autofluorescence Reduction Technology" (ART™, PerkinElmer) technique is possible with the Inform® software (PerkinElmer). Of course, the technologies developed for a specific type of cancer are subsequently transposable to the majority of other tumor proliferations or inflammatory diseases. Finally, virtual slides can be analyzed automatically (cell counting, surface measurements, etc.) using dedicated image analysis software (Figure 8). In particular, some software enables the quantification of weakly expressing and overlapping biomarkers within cells and cellular compartments.

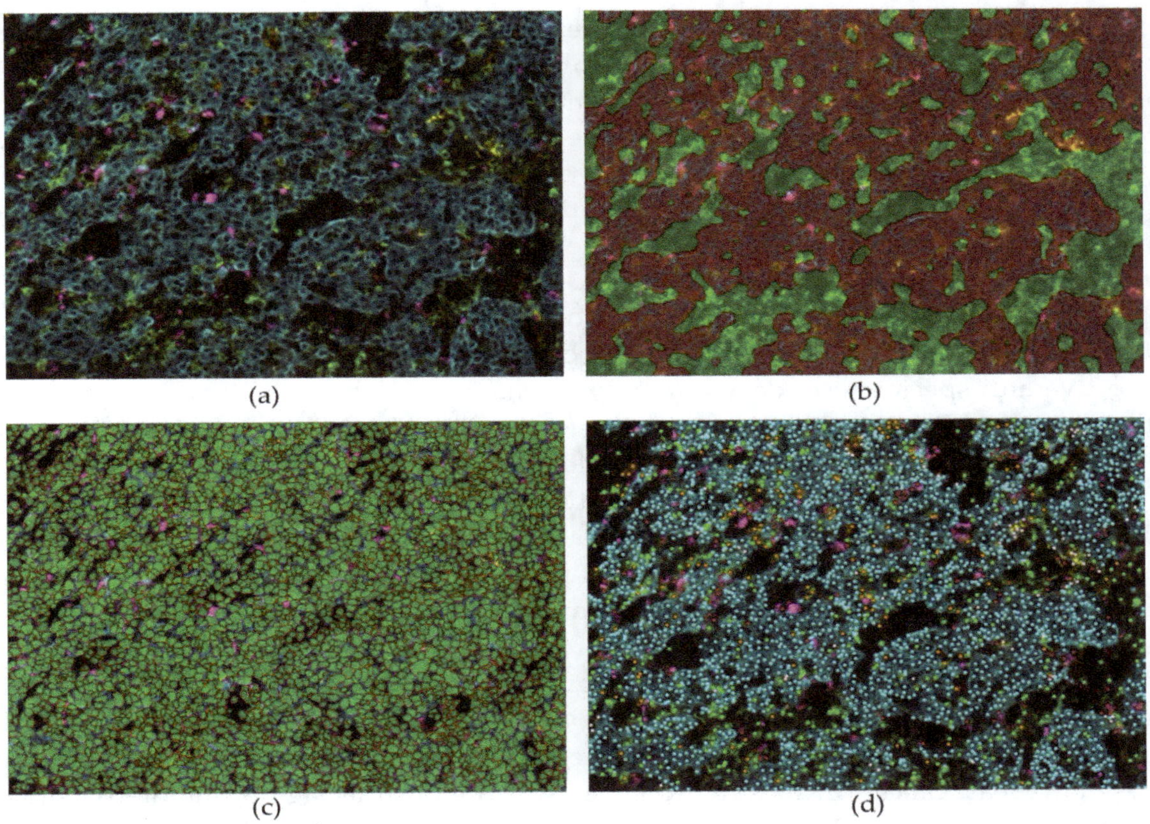

Figure 8. Automated digital analysis of fluorescent multiplexing using Inform software in tonsil tissue (20× magnification). (**a**) Multiparametric fluorescent staining Pan-Cytokeratin (turquoise), CD4 (green), CD68 (purple), PD-1 (red), PD-L1 (yellow) and dapi (blue). (**b**) Tissue segmentation: identification and recognition of tumor areas (red) or stroma (green). (**c**) Individual cells identification and segmentation, with nuclear, membranous and cytoplasmic segmentation. (**d**) Phenotyping: identification of the cells on the slide, with their phenotypes, among all the cells present in the image, or among the cells stained.

These new approaches allow us to explore cellular interactions to find biomarkers in a non-supervised manner. The education of the software remains long and tedious, with a phase of learning or "teaching". However, an approach without *a priori* knowledge can also be developed in parallel. Several companies developed such software (e.g., Definiens AG, Munich, Germany; TRIBVN Healthcare, Châtillon, France; Owkin, Paris, France; Imstar, Paris, France; Indica Labs; PerkinElmer). These software systems are becoming more and more efficient, and they can differentiate anatomical structures, such as glands [86], but the recognition of cell units is more delicate. The results obtained in the context of cross-sectional research studies are, however, very impressive and we must expect a change in diagnostic habits with the implementation of deep learning [87].

Finally, an important issue for mIHC digital analysis and relevant data extraction is the calibration of the signal acquisition technology and the control of variations caused by the different staining techniques when several batches are required to analyze large clinical series (e.g., for biomarker validation). These controls are also necessary for the valid comparison of different series or studies and ultimately for clinical application [88].

5. Advantages and Current Limitations of Multiplexed Immunohistochemistry

Recently developed multiplexing platforms exhibit compelling advantages. The major advantage of mIHC, which may also warrant its implementation in the routine clinical workflow, is related to maximal data harvesting per tissue section, improvement in the quality and detail of pathology analysis and efficient tissue utilization, which is crucial when the availability of sample is limited [89]. Approaches like mIHC enable pathologists to gather a wealth of data from a limited amount of tissue. This is especially promising for NSCLC patients whose tumors are in a difficult-to-access location, where only a small needle or cytology sample can be obtained. It also enables more research to be conducted with less material than is often required [89]. Unlike other multiplex approaches, such as next generation sequencing or mass spectrometry, mIHC gives an edge to analyze co-expression and to quantify single-cell expression with the spatial relationships of many targets while preserving tissue integrity. Several studies have shown that the proximity of certain immune cells within a tumor microenvironment correlates with patient outcome [41,85,90].

Recently developed strategies in the field of brightfield chromogenic mIHC have enabled automation of mIHC assays through the use of commercially available primary antibodies with their respective anti-species secondary antibody to ensure staining reliability and reproducibility, toward the clinical application [22]. Moreover, conventional brightfield microscopes and scanners can accommodate image acquisition of the stained slides [78].

However, multiple pre-analytical and analytical challenges arise when using chromogens for high-level mIHC analysis. The limited number of available chromogens, compared to highly multiplexed fluorescent assays, limits the degree of flexibility for biomarker research. As chromogenic mIHC is technically similar, in some ways, to conventional IHC it is subjected to the same critical hurdles [91]. The lack of standardization due to pre-analytic variables, including fixation time, type of fixative, dehydration, clearing, paraffin impregnation, and drying and storage of the slides, still represents a major potential challenge [92]. Similarly, poorly characterized or cross-reactive antibodies will give non-reproducible results [93]. For instance, despite numerous efforts to standardize the IHC markers used in breast cancer (ER/PR/HER2), they still demonstrate significant inter-laboratory and intra-laboratory variability [94]. If such issues cannot be overreached for these "conventional" IHC biomarkers, the multiplexing of several markers will need sufficient robustness prior to a clinical use. As for the clinical single IHC assays, a positive tissue control previously validated and characterized should be run on each same slide tested with mIHC. This would allow "real-time" validation of the multiplexed staining along with the quality control of data generated by the mIHC assay.

As tumors frequently harbor significant cellular and spatial heterogeneity (e.g., stroma, tumor-stroma interface, intratumoral), in particular for immune markers such as PD-L1 or CD8 infiltrates [95], it is essential to perform high-resolution multiplexed analysis across whole tumor sections. It has been demonstrate that the analysis of small ROIs generates significant variation and errors in the assessment of tumor and immune markers in cancer [96,97]. Hence, there is a need for integrated mIHC systems enabling high-degree of multiplexing coupled with digital analysis for high-resolution analyses on whole tumor slides [98].

Moreover, mIHC is the only technology enabling quantitative information on multiple distinct subtypes of tumor-infiltrating immune cells within a preserved tissue architecture, hence allowing the analysis of the topology and proximity between specific cell populations [99]. Ultimately, the quantitative spatial profiling of key tumor-immune pathways could improve the stratification of cancer patients for immunotherapy [100]. In addition, the explosion of potentially important or actionable biomarkers poses both cost and selection challenges. The increase in the number of developed chromogens could make this challenge somewhat easier to handle [16]. However, the current cost of the primary antibodies or different chromogens and the instrumentation requirements are still high. More than four antibodies can be sequentially incubated on autostainers, reducing the difficulty, delay and therefore cost to perform the mIHC analysis in a clinical setting, although, as noted above, pre-analytical variability and antigen retrieval methods will first need to be critically evaluated. Moreover, evaluation of multiple targets per tissue slide will require digital image viewing with analysis tools for computer-assisted interpretation that are yet to be readily integrated in the clinical workflow [78]. For a wide clinical implementation and pathologists' acceptance, regulatory and reimbursement rules should be planned in the near future. Nevertheless, the extraordinary value of such a technological approach to improve pathology interpretation and to yield new insights into understanding cancer phenotypes with direct clinical impacts warrants further effort.

The different considerations presented above could be declined for the fluorescent mIHC. The specificity of the staining has been improved with the use of tyramide techniques allowing simultaneous staining with 7 to 9 colors in a same slide. The different technical implementations described in this article have to reinforce the efforts made to increase the knowledge about microenvironment. Fluorescent staining keeps an advantage in research for the observation of very rare events, rare cells, co-localization and still allows a better study of the different cell compartments. Nevertheless, this technique is still difficult to be used in routine; the signal reproducibility is difficult to be obtained, even with an automation of the staining.

Several alternative multiplexed technologies for a use on FFPE samples have recently been developed (e.g. multiplexed ion beam imaging-MIBI, IONpath, Inc., Menlo Park, CA, USA; imaging mass cytometry, Fluidigm, South San Francisco, CA, USA; digital spatial profiling technology, NanoString Technologies, Inc., Seattle, WA, USA; InSituPlex, Ultivue, Cambridge MA, USA) demonstrating a high degree of multiplexing, and could be complementary to mIHC approaches described herein [89,101–103].

6. Conclusions

Technological advances in mIHC and the introduction of automated slide scanners has allowed for huge amounts of data to be generated in a single experiment. Combining this with automated digital analysis means the data can be analyzed in a quantitative and efficient manner, producing a high-throughput workflow for molecular and immune profiling with the promise of discovering novel biomarkers and improving clinical management of patients with NSCLC.

Author Contributions: Conceptualization, P.H., C.B. and M.I.; methodology, P.H., E.T., F.H., C.B., and M.I.; software, E.T., F.H., C.B., and M.I.; validation, P.H., E.T., F.H., C.B., and M.I.; formal analysis, P.H., E.T., F.H., C.B., and M.I.; investigation, P.H., E.T., F.H., L.B., E.L-M., S.L., H.R., V.H., C.B., and M.I.; resources, P.H., E.T., F.H., L.B., E.L-M., S.L., H.R., V.H., C.B., and M.I.; data curation, P.H., E.T., F.H., L.B., E.L-M., S.L., H.R., V.H., C.B., and M.I.; writing—original draft preparation, P.H., E.T., F.H., C.B., and M.I.; writing—review and editing, P.H., E.T., F.H., L.B., E.L-M., S.L., H.R., V.H., C.B., and M.I.; visualization, P.H., E.T., F.H., C.B., and M.I.; supervision, P.H., E.T., F.H., C.B., and M.I.; project administration, P.H., E.T., F.H., C.B., and M.I.; funding acquisition, P.H., E.T., F.H., C.B., and M.I.

Acknowledgments: To Julien Fayada and Marion Mandavit for their technical support.

References

1. Bray, F.; Ferlay, J.; Soerjomataram, I.; Siegel, R.L.; Torre, L.A.; Jemal, A. Global cancer statistics 2018: GLOBOCAN estimates of incidence and mortality worldwide for 36 cancers in 185 countries. *CA Cancer J. Clin.* **2018**, *68*, 394–424. [CrossRef] [PubMed]
2. Scagliotti, G.V.; Bironzo, P.; Vansteenkiste, J.F. Addressing the unmet need in lung cancer: The potential of immuno-oncology. *Cancer Treat. Rev.* **2015**, *41*, 465–475. [CrossRef] [PubMed]
3. Lee, C.K.; Brown, C.; Gralla, R.J.; Hirsh, V.; Thongprasert, S.; Tsai, C.M.; Tan, E.H.; Ho, J.C.; Chu da, T.; Zaatar, A.; et al. Impact of EGFR inhibitor in non-small cell lung cancer on progression-free and overall survival: A meta-analysis. *J. Natl. Cancer Inst.* **2013**, *105*, 595–605. [CrossRef] [PubMed]
4. Shaw, A.T.; Engelman, J.A. ALK in lung cancer: Past, present, and future. *J. Clin. Oncol.* **2013**, *31*, 1105–1111. [CrossRef] [PubMed]
5. Schiller, J.H.; Harrington, D.; Belani, C.P.; Langer, C.; Sandler, A.; Krook, J.; Zhu, J.; Johnson, D.H. Comparison of four chemotherapy regimens for advanced non-small-cell lung cancer. *N. Engl. J. Med.* **2002**, *346*, 92–98. [CrossRef] [PubMed]
6. Forde, P.M.; Chaft, J.E.; Smith, K.N.; Anagnostou, V.; Cottrell, T.R.; Hellmann, M.D.; Zahurak, M.; Yang, S.C.; Jones, D.R.; Broderick, S.; et al. Neoadjuvant PD-1 Blockade in Resectable Lung Cancer. *N. Engl. J. Med.* **2018**, *378*, 1976–1986. [CrossRef] [PubMed]
7. Reck, M.; Rodriguez-Abreu, D.; Robinson, A.G.; Hui, R.; Csoszi, T.; Fulop, A.; Gottfried, M.; Peled, N.; Tafreshi, A.; Cuffe, S.; et al. Pembrolizumab versus Chemotherapy for PD-L1-Positive Non-Small-Cell Lung Cancer. *N. Engl. J. Med.* **2016**, *375*, 1823–1833. [CrossRef] [PubMed]
8. Reck, M.; Popat, S.; Reinmuth, N.; De Ruysscher, D.; Kerr, K.M.; Peters, S.; Group, E.G.W. Metastatic non-small-cell lung cancer (NSCLC): ESMO Clinical Practice Guidelines for diagnosis, treatment and follow-up. *Ann. Oncol.* **2014**, *25*, iii27–iii39. [CrossRef] [PubMed]
9. Ribas, A.; Wolchok, J.D. Cancer immunotherapy using checkpoint blockade. *Science* **2018**, *359*, 1350–1355. [CrossRef] [PubMed]
10. Planchard, D.; Popat, S.; Kerr, K.; Novello, S.; Smit, E.F.; Faivre-Finn, C.; Mok, T.S.; Reck, M.; Van Schil, P.E.; Hellmann, M.D.; et al. Metastatic non-small cell lung cancer: ESMO Clinical Practice Guidelines for diagnosis, treatment and follow-up. *Ann. Oncol.* **2018**, *29*, iv192–iv237. [CrossRef] [PubMed]
11. Dietel, M.; Bubendorf, L.; Dingemans, A.M.; Dooms, C.; Elmberger, G.; Garcia, R.C.; Kerr, K.M.; Lim, E.; Lopez-Rios, F.; Thunnissen, E.; et al. Diagnostic procedures for non-small-cell lung cancer (NSCLC): Recommendations of the European Expert Group. *Thorax* **2016**, *71*, 177–184. [CrossRef] [PubMed]
12. Travis, W.D.; Brambilla, E.; Nicholson, A.G.; Yatabe, Y.; Austin, J.H.; Beasley, M.B.; Chirieac, L.R.; Dacic, S.; Duhig, E.; Flieder, D.B.; et al. The 2015 World Health Organization Classification of Lung Tumors: Impact of Genetic, Clinical and Radiologic Advances Since the 2004 Classification. *J. Thorac. Oncol.* **2015**, *10*, 1243–1260. [CrossRef] [PubMed]
13. Inamura, K. Update on Immunohistochemistry for the Diagnosis of Lung Cancer. *Cancers* **2018**, *10*, 72. [CrossRef] [PubMed]
14. Giraldo, N.A.; Peske, J.D.; Sautes-Fridman, C.; Fridman, W.H. Integrating histopathology, immune biomarkers, and molecular subgroups in solid cancer: The next step in precision oncology. *Virchows Arch.* **2019**. [CrossRef] [PubMed]
15. Coghlin, C.L.; Smith, L.J.; Bakar, S.; Stewart, K.N.; Devereux, G.S.; Nicolson, M.C.; Kerr, K.M. Quantitative analysis of tumor in bronchial biopsy specimens. *J. Thorac. Oncol.* **2010**, *5*, 448–452. [CrossRef] [PubMed]
16. Levenson, R.M.; Borowsky, A.D.; Angelo, M. Immunohistochemistry and mass spectrometry for highly multiplexed cellular molecular imaging. *Lab. Investig.* **2015**, *95*, 397–405. [CrossRef] [PubMed]
17. Parra, E.R.; Francisco-Cruz, A.; Wistuba, I.I. State-of-the-Art of Profiling Immune Contexture in the Era of Multiplexed Staining and Digital Analysis to Study Paraffin Tumor Tissues. *Cancers* **2019**, *11*. [CrossRef] [PubMed]

18. Blom, S.; Paavolainen, L.; Bychkov, D.; Turkki, R.; Maki-Teeri, P.; Hemmes, A.; Valimaki, K.; Lundin, J.; Kallioniemi, O.; Pellinen, T. Systems pathology by multiplexed immunohistochemistry and whole-slide digital image analysis. *Sci. Rep.* **2017**, *7*, 15580. [CrossRef] [PubMed]
19. Gorris, M.A.J.; Halilovic, A.; Rabold, K.; van Duffelen, A.; Wickramasinghe, I.N.; Verweij, D.; Wortel, I.M.N.; Textor, J.C.; de Vries, I.J.M.; Figdor, C.G. Eight-Color Multiplex Immunohistochemistry for Simultaneous Detection of Multiple Immune Checkpoint Molecules within the Tumor Microenvironment. *J. Immunol.* **2018**, *200*, 347–354. [CrossRef] [PubMed]
20. Tsujikawa, T.; Kumar, S.; Borkar, R.N.; Azimi, V.; Thibault, G.; Chang, Y.H.; Balter, A.; Kawashima, R.; Choe, G.; Sauer, D.; et al. Quantitative Multiplex Immunohistochemistry Reveals Myeloid-Inflamed Tumor-Immune Complexity Associated with Poor Prognosis. *Cell Rep.* **2017**, *19*, 203–217. [CrossRef] [PubMed]
21. Remark, R.; Merghoub, T.; Grabe, N.; Litjens, G.; Damotte, D.; Wolchok, J.D.; Merad, M.; Gnjatic, S. In-depth tissue profiling using multiplexed immunohistochemical consecutive staining on single slide. *Sci. Immunol.* **2016**, *1*, aaf6925. [CrossRef] [PubMed]
22. Ilie, M.; Beaulande, M.; Hamila, M.; Erb, G.; Hofman, V.; Hofman, P. Automated chromogenic multiplexed immunohistochemistry assay for diagnosis and predictive biomarker testing in non-small cell lung cancer. *Lung Cancer* **2018**, *124*, 90–94. [CrossRef] [PubMed]
23. Gibney, G.T.; Weiner, L.M.; Atkins, M.B. Predictive biomarkers for checkpoint inhibitor-based immunotherapy. *Lancet Oncol.* **2016**, *17*, e542–e551. [CrossRef]
24. Stack, E.C.; Wang, C.; Roman, K.A.; Hoyt, C.C. Multiplexed immunohistochemistry, imaging, and quantitation: A review, with an assessment of Tyramide signal amplification, multispectral imaging and multiplex analysis. *Methods* **2014**, *70*, 46–58. [CrossRef] [PubMed]
25. Osman, T.A.; Oijordsbakken, G.; Costea, D.E.; Johannessen, A.C. Successful triple immunoenzymatic method employing primary antibodies from same species and same immunoglobulin subclass. *Eur. J. Histochem.* **2013**, *57*, e22. [CrossRef] [PubMed]
26. Feng, Z.; Puri, S.; Moudgil, T.; Wood, W.; Hoyt, C.C.; Wang, C.; Urba, W.J.; Curti, B.D.; Bifulco, C.B.; Fox, B.A. Multispectral imaging of formalin-fixed tissue predicts ability to generate tumor-infiltrating lymphocytes from melanoma. *J. Immunother. Cancer* **2015**, *3*, 47. [CrossRef] [PubMed]
27. Pirici, D.; Mogoanta, L.; Kumar-Singh, S.; Pirici, I.; Margaritescu, C.; Simionescu, C.; Stanescu, R. Antibody elution method for multiple immunohistochemistry on primary antibodies raised in the same species and of the same subtype. *J. Histochem. Cytochem.* **2009**, *57*, 567–575. [CrossRef] [PubMed]
28. Gendusa, R.; Scalia, C.R.; Buscone, S.; Cattoretti, G. Elution of High-affinity (>10–9 KD) Antibodies from Tissue Sections: Clues to the Molecular Mechanism and Use in Sequential Immunostaining. *J. Histochem. Cytochem.* **2014**, *62*, 519–531. [CrossRef] [PubMed]
29. Glass, G.; Papin, J.A.; Mandell, J.W. SIMPLE: A sequential immunoperoxidase labeling and erasing method. *J. Histochem. Cytochem.* **2009**, *57*, 899–905. [CrossRef] [PubMed]
30. Zhang, W.; Hubbard, A.; Jones, T.; Racolta, A.; Bhaumik, S.; Cummins, N.; Zhang, L.; Garsha, K.; Ventura, F.; Lefever, M.R.; et al. Fully automated 5-plex fluorescent immunohistochemistry with tyramide signal amplification and same species antibodies. *Lab. Investig.* **2017**, *97*, 873–885. [CrossRef] [PubMed]
31. Buchwalow, I.; Samoilova, V.; Boecker, W.; Tiemann, M. Multiple immunolabeling with antibodies from the same host species in combination with tyramide signal amplification. *Acta Histochem.* **2018**, *120*, 405–411. [CrossRef] [PubMed]
32. Prichard, J.W. Overview of automated immunohistochemistry. *Arch. Pathol. Lab. Med.* **2014**, *138*, 1578–1582. [CrossRef] [PubMed]
33. Ilie, M.; Beaulande, M.; Ben Hadj, S.; Chamorey, E.; Schiappa, R.; Long-Mira, E.; Lassalle, S.; Butori, C.; Cohen, C.; Leroy, S.; et al. Chromogenic Multiplex Immunohistochemistry Reveals Modulation of the Immune Microenvironment Associated with Survival in Elderly Patients with Lung Adenocarcinoma. *Cancers* **2018**, *10*. [CrossRef] [PubMed]
34. Dixon, A.R.; Bathany, C.; Tsuei, M.; White, J.; Barald, K.F.; Takayama, S. Recent developments in multiplexing techniques for immunohistochemistry. *Expert Rev. Mol. Diagn.* **2015**, *15*, 1171–1186. [CrossRef] [PubMed]
35. Chen, T.; Srinivas, C. Group sparsity model for stain unmixing in brightfield multiplex immunohistochemistry images. *Comput. Med. Imaging Graph.* **2015**, *46*, 30–39. [CrossRef] [PubMed]

36. Galon, J.; Costes, A.; Sanchez-Cabo, F.; Kirilovsky, A.; Mlecnik, B.; Lagorce-Pages, C.; Tosolini, M.; Camus, M.; Berger, A.; Wind, P.; et al. Type, density, and location of immune cells within human colorectal tumors predict clinical outcome. *Science* **2006**, *313*, 1960–1964. [CrossRef] [PubMed]
37. Salama, P.; Phillips, M.; Grieu, F.; Morris, M.; Zeps, N.; Joseph, D.; Platell, C.; Iacopetta, B. Tumor-infiltrating FOXP3 + T regulatory cells show strong prognostic significance in colorectal cancer. *J. Clin. Oncol.* **2009**, *27*, 186–192. [CrossRef] [PubMed]
38. Badoual, C.; Hans, S.; Rodriguez, J.; Peyrard, S.; Klein, C.; Agueznay Nel, H.; Mosseri, V.; Laccourreye, O.; Bruneval, P.; Fridman, W.H.; et al. Prognostic value of tumor-infiltrating CD4 + T-cell subpopulations in head and neck cancers. *Clin. Cancer Res.* **2006**, *12*, 465–472. [CrossRef] [PubMed]
39. Granier, C.; Vinatier, E.; Colin, E.; Mandavit, M.; Dariane, C.; Verkarre, V.; Biard, L.; El Zein, R.; Lesaffre, C.; Galy-Fauroux, I.; et al. Multiplexed Immunofluorescence Analysis and Quantification of Intratumoral PD-1 + Tim-3 + CD8 + T Cells. *J. Vis. Exp.* **2018**. [CrossRef] [PubMed]
40. Anichini, A.; Tassi, E.; Grazia, G.; Mortarini, R. The non-small cell lung cancer immune landscape: Emerging complexity, prognostic relevance and prospective significance in the context of immunotherapy. *Cancer Immunol. Immunother.* **2018**, *67*, 1011–1022. [CrossRef] [PubMed]
41. Remark, R.; Becker, C.; Gomez, J.E.; Damotte, D.; Dieu-Nosjean, M.C.; Sautes-Fridman, C.; Fridman, W.H.; Powell, C.A.; Altorki, N.K.; Merad, M.; et al. The non-small cell lung cancer immune contexture. A major determinant of tumor characteristics and patient outcome. *Am. J. Respir. Crit. Care Med.* **2015**, *191*, 377–390. [CrossRef] [PubMed]
42. Rakaee, M.; Busund, L.T.; Paulsen, E.E.; Richardsen, E.; Al-Saad, S.; Andersen, S.; Donnem, T.; Bremnes, R.M.; Kilvaer, T.K. Prognostic effect of intratumoral neutrophils across histological subtypes of non-small cell lung cancer. *Oncotarget* **2016**, *7*, 72184–72196. [CrossRef] [PubMed]
43. Ilie, M.; Hofman, V.; Ortholan, C.; Bonnetaud, C.; Coelle, C.; Mouroux, J.; Hofman, P. Predictive clinical outcome of the intratumoral CD66b-positive neutrophil-to-CD8-positive T-cell ratio in patients with resectable nonsmall cell lung cancer. *Cancer* **2012**, *118*, 1726–1737. [CrossRef] [PubMed]
44. Donnem, T.; Kilvaer, T.K.; Andersen, S.; Richardsen, E.; Paulsen, E.E.; Hald, S.M.; Al-Saad, S.; Brustugun, O.T.; Helland, A.; Lund-Iversen, M.; et al. Strategies for clinical implementation of TNM-Immunoscore in resected nonsmall-cell lung cancer. *Ann. Oncol.* **2016**, *27*, 225–232. [CrossRef] [PubMed]
45. Pages, F.; Mlecnik, B.; Marliot, F.; Bindea, G.; Ou, F.S.; Bifulco, C.; Lugli, A.; Zlobec, I.; Rau, T.T.; Berger, M.D.; et al. International validation of the consensus Immunoscore for the classification of colon cancer: A prognostic and accuracy study. *Lancet* **2018**, *391*, 2128–2139. [CrossRef]
46. Chiari, R.; Sidoni, A.; Metro, G. Early stage resectable non-small cell lung cancer: Is neoadjuvant immunotherapy the right way forward? *J. Thorac. Dis.* **2018**, *10*, S3890–S3894. [CrossRef] [PubMed]
47. Cottrell, T.R.; Thompson, E.D.; Forde, P.M.; Stein, J.E.; Duffield, A.S.; Anagnostou, V.; Rekhtman, N.; Anders, R.A.; Cuda, J.D.; Illei, P.B.; et al. Pathologic features of response to neoadjuvant anti-PD-1 in resected non-small-cell lung carcinoma: A proposal for quantitative immune-related pathologic response criteria (irPRC). *Ann. Oncol.* **2018**, *29*, 1853–1860. [CrossRef] [PubMed]
48. Remon, J.; Vilarino, N.; Reguart, N. Immune checkpoint inhibitors in non-small cell lung cancer (NSCLC): Approaches on special subgroups and unresolved burning questions. *Cancer Treat. Rev.* **2018**, *64*, 21–29. [CrossRef] [PubMed]
49. Zinger, A.; Cho, W.C.; Ben-Yehuda, A. Cancer and Aging—The Inflammatory Connection. *Aging Dis.* **2017**, *8*, 611–627. [CrossRef] [PubMed]
50. Shah, W.; Yan, X.; Jing, L.; Zhou, Y.; Chen, H.; Wang, Y. A reversed CD4/CD8 ratio of tumor-infiltrating lymphocytes and a high percentage of CD4 (+) FOXP3 (+) regulatory T cells are significantly associated with clinical outcome in squamous cell carcinoma of the cervix. *Cell Mol. Immunol.* **2011**, *8*, 59–66. [CrossRef] [PubMed]
51. Chee, S.J.; Lopez, M.; Mellows, T.; Gankande, S.; Moutasim, K.A.; Harris, S.; Clarke, J.; Vijayanand, P.; Thomas, G.J.; Ottensmeier, C.H. Evaluating the effect of immune cells on the outcome of patients with mesothelioma. *Br. J. Cancer* **2017**, *117*, 1341–1348. [CrossRef] [PubMed]
52. Han, S.; Zhang, C.; Li, Q.; Dong, J.; Liu, Y.; Huang, Y.; Jiang, T.; Wu, A. Tumour-infiltrating CD4 (+) and CD8 (+) lymphocytes as predictors of clinical outcome in glioma. *Br. J. Cancer* **2014**, *110*, 2560–2568. [CrossRef] [PubMed]

53. Ilie, M.; Hofman, V.; Dietel, M.; Soria, J.C.; Hofman, P. Assessment of the PD-L1 status by immunohistochemistry: Challenges and perspectives for therapeutic strategies in lung cancer patients. *Virchows Arch.* **2016**, *468*, 511–525. [CrossRef] [PubMed]
54. Kayser, G.; Csanadi, A.; Otto, C.; Plones, T.; Bittermann, N.; Rawluk, J.; Passlick, B.; Werner, M. Simultaneous multi-antibody staining in non-small cell lung cancer strengthens diagnostic accuracy especially in small tissue samples. *PLoS ONE* **2013**, *8*, e56333. [CrossRef] [PubMed]
55. Selves, J.; Long-Mira, E.; Mathieu, M.C.; Rochaix, P.; Ilie, M. Immunohistochemistry for Diagnosis of Metastatic Carcinomas of Unknown Primary Site. *Cancers* **2018**, *10*, 108. [CrossRef] [PubMed]
56. Cruz, A.F.; Parra, E.R.; Jiang, M.; Fujimoto, J.; Chow, C.W.; Rodriguez-Canales, J.; Behrens, C.; Kalhor, N.; Weissferdt, A.; Heymach, J.; et al. Characterization of the Immunologic Intra-Tumor Heterogeneity in Early Stages of Non-Small Cell Lung. Cancer by Multiplex Immunofluorescence. In Proceedings of the IASLC 19th World Conference on Lung Cancer, Toronto, ON, Canada, 23–26 September 2018; pp. S325–S326.
57. Schalper, K.A.; Carvajal-Hausdorf, D.; McLaughlin, J.; Altan, M.; Velcheti, V.; Gaule, P.; Sanmamed, M.F.; Chen, L.; Herbst, R.S.; Rimm, D.L. Differential Expression and Significance of PD-L1, IDO-1, and B7-H4 in Human Lung Cancer. *Clin. Cancer Res.* **2017**, *23*, 370–378. [CrossRef] [PubMed]
58. Spranger, S.; Spaapen, R.M.; Zha, Y.; Williams, J.; Meng, Y.; Ha, T.T.; Gajewski, T.F. Up-regulation of PD-L1, IDO, and T(regs) in the melanoma tumor microenvironment is driven by CD8 (+) T cells. *Sci. Transl. Med.* **2013**, *5*, 200ra116. [CrossRef] [PubMed]
59. Schalper, K.A.; Brown, J.; Carvajal-Hausdorf, D.; McLaughlin, J.; Velcheti, V.; Syrigos, K.N.; Herbst, R.S.; Rimm, D.L. Objective measurement and clinical significance of TILs in non-small cell lung cancer. *J. Natl. Cancer Instig.* **2015**, *107*. [CrossRef] [PubMed]
60. Parra, E.R.; Villalobos, P.; Behrens, C.; Jiang, M.; Pataer, A.; Swisher, S.G.; William, W.N., Jr.; Zhang, J.; Lee, J.; Cascone, T.; et al. Effect of neoadjuvant chemotherapy on the immune microenvironment in non-small cell lung carcinomas as determined by multiplex immunofluorescence and image analysis approaches. *J. Immunother. Cancer* **2018**, *6*, 48. [CrossRef] [PubMed]
61. Mami-Chouaib, F.; Blanc, C.; Corgnac, S.; Hans, S.; Malenica, I.; Granier, C.; Tihy, I.; Tartour, E. Resident memory T cells, critical components in tumor immunology. *J. Immunother. Cancer* **2018**, *6*, 87. [CrossRef] [PubMed]
62. Nizard, M.; Roussel, H.; Diniz, M.O.; Karaki, S.; Tran, T.; Voron, T.; Dransart, E.; Sandoval, F.; Riquet, M.; Rance, B.; et al. Induction of resident memory T cells enhances the efficacy of cancer vaccine. *Nat. Commun.* **2017**, *8*, 15221. [CrossRef] [PubMed]
63. Ganesan, A.P.; Clarke, J.; Wood, O.; Garrido-Martin, E.M.; Chee, S.J.; Mellows, T.; Samaniego-Castruita, D.; Singh, D.; Seumois, G.; Alzetani, A.; et al. Tissue-resident memory features are linked to the magnitude of cytotoxic T cell responses in human lung cancer. *Nat. Immunol.* **2017**. [CrossRef] [PubMed]
64. Djenidi, F.; Adam, J.; Goubar, A.; Durgeau, A.; Meurice, G.; de Montpreville, V.; Validire, P.; Besse, B.; Mami-Chouaib, F. CD8 + CD103 + tumor-infiltrating lymphocytes are tumor-specific tissue-resident memory T cells and a prognostic factor for survival in lung cancer patients. *J. Immunol.* **2015**, *194*, 3475–3486. [CrossRef] [PubMed]
65. Mezheyeuski, A.; Bergsland, C.H.; Backman, M.; Djureinovic, D.; Sjoblom, T.; Bruun, J.; Micke, P. Multispectral imaging for quantitative and compartment-specific immune infiltrates reveals distinct immune profiles that classify lung cancer patients. *J. Pathol.* **2018**, *244*, 421–431. [CrossRef] [PubMed]
66. Granier, C.; De Guillebon, E.; Blanc, C.; Roussel, H.; Badoual, C.; Colin, E.; Saldmann, A.; Gey, A.; Oudard, S.; Tartour, E. Mechanisms of action and rationale for the use of checkpoint inhibitors in cancer. *ESMO Open* **2017**, *2*, e000213. [CrossRef] [PubMed]
67. Song, Z.; Yu, X.; Zhang, Y. Altered expression of programmed death-ligand 1 after neo-adjuvant chemotherapy in patients with lung squamous cell carcinoma. *Lung Cancer* **2016**, *99*, 166–171. [CrossRef] [PubMed]
68. Mesnage, S.J.L.; Auguste, A.; Genestie, C.; Dunant, A.; Pain, E.; Drusch, F.; Gouy, S.; Morice, P.; Bentivegna, E.; Lhomme, C.; et al. Neoadjuvant chemotherapy (NACT) increases immune infiltration and programmed death-ligand 1 (PD-L1) expression in epithelial ovarian cancer (EOC). *Ann. Oncol.* **2017**, *28*, 651–657. [CrossRef] [PubMed]
69. Roussel, H.; De Guillebon, H.; Biard, L.; Mandavit, M.; Gibault, L.; Fabre, E.; Antoine, M.; Hofman, P.; Beau-Faller, M.; Blons, H.; et al. Composite biomarkers defined by multiparametric immunofluorescence

analysis identify ALK-positive adenocarcinoma as a potential target for immunotherapy. *Oncoimmunology* **2017**, *6*, e1286437. [CrossRef] [PubMed]

70. Remon, J.; Hendriks, L.E.; Cabrera, C.; Reguart, N.; Besse, B. Immunotherapy for oncogenic-driven advanced non-small cell lung cancers: Is the time ripe for a change? *Cancer Treat. Rev.* **2018**, *71*, 47–58. [CrossRef] [PubMed]
71. Gainor, J.F.; Shaw, A.T.; Sequist, L.V.; Fu, X.; Azzoli, C.G.; Piotrowska, Z.; Huynh, T.G.; Zhao, L.; Fulton, L.; Schultz, K.R.; et al. EGFR Mutations and ALK Rearrangements Are Associated with Low Response Rates to PD-1 Pathway Blockade in Non-Small Cell Lung Cancer: A Retrospective Analysis. *Clin. Cancer Res.* **2016**, *22*, 4585–4593. [CrossRef] [PubMed]
72. Liu, S.Y.; Dong, Z.Y.; Wu, S.P.; Xie, Z.; Yan, L.X.; Li, Y.F.; Yan, H.H.; Su, J.; Yang, J.J.; Zhou, Q.; et al. Clinical relevance of PD-L1 expression and CD8 + T cells infiltration in patients with EGFR-mutated and ALK-rearranged lung cancer. *Lung Cancer* **2018**, *125*, 86–92. [CrossRef] [PubMed]
73. Badoual, C.; Hans, S.; Merillon, N.; Van Ryswick, C.; Ravel, P.; Benhamouda, N.; Levionnois, E.; Nizard, M.; Si-Mohamed, A.; Besnier, N.; et al. PD-1-expressing tumor-infiltrating T cells are a favorable prognostic biomarker in HPV-associated head and neck cancer. *Cancer Res.* **2013**, *73*, 128–138. [CrossRef] [PubMed]
74. Granier, C.; Dariane, C.; Combe, P.; Verkarre, V.; Urien, S.; Badoual, C.; Roussel, H.; Mandavit, M.; Ravel, P.; Sibony, M.; et al. Tim-3 Expression on Tumor-Infiltrating PD-1 + CD8 + T Cells Correlates with Poor Clinical Outcome in Renal Cell Carcinoma. *Cancer Res.* **2017**, *77*, 1075–1082. [CrossRef] [PubMed]
75. Gettinger, S.N.; Choi, J.; Mani, N.; Sanmamed, M.F.; Datar, I.; Sowell, R.; Du, V.Y.; Kaftan, E.; Goldberg, S.; Dong, W.; et al. A dormant TIL phenotype defines non-small cell lung carcinomas sensitive to immune checkpoint blockers. *Nat. Commun.* **2018**, *9*, 3196. [CrossRef] [PubMed]
76. Parra, E.R.; Behrens, C.; Rodriguez-Canales, J.; Lin, H.; Mino, B.; Blando, J.; Zhang, J.; Gibbons, D.L.; Heymach, J.V.; Sepesi, B.; et al. Image Analysis-based Assessment of PD-L1 and Tumor-Associated Immune Cells Density Supports Distinct Intratumoral Microenvironment Groups in Non-small Cell Lung Carcinom Patients. *Clin. Cancer Res.* **2016**, *22*, 6278–6289. [CrossRef] [PubMed]
77. Seyed Jafari, S.M.; Hunger, R.E. IHC Optical Density Score: A New Practical Method for Quantitative Immunohistochemistry Image Analysis. *Appl. Immunohistochem. Mol. Morphol.* **2017**, *25*, e12–e13. [CrossRef] [PubMed]
78. Koelzer, V.H.; Sirinukunwattana, K.; Rittscher, J.; Mertz, K.D. Precision immunoprofiling by image analysis and artificial intelligence. *Virchows Arch.* **2018**. [CrossRef] [PubMed]
79. Ruifrok, A.C.; Johnston, D.A. Quantification of histochemical staining by color deconvolution. *Anal. Quant. Cytol. Histol.* **2001**, *23*, 291–299. [PubMed]
80. Thommen, D.S.; Koelzer, V.H.; Herzig, P.; Roller, A.; Trefny, M.; Dimeloe, S.; Kiialainen, A.; Hanhart, J.; Schill, C.; Hess, C.; et al. A transcriptionally and functionally distinct PD-1(+) CD8(+) T cell pool with predictive potential in non-small-cell lung cancer treated with PD-1 blockade. *Nat. Med.* **2018**, *24*, 994–1004. [CrossRef] [PubMed]
81. Huang, W.; Hennrick, K.; Drew, S. A colorful future of quantitative pathology: Validation of Vectra technology using chromogenic multiplexed immunohistochemistry and prostate tissue microarrays. *Hum. Pathol.* **2013**, *44*, 29–38. [CrossRef] [PubMed]
82. Ribas, A.; Dummer, R.; Puzanov, I.; VanderWalde, A.; Andtbacka, R.H.I.; Michielin, O.; Olszanski, A.J.; Malvehy, J.; Cebon, J.; Fernandez, E.; et al. Oncolytic Virotherapy Promotes Intratumoral T Cell Infiltration and Improves Anti-PD-1 Immunotherapy. *Cell* **2017**, *170*, 1109.e1110–1119.e1110. [CrossRef] [PubMed]
83. Steele, K.E.; Tan, T.H.; Korn, R.; Dacosta, K.; Brown, C.; Kuziora, M.; Zimmermann, J.; Laffin, B.; Widmaier, M.; Rognoni, L.; et al. Measuring multiple parameters of CD8+ tumor-infiltrating lymphocytes in human cancers by image analysis. *J. Immunother. Cancer* **2018**, *6*, 20. [CrossRef] [PubMed]
84. Rojo, M.G.; Bueno, G.; Slodkowska, J. Review of imaging solutions for integrated quantitative immunohistochemistry in the Pathology daily practice. *Folia Histochem. Cytobiol.* **2009**, *47*, 349–354. [CrossRef] [PubMed]
85. Tumeh, P.C.; Harview, C.L.; Yearley, J.H.; Shintaku, I.P.; Taylor, E.J.; Robert, L.; Chmielowski, B.; Spasic, M.; Henry, G.; Ciobanu, V.; et al. PD-1 blockade induces responses by inhibiting adaptive immune resistance. *Nature* **2014**, *515*, 568–571. [CrossRef] [PubMed]
86. Sirinukunwattana, K.; Snead, D.R.; Rajpoot, N.M. A Stochastic Polygons Model for Glandular Structures in Colon Histology Images. *IEEE Trans. Med. Imaging* **2015** *34*, 2366–2378. [CrossRef] [PubMed]

87. Litjens, G.; Kooi, T.; Bejnordi, B.E.; Setio, A.A.A.; Ciompi, F.; Ghafoorian, M.; van der Laak, J.; van Ginneken, B.; Sanchez, C.I. A survey on deep learning in medical image analysis. *Med. Image Anal.* **2017**, *42*, 60–88. [CrossRef] [PubMed]
88. Pantanowitz, L.; Sinard, J.H.; Henricks, W.H.; Fatheree, L.A.; Carter, A.B.; Contis, L.; Beckwith, B.A.; Evans, A.J.; Lal, A.; Parwani, A.V. Validating whole slide imaging for diagnostic purposes in pathology: Guideline from the College of American Pathologists Pathology and Laboratory Quality Center. *Arch. Pathol. Lab. Med.* **2013**, *137*, 1710–1722. [CrossRef] [PubMed]
89. Decalf, J.; Albert, M.L.; Ziai, J. New tools for pathology: A user's review of a highly multiplexed method for in situ analysis of protein and RNA expression in tissue. *J. Pathol.* **2018**. [CrossRef] [PubMed]
90. Charoentong, P.; Finotello, F.; Angelova, M.; Mayer, C.; Efremova, M.; Rieder, D.; Hackl, H.; Trajanoski, Z. Pan-cancer Immunogenomic Analyses Reveal Genotype-Immunophenotype Relationships and Predictors of Response to Checkpoint Blockade. *Cell Rep.* **2017**, *18*, 248–262. [CrossRef] [PubMed]
91. Rimm, D.L. Next-gen immunohistochemistry. *Nat. Methods* **2014**, *11*, 381–383. [CrossRef] [PubMed]
92. Magaki, S.; Hojat, S.A.; Wei, B.; So, A.; Yong, W.H. An Introduction to the Performance of Immunohistochemistry. *Methods Mol. Biol.* **2019**, *1897*, 289–298. [CrossRef] [PubMed]
93. Torlakovic, E.E.; Cheung, C.C.; D'Arrigo, C.; Dietel, M.; Francis, G.D.; Gilks, C.B.; Hall, J.A.; Hornick, J.L.; Ibrahim, M.; Marchetti, A.; et al. Evolution of Quality Assurance for Clinical Immunohistochemistry in the Era of Precision Medicine. Part 3: Technical Validation of Immunohistochemistry (IHC) Assays in Clinical IHC Laboratories. *Appl. Immunohistochem. Mol. Morphol.* **2017**, *25*, 151–159. [CrossRef] [PubMed]
94. Lin, C.Y.; Carneal, E.E.; Lichtensztajn, D.Y.; Gomez, S.L.; Clarke, C.A.; Jensen, K.C.; Kurian, A.W.; Allison, K.H. Regional Variability in Percentage of Breast Cancers Reported as Positive for HER2 in California: Implications of Patient Demographics on Laboratory Benchmarks. *Am. J. Clin. Pathol.* **2017**, *148*, 199–207. [CrossRef] [PubMed]
95. Ilie, M.; Long-Mira, E.; Bence, C.; Butori, C.; Lassalle, S.; Bouhlel, L.; Fazzalari, L.; Zahaf, K.; Lalvee, S.; Washetine, K.; et al. Comparative study of the PD-L1 status between surgically resected specimens and matched biopsies of NSCLC patients reveal major discordances: A potential issue for anti-PD-L1 therapeutic strategies. *Ann. Oncol.* **2016**, *27*, 147–153. [CrossRef] [PubMed]
96. Barnes, M.; Srinivas, C.; Bai, I.; Frederick, J.; Liu, W.; Sarkar, A.; Wang, X.; Nie, Y.; Portier, B.; Kapadia, M.; et al. Whole tumor section quantitative image analysis maximizes between-pathologists' reproducibility for clinical immunohistochemistry-based biomarkers. *Lab. Investig.* **2017**, *97*, 1508–1515. [CrossRef] [PubMed]
97. Christgen, M.; von Ahsen, S.; Christgen, H.; Langer, F.; Kreipe, H. The region-of-interest size impacts on Ki67 quantification by computer-assisted image analysis in breast cancer. *Hum. Pathol.* **2015**, *46*, 1341–1349. [CrossRef] [PubMed]
98. Klauschen, F.; Muller, K.R.; Binder, A.; Bockmayr, M.; Hagele, M.; Seegerer, P.; Wienert, S.; Pruneri, G.; de Maria, S.; Badve, S.; et al. Scoring of tumor-infiltrating lymphocytes: From visual estimation to machine learning. *Semin. Cancer Biol.* **2018**, *52*, 151–157. [CrossRef] [PubMed]
99. Carey, C.D.; Gusenleitner, D.; Lipschitz, M.; Roemer, M.G.M.; Stack, E.C.; Gjini, E.; Hu, X.; Redd, R.; Freeman, G.J.; Neuberg, D.; et al. Topological analysis reveals a PD-L1-associated microenvironmental niche for Reed-Sternberg cells in Hodgkin lymphoma. *Blood* **2017**, *130*, 2420–2430. [CrossRef] [PubMed]
100. Johnson, D.B.; Bordeaux, J.; Kim, J.Y.; Vaupel, C.; Rimm, D.L.; Ho, T.H.; Joseph, R.W.; Daud, A.I.; Conry, R.M.; Gaughan, E.M.; et al. Quantitative Spatial Profiling of PD-1/PD-L1 Interaction and HLA-DR/IDO-1 Predicts Improved Outcomes of Anti-PD-1 Therapies in Metastatic Melanoma. *Clin. Cancer Res.* **2018**, *24*, 5250–5260. [CrossRef] [PubMed]
101. Giesen, C.; Wang, H.A.; Schapiro, D.; Zivanovic, N.; Jacobs, A.; Hattendorf, B.; Schuffler, P.J.; Grolimund, D.; Buhmann, J.M.; Brandt, S.; et al. Highly multiplexed imaging of tumor tissues with subcellular resolution by mass cytometry. *Nat. Methods* **2014**, *11*, 417–422. [CrossRef] [PubMed]
102. Angelo, M.; Bendall, S.C.; Finck, R.; Hale, M.B.; Hitzman, C.; Borowsky, A.D.; Levenson, R.M.; Lowe, J.B.; Liu, S.D.; Zhao, S.; et al. Multiplexed ion beam imaging of human breast tumors. *Nat. Med.* **2014**, *20*, 436–442. [CrossRef] [PubMed]
103. Nir, G.; Farabella, I.; Perez Estrada, C.; Ebeling, C.G.; Beliveau, B.J.; Sasaki, H.M.; Lee, S.D.; Nguyen, S.C.; McCole, R.B.; Chattoraj, S.; et al. Walking along chromosomes with super-resolution imaging, contact maps, and integrative modeling. *PLoS Genet.* **2018**, *14*, e1007872. [CrossRef] [PubMed]

12

State-of-the-Art of Profiling Immune Contexture in the Era of Multiplexed Staining and Digital Analysis to Study Paraffin Tumor Tissues

Edwin Roger Parra *, Alejandro Francisco-Cruz and Ignacio Ivan Wistuba

Department of Translational Molecular Pathology, The University of Texas MD Anderson Cancer Center, 2130 West Holcombe Blvd, Houston, TX 77030, USA; AFrancisco@mdanderson.org (A.F.-C.); iiwistuba@mdanderson.org (I.I.W.)

* Correspondence: erparra@mdanderson.org

Abstract: Multiplexed platforms for multiple epitope detection have emerged in the last years as very powerful tools to study tumor tissues. These revolutionary technologies provide important visual techniques for tumor examination in formalin-fixed paraffin-embedded specimens to improve the understanding of the tumor microenvironment, promote new treatment discoveries, aid in cancer prevention, as well as allowing translational studies to be carried out. The aim of this review is to highlight the more recent methodologies that use multiplexed staining to study simultaneous protein identification in formalin-fixed paraffin-embedded tumor tissues for immune profiling, clinical research, and potential translational analysis. New multiplexed methodologies, which permit the identification of several proteins at the same time in one single tissue section, have been developed in recent years with the ability to study different cell populations, cells by cells, and their spatial distribution in different tumor specimens including whole sections, core needle biopsies, and tissue microarrays. Multiplexed technologies associated with image analysis software can be performed with a high-quality throughput assay to study cancer specimens and are important tools for new discoveries. The different multiplexed technologies described in this review have shown their utility in the study of cancer tissues and their advantages for translational research studies and application in cancer prevention and treatments.

Keywords: immune profiling; cancer tissues; multiplexed methodologies; image analysis; spatial analysis

1. Introduction

Despite the recent advances in immunotherapy strategies in recent years in cancer treatment and clinical responses, the study of immune cell phenotypes and their spatial distribution at the tumor site has prompted the need for multiplexed analyses of tumor tissues. To address this necessity, in recent years, multiplexed imaging platforms have arisen as important tools that can provide critical information about the cancer microenvironment, prognosis, therapy, and relapse [1–5]. Different components of the tumor microenvironment can be examined simultaneously using multiplexed methodologies, providing an insight into the biological cross-talk present at the tumor–host interface, and providing information from the subcellular level to the cell population level. Indeed, the most important factor is the precision with these new techniques can evaluate the special localization of multiple, simultaneously-detected biomarkers and their co-expressions or interactions between cells [5]. Attempts are presently being made to develop even more comprehensive multiplexed technologies that allow simultaneous visualization of an even larger number of biomarkers from a single tissue section, as well as to streamline, automate, and reduce the time expended on tissue staining and processing. Multiplexed methods can help to achieve these technological goals to ultimately enhance disease diagnosis and better inform timely patient care [6].

Multiplexed technologies are being used to identify the presence of multiple biological markers on a single tissue sample or an ensemble of different tissue samples [7]. The multiplexed imagining techniques provide unique biological information that, in many cases, cannot be attained by other non-imaging methods or by single immunohistochemistry (IHC) techniques. As mentioned, individual cells can be accessed with extraordinary fidelity equal to that achievable in the bulk population, such than even rare cell populations can be studied, showing their important role in translational research. This knowledge can be applied in cancer prevention. In this review, we discuss the most recent multiplexed methodologies that can be used to identify simultaneous biomarkers in formalin-fixed, paraffin-embedded (FFPE) tumor tissue samples as well as imaging analysis platforms with potential application for future cancer immunotherapy biomarker discoveries.

2. Non-Fluorescence-Based Platforms

2.1. *Multiplexed Immunohistochemical Consecutive Staining on Single Slide*

The multiplexed immunohistochemical consecutive staining on single slide (MICSSS) [8] method is a series of sequential cycles of staining, image scanning, and destaining of chromogenic substrate than can be performed on FFPE tissue samples. This multiplex staining approach uses conventional chromogenic-immunohistochemistry staining, followed by a scanning process by the destained chromogenic substrate in organic solvent [8] that can completely remove the staining. The MICSS method can allow up to 10 different antibodies on one single tissue section using sequential cycles without any damage to the tissue antigenicity or architecture. The relatively slow process of the technique is the main limitation of the MICSSS, but as the authors mentioned, this limitation could be easily resolved with the automation of the process. However, although this methodology was tested on limited data, it showed the versatility and potential of the process to study and analyze the complexity of the tumor microenvironment.

2.2. *Sequential Immunoperoxidase Labeling and Erasing*

Sequential immunoperoxidase labeling and erasing (SIMPLE) is a multiplex immuno-histochemistry approach with a sequential labeling bleaching technique that enables simultaneous marker visualization [9]. The SIMPLE approach can combine five to twelve markers using the alcohol-soluble peroxidase substrate 3-amino-9-ethylcarbazole with a fast, non-destructive method for antibody–antigen separation. Then, in each round of labeling, a given precipitate is gave a pseudocolor, and all colors are overlapped at the end of the process to visualize all of the target antigens used. This method has shown the ability to erase the results of a single stain while preserving tissue antigenicity for repeated rounds of labeling [9]. Using the SIMPLE platform in a head and neck squamous cell carcinoma cohort, differential immune complexity of lymphoid- and myeloid-inflamed tumors has been demonstrated, correlating with clinical outcomes and tumor subclassification. In addition, geometrical mapping analysis revealed that the immune complexity status is associated with the therapeutic response to vaccination therapy in pancreatic ductal adenocarcinoma, where myeloid-inflamed and T cell exhaustion status are correlated with a shorter overall survival time [10].

3. Fluorescence-Based Platforms

3.1. *Bleaching Techniques without Signal Amplification System*

Multiplexed staining bleaching techniques were created with different platforms to study tumor tissue specimens. The basic concept of these techniques is to erase the staining marker when it is done to initiate the next biomarker in a consecutive cycle of desired biomarkers to identify multiple antigens in a single sample.

3.2. Multi-Epitope-Ligand Cartography

Multi-epitope-ligand cartography (MELC) [11,12], is a bleaching or erasure technique that is capable of co-localizing the locations of different proteins in one single tissue sample using consecutives rounds of conjugate biomarkers with fluorescent detection [13]. A couple of antibodies are added during each staining cycle, followed by image acquisition of the sample using a high-sensitivity digital camera. Then, the sample is bleached with phosphate buffer saline to eliminate the excitation wavelengths, and a new cycle of staining is started. One limitation of the MELC technique is that the photobleaching step can only be applied to the microscope's field of view, meaning that the multiprobe image is limited to a single microscopic medium-to-high power field [9]. MELC can be applied on FFPE and frozen tissue sections, and it has been coupled to RNA extraction to combine RNA and protein expression analysis [14]. MELC has been used as a very efficient methodology to study immune cell markers and intracellular signaling pathways in an infectious context [15,16] and to perform systematic high-content proteomic analysis of colorectal cancer, and the T cell-related protein expression patterns and their modification in the tissue of Barrett's esophagus and esophageal adenocarcinoma patients [17,18].

3.3. MultiOmyx^{TM} Staining or Hyperplexed Immunofluorescence Assay

General Electric Healthcare (Niskayuna, NY, USA) has developed an erase methodology platform called MultiOmyx^{TM}, which is a multiplex direct immunofluorescence approach where up to 50 antibodies can be interrogated from a single FFPE section. It uses primary conjugated antibodies with fluorochromes to stain different biomarkers of interest in batches of two or four at one time. After deactivating the tissue autofluorescence and completing the first cycle of staining, the tissue is imaged and deactivation of the fluorochromes via alkaline oxidation is done to start a new cycle of staining. The MultiOmyx^{TM} platform can stain multiplex rounds of biomarkers by repeating the same procedure several times until all desired targets have been reached in a multiplexed iterative manner [19,20]. The MultiOmyx^{TM} platform has been used to evaluate the epithelial-to-mesenchymal transition in medullary colorectal cancer tissue where coexpression of CK, CDH3, VIM, and Cyt-PLAC8 provided evidence that excess PLAC8 is involved in the epithelial-to-mesenchymal transition [21]. An interesting field of application of this technology is in hematopathology where the routine diagnosis of hematological neoplasms includes several IHC markers, for example, CD30, CD15, PAX-5, CD20, CD79a, CD45, BOB.1, OCT-2, and CD3 antibodies in the diagnosis of classical Hodgkin lymphoma. It was demonstrated that the use of MultiOmyx^{TM} is equivalent to routine morphological and IHC evaluation of cases in which classical Hodgkin lymphoma was included within the differential diagnoses [12].

4. Tissue-Based Cyclic Immunofluorescence (t-CyCIF) Method

Recently described in the literature, the tissue-based cyclic immunofluorescence (t-CyCIF) [22] method can create highly multiplexed images using an iterative process in which conventional low-plex fluorescence images are repeatedly collected from the same sample and then assembled into a high-dimensional representation. The t-CyCIF cycles involve antibody staining against protein antigens, nuclear staining (same fluorophore per cycle), image scanning (low and high magnification) and fluorophore bleaching steps. According to the authors, the cycles can be repeated more than 15 times without any problem with cell preservation or tissue morphology to complete all the desired targets. However, each t-CyCIF cycle involves a relatively slow process (each cycle is 6–8 h); a single operator can process 30 slides in parallel with relative flexibility. Recently, Bolognesi and colleagues [23] described multiplex staining by sequential immunostaining involving 30 markers using beta-mercaptoethanol/sodium dodecyl sulfate for the stripping procedure during each cycle of staining and scanning with very good results.

Co-Detection by Indexing or Fluorescent Immunohisto-PCR

CO-Detection by indEXing (CODEX) is a fluorescent-based imaging approach that uses oligo-DNA conjugated antibodies. The oligonucleotide duplexes encodes uniquely designed sequences with 5′ overhangs [24]. Fresh frozen tissue and isolated cells were used to validate this methodology, but its application on FFPE tissue is under development. Cells or fresh frozen tissue are stained with a cocktail containing all conjugated antibodies (up to 50 antibodies) at the same time. This methodology is based on secondary detection index cycles where tags are iteratively revealed in situ by using indexing nucleotides (adenine and guanine) and rendering fluorophores-conjugated nucleotides (uracil and cytidine) with the combination of a polymerization cycle and a fluorescent channel, at which a given DNA tag incorporates one of two fluorescently labeled dNTP species. Specifically, the antibody-matched overhangs (indexes) include a region to be filled by blank letters and a dedicated position for a dye labeled nucleotide at the end. The antibodies to be revealed first generally have shorter overhangs than the antibodies to be visualized later (Figure 1). Each extension and bleaching (with TCEP) cycle takes 10 min. Imaging in each cycle takes min to hours depending on sample dimensions, resolution, and the microscope used (a standard fluorescence microscope). The platform can be performed on any three-color fluorescence microscope enabling the conversion of a regular fluorescence microscope into a tool for multidimensional tissue rendering and cell cytometry [24], giving a good advantage to users of this platform. CODEX is an innovate platform that has achieved and reported deep immune profiling of the mouse splenic architecture by comparing normal murine spleens to spleens from animals with systemic autoimmune disease [14]. Another barcoding platform is the DNA exchange imaging (DEI) technique [25] that overcomes speed restrictions by allowing for single-round immunostaining with DNA-barcoded antibodies. The DEI is the new generation of exchange-PAINT described by the same group [26]. According to the authors, it is an easy multiplexed technique that can be adapted to diverse imaging platforms, including standard resolution Exchange-Confocal and various super-resolution methods. There are no cancer-related study publications using these methods, but they are promising techniques and highly efficient methodology to study the tumor-associated immune contexture.

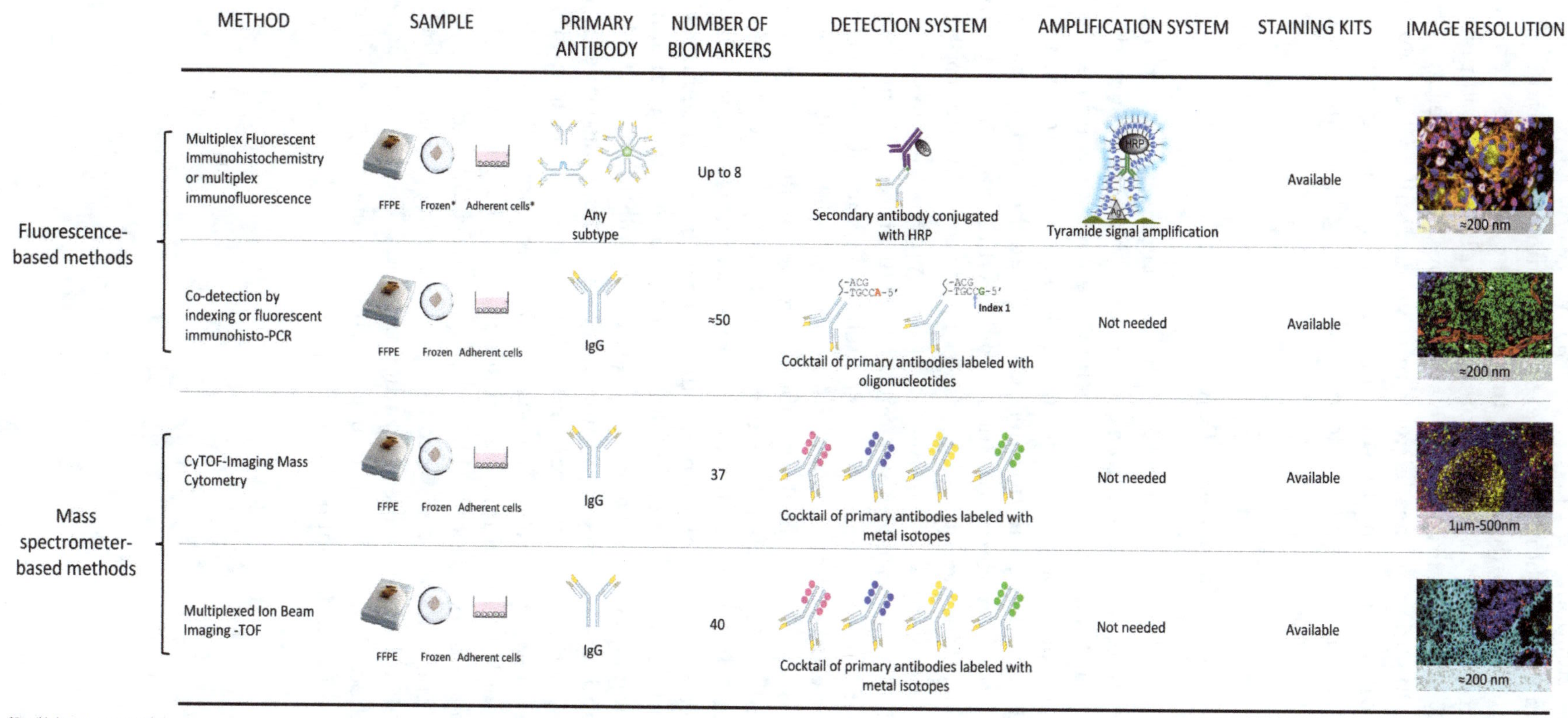

*Possible but not recommended

**Images published in webpages https://www.akoyabio.com/codextm/technology, https://www.ionpath.com/mibi-technology/

Figure 1. Technical comparison of fluorescent-based platforms and mass spectrometer-based platforms for digital image analysis. Digital image analysis for cancer research applications can be achieved with several methodologies. Some of them have advantages over others depending on the sample available, the specific antibodies against biological markers of interest, the detection system needed, and in some cases, the amplification of the signal for poorly expressed markers.

5. Amplification of the Epitope Detection

5.1. Multiplex Modified Hapten-Based Technology

Modified-hapten based technology is a recent technique that allows simultaneous detection of multiplex biomarkers using a standard two-step procedure. The technique is antibody species independent and the signals of the markers can be stronger than those usually observed with direct flour-labeled secondary antibody detection of multiplex. Created by the company Cell IDx (San Diego, CA, USA), primary antibodies are combined in cocktails and then detected with a panel of anti-hapten secondary antibodies, each labeled with a different fluorochrome. The procedure takes two hours [27], which is a principal advantage of this multiplexed method.

5.2. Tyramide Signal Amplification and Fluorescent Multiplex Immunohistochemistry

Tyramide signal amplification (TSA) was described in the 1990s by Bobrow and colleagues [28,29]. It is an enzyme-linked signal amplification method that is using to detect and localize the low copy number of proteins present in tissue by the conventional IHC protocol, using, most commonly, the alkaline phosphatase or horseradish peroxidase (HRP) enzymatic reaction to catalyse the deposition of tyramide labelled molecules at the site of the probe or epitope detection. Tyramides are conjugated to biotin or fluorescent labels and revealed by the streptavidin–HRP system [6,30]. The HRP catalyzes the formation of tyramide into highly reactive tyramide radicals that covalently bind to electron-rich tyrosine moieties close to the epitope of interest on FFPE tissue. Tissue surfaces with anchored biotinylated tyramide must be further treated with fluorescent or enzyme tagged proteins that have a high affinity for biotin, such as streptavidin, before microscopic visualization [6,30]. The detection of the proteins is more than 10-times greater than standard biotin-based staining methods [31].

Akoya/PerkinElmer (Waltham, MA, USA) developed the Opal™ workflow (Figure 1), which allows simultaneous staining of multiple biomarkers within a single paraffin tissue section. Fluorescent Multiplex Immunohistochemistry (fmIHC) allows researchers to use antibodies raised in the same species, and different panels combining different targets can be created using this technology [4,30]. The manual protocol approach involves detection with fluorescent TSA reagents, followed by microwave treatment that removes the primary and secondary antibodies between cycles and any nonspecific staining that reduces tissue autofluorescence for each antibody cycle. In the automated protocol using Leica Bond RX or another autostainer, the time is reduced drastically as compared with manual staining. The possibilities for fmIHC are expanding our knowledge of tumor immune contexture. Mapping the tumor microenvironment and the predictive and/or prognostic value of immune checkpoint expression on malignant cells and tumor infiltrating immune cells has been characterized in patients with melanoma, lung cancer, breast cancer, gastric cancer, Hodgkin lymphoma, and others by fmIHC [32–36].

5.3. Nanocrystal Quantum Dots

The method uses specially coated nanocrystals (around 1–10 nm in diameter) called quantum dots instead of the chromogen [37,38]. Nanocrystal quantum dots have the property of being excited by any type or wavelength of light to emit light in a very thin fluorescence spectrum. The use of these fluorescent markers in combination with multispectral imaging technology has been a particular utility for multiplexed detection when used as a fluorescent probe bound to different antibody markers [39,40]. Despite the favorable optical properties of nanocrystal quantum dots, as a fluorescence-based method, they can avoid the endogenous autofluorescence associated with tissue sections [41], have high photostability [42], and have a symmetric emission spectrum [43]. An important reported limitation of using nanocrystal quantum dots is the limited number of nanocrystals that possess the proper chemistry to attach themselves to their targeted molecules. Nanotechnology is a promising platform in cancer nanodiagnostics and nanotherapy because of the unique optical and electronic features. When conjugated with antibodies, QD-based probes can be used to target cancer molecules with high specificity and sensitivity [36]. In addition, the use of QD-based multifunctional probes has been proposed for multiplexed molecular cancer diagnosis, and in vivo imaging [36,44].

6. Fundamentals of Multiplexed Techniques Based on Mass Spectrometry

6.1. Imaging Mass Spectrometry

Imaging mass spectrometry (IMS) is defined as the visual representation of the elemental or molecular component of fixed cells or tissues by mass spectrometry (Figure 2) [27]. IMS is a technique that uses a mass spectrometer (MS) to visualize the spatial distribution of compounds, biomarkers, metabolites, proteins, peptides, or small molecules by their molecular masses [45]. The incorporation of a computer data system to mass spectrometry started the path of IMS. In 1967, two computational systems were applied to MS [28]. The Massachusetts Institute of Technology system was the first computer-assisted digital data acquisition system for this purpose. The software identifies the mass spectral peaks and assigns them mass values and intensities to transform the results in numerical and graphical form [46]. The Stanford system was the second system created. It uses computer software that controls the data acquisition from a quadrupole MS interfaced to a gas chromatograph that scans each spectrum from peak to peak each spectrum to predetermine the total ion current [46].

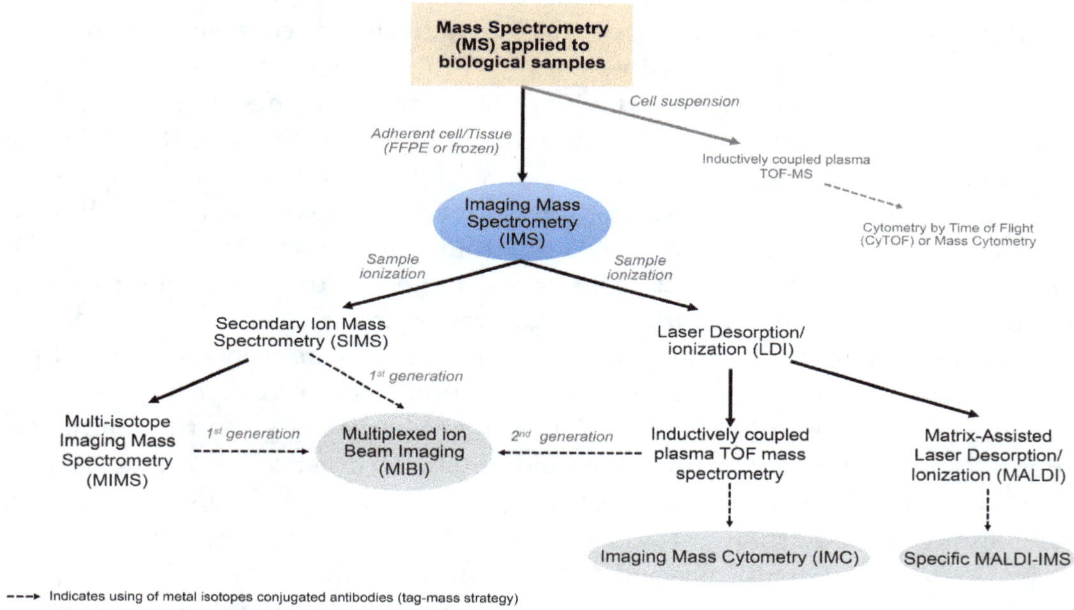

Figure 2. Byproducts and fundamentals of the imaging mass spectrometer. The application of mass spectrometry to biological research began in the last half century and it represents the conjunction of biological and deep physical and technological knowledge in biomedicine. Imaging Mass Spectrometry (IMS) came from the idea of building a 2D image with the elemental composition of a biological surface. The way that the surface is evaporated allowed the generation of two methods: one based on an ion beam and the second using a laser. The application of a tag-mass strategy to IMS is the most recent efficient and highly multiplexed platform for the digital image analysis of biological samples.

IMS is applied to biological and non-biological samples such as cells, tissues, polymers, and minerals [47–49]. In general, the methodology can be applied to all systems mentioned; it analyzes a thin section of the sample placed on a target-plate. The sample is introduced into the source region of the MS where the surface is subjected to bombarding ions, photons, and/or atomic or molecular beams. Then, compounds present in the sample are ionized and mass analyzed. This process is then repeated as necessary in a raster over a selected region of interest until the complete desired area has been sampled. The intensity of any given ion may be plotted as a function of its x and y positions, thus generating specific two-dimensional molecular/ion images of the sample [46].

6.2. Secondary Ion Mass Spectrometry

Secondary Ion Mass Spectrometry (SIMS) achieves chemical or elemental analysis of surface constituents, rather than being excited to emit some characteristic secondary signals, such as fluorescence-based techniques. A light (static SIMS) or heavy (dynamic SIMS) energetic primary ion causes a collision cascade. Those ionized particles from the surface are subsequently identified with MS [46,50]. This is one of the most destructive methods of surface analysis, but the it is the most sensitive as all elements are detectable, including hydrogen [50]. During the analysis, the sample surface is gradually eroded away [50].

SIMS was developed for the elemental analysis of non-biological and biological surfaces, such as the study of a lunar basalt from the Apolo 11 in the 1970s and the study of the insect abdomen tissue morphology in 1975 [49,51]. The sources of the primary ion beam that have been used more frequently are Ar^+, $O_2{}^+$, N^+, O^-, and Cs^+; however, in principle, the primary ion may be a positive or negative ion. Noble or reactive gas ions are usually extracted from discharged plasma. The secondary ion beam detection includes stable and radio isotopes like ^{2}D, ^{15}N, ^{13}C, ^{18}O, ^{33}S, ^{74}Se ^{90}Zr, ^{56}Fe, ^{40}Ca, and ^{14}C. Since 1960, there have been two ways to acquire the secondary ion content: an ion microscope instrument mode (Cameca, Gennevilliers, Paris, France) and a scanner ion microprobe mass analyzer (IMMA) mode (Applied Research Laboratories, Austin, TX, USA) [52]. In microscope mode, the MS analyzes one ion per time, and its position is mirrored on the detector, and each ion image is generated independently. In the microprobe mode, the primary ion beam rasters the sample to produce a mass spectrum at small locations on the sample surface. An entire mass spectrum is obtained at each position or pixel, and the images may be constructed by plotting the ion intensities across the sample in a two-dimensional fashion [46].

SIMS has been compared with electron microscopy because of the resolution of its images; however, an ideal instrument should have a lateral resolution of 100 A, a mass resolution for secondary ions better than 10,000 A, a secondary ion transmission of close to 100%, and simultaneous detection of all secondary ions [50].

Time-of-Flight (TOF) Secondary Ion Mass Spectrometry started to be applied to biological cells as a chemometric methodology to study the cellular surface composition and the discriminations between normal and neoplastic cells, an issue that can be challenging in cases where neoplastic morphological features may not be evident, such as low grade prostate cancer and bladder cancer [53,54], or to study the chemical composition that can differentiate subtypes of well-defined neoplasia, such as estrogen-receptor-positive (ER+) and estrogen-receptor-negative (ER−) breast cancers [55].

6.3. Laser Desorption/Ionization

Laser desorption/ionization (LDI) is another IMS platform created in the 1960s that nebulizes a solid surface in order to obtain free ions or ion clusters for imaging. It involves the use of lasers, UV or IR, instead of an ion beam. The coupling of LDI to Time-Of-Flight (TOF) mass analyzer was possible in the 1970s, and the first report of metal bioimaging by laser ablation inductively coupled plasma mass spectrometry (LA-ICP) was reported in 2010 to have high sensitivity and quantitative abilities. One of the first biological reports of these methodologies involved the quantitative imaging of copper in the human hippocampus and substantia nigra [46]. One of the most interesting applications of this platform is to test the efficacy of metal-based anticancer agents into tumor models, such as the distribution of platinum-based anticancer compounds in a human colorectal cancer spheroid model [56].

6.4. Matrix-Assisted Laser Desorption/Ionization

Matrix-Assisted Laser Desorption/Ionization (MALDI), a type of molecular imaging technology, was evolving in the same way as SIMS and LDI, with improved resolution and sensitivity. MALDI imaging initially applied TOF-MS, but other platforms were coupled to MALDI later on with the objective of localizing small pharmaceutical molecules directly on tissue sections [46,57]. MALDI is a soft ionization technique that uses an organic compound matrix such as 2.5-dihydroxy benzoic acid (DHB) that, when combined with pulsed UV or N_2 laser irradiation, promotes the efficient desorption and ionization of molecules from the vaporization of the matrix [57–59]. In general, this technology is used in clinical and research applications to study bacterial and fungal identification from a single colony [60], mutational identification, polymorphisms, insertion/deletion, splicing, quantitative changes variation, gene expression, and allele expression, as well as DNA methylation, and post-transcriptional modification of tRNAs and rRNAs [61,62].

One of the most exciting applications of MALDI is the analysis of the proteomic pattern composition of tumor cells and the determination of unique profiles that can actually differentiate normal cells from neoplastic cells, even between different subtypes of tumor cells and between primary and metastatic tumors, an approach that has already been explored in non-small cell lung cancer (NSCLC) [63]. SIMS, LDI, and MALDI are looking to minimize the analysis time of the imaging experiment.

6.5. Multiplexed Ion Beam Imaging and Imaging Mass Cytometry: The Antibody-Based Tag-Mass IMS Strategy

The tag-mass strategy is an affinity-based strategy where a probe, such as an antibody or an oligonucleotide, is directed against a specific target using a probe that can be imaged by any IMS strategy (Figure 2). The tag-mass needs a reporter group or element where the reporter is used to indirectly obtain the image from the probe attached to the target. The reporter must be designed to be an atom or molecule of known molecular mass that is easily detectable by MS, taking care to use a molecule that is not biologically active in the tissue to be analyzed. For SIMS or LA-ICP, metal isotopes conjugated to antibodies directly contain a monoatomic element that is easily detectable in biological studies. Where the element is not present naturally on the study surface, the former receives the name Multiplexed Ion Beam Imaging (MIBI) and the latter is named Imaging Mass Cytometry (IMC). The tag-mass IMS strategy is overwhelmingly expanding the possibilities of applications of mass-spectrometry to biological systems and biological samples. It is leading a revolutionary new wave of molecular and digital imaging, and it is the most powerful platform for multiplexing in the era of *theranostics*.

6.6. Multiplexed Ion Beam Imaging

Multiplexed ion beam imaging (MIBI) applies the principles of multi-isotope imaging mass spectrometry (MIMS) and the mass-tag strategy with metal-chelated isotopes conjugated to antibodies that will be incubated on the tissue of analysis (Figure 2) [64]. It allows subcellular imaging resolution. Instead of direct isotope labeling of the target cell or tissue, as described in the previous platforms, MIBI uses specific antibodies to "deliver" a specific mass to the targeted antigen. MIBI combines SIMS fundamentals, stable isotope reporters, specific antibodies, and intensive computation.

MIBI is based on SIMS. An ionic beam erodes the surface or atomic layer of the sample, resulting in ionization of a small atomic fraction. In a SIMS instrument, a magnetic sector mass analyzer must filter the collected secondary ion beam; secondary ions are separated by mass and then used to derive a quantitative atomic mass image of the surface to be analyzed. Up to seven parallel masses of different elements or isotopes can be simultaneously analyzed, but by moving six of the seven detectors, the instrument can measure more data from multiple isotopes from the same region. The data are reconstructed into a grey scale image in which the pixel intensity is derived from the total number of counts of a given secondary ion within the area representing a given pixel (Figure 3). The lateral resolution is dependent on factors including the beam size and the number of pixels per image acquisition area [64].

Instead of fluorophores or enzyme-conjugated reagents, biological specimens for MIBI analysis are incubated with primary antibodies coupled to stable lanthanides that are highly enriched for a single isotope. The prepared specimens are mounted in a sample receptacle and subjected to a rasterized oxygen duoplasmatron primary ion beam. The coupling of MIBI to SIMS and TOF-MS allows the study of more than 50 metal-isotope labeled antibodies at the same time with a speed of 20–200 fields-of-view per day collected automatically. Depending on the element of interest, MIBI can achieve as low as parts-per-billion sensitivity with a dynamic range of 10^5 and a resolution comparable to high-magnification light microscopy or close to 200 nm of resolution (Figure 1). MIBI is capable of analyzing standard FFPE tissue sections, fresh frozen tissue, and adherent cell samples [65,66]. The platform has a number of advantages over conventional multiplexed techniques, as there is no background because of the absence of autofluorescence and the very good definition of the signals for the image [67]. MIBI has been applied to demonstrate that it is a useful surrogate for standard IHC for diagnostics of molecular subtypes of breast cancer. In addition, through this platform, it could be possible to quantify the protein expression of markers [5,65], and as shown by Keren and colleagues [68] through the analysis of 36 proteins in 41 triple-negative breast cancer patients, the methodology has the capacity to provide data for application in immune oncology.

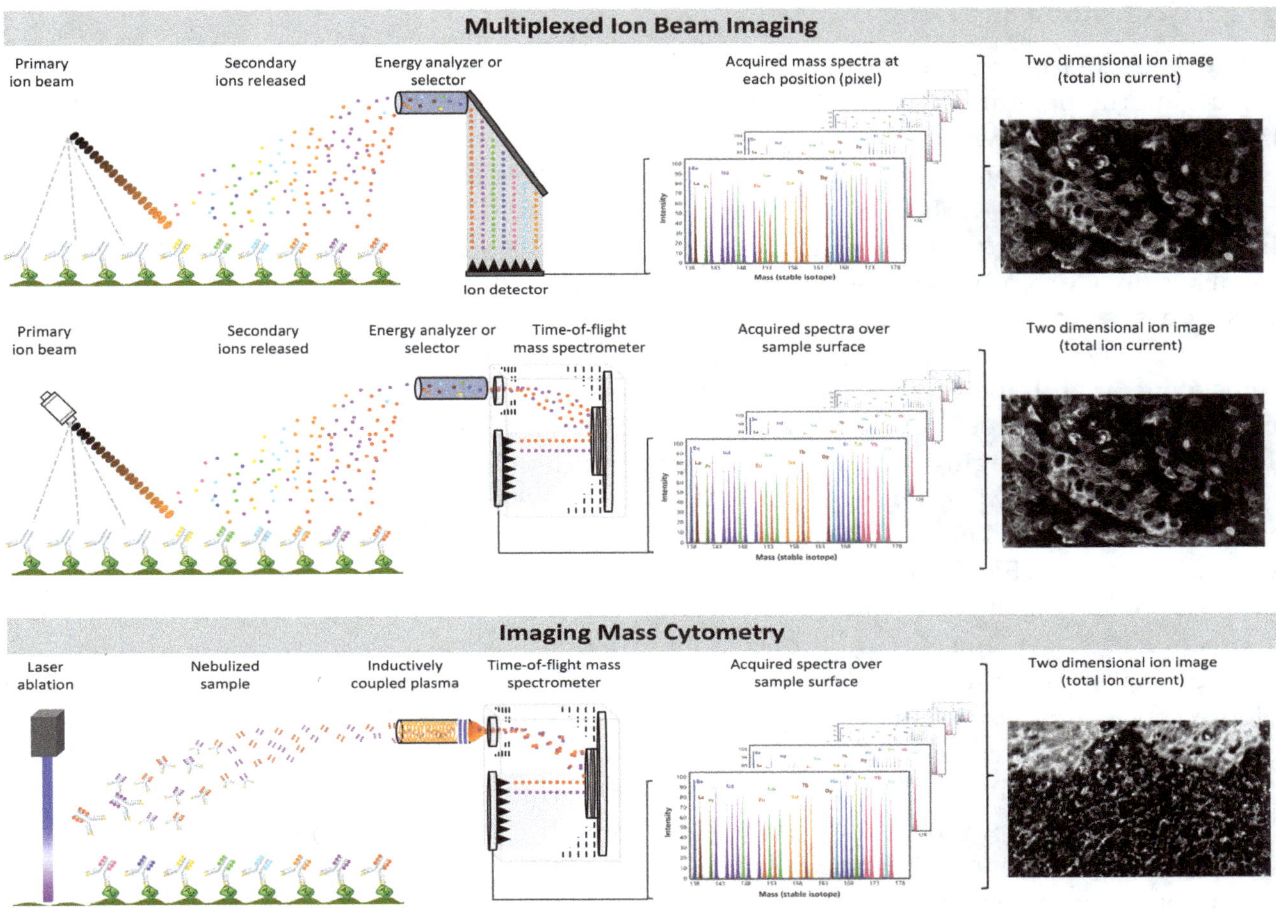

Figure 3. Basic fundamentals and similarities between multiplexed ion beam imaging and imaging mass cytometry. Characterization of multiplexed ion beam imaging and imaging mass cytometry.

6.7. Imaging Mass Cytometry

Imaging Mass Cytometry (IMC) is a tag-mass IMS strategy coupled to Mass Cytometry by TOF (CyTOF). It uses LA-ICP and TOF MS fundamentals, in which antibodies are labeled with metal ion isotopes tags rather than fluorochromes [69] (Figures 1–3). This allows the combination of many more antibody specificities (up to 50) in a single tissue sample (fresh frozen or FFPE) or adherent cell sample, without significant spillover between channels with a resolution from 1 μm up to 500 nm. Traditional labeling techniques can be used in this technique with minimal change to current protocols, allowing the panel design to be performed more easily and avoiding autofluorescence issues [70]. Although slower acquisition is observed (~1 h/mm^2) and complete biological material is ablated, the IMC-CyTOF represents a new way of quantifying several phenotypes of cells at the same time, allowing the detection of up to 50 markers at the same time [71].

Currently, IMC has been used more often than MIBI in biological research. It is probably the most powerful platform for multiplex digital image analysis and together with MIBI, it is still undergoing development and improvement. IMC was developed on breast tumor tissue, and it is able to analyze cell-type markers, signaling activity, and hypoxia on FFPE samples, opening the possibility of carrying out deep analyses of tumor biology and heterogeneity [72]. Recently, the simultaneous multiplexed imaging of mRNA and protein expressions with subcellular resolution has been developed in breast cancer tissue samples by IMC, representing the first IMS platform that is able to study transcriptomic and protein expression with a high quality resolution, which expands the possibilities for applications to cancer research and overcomes the difficulties of the study of soluble proteins by conventional IHC [73].

7. Image Acquisition and Data Analysis

The main reason for performing a multiplexed assay is to obtain a high volume of tumor biological information through multidimensional data related to tissue architecture, spatial distribution of multiple cell phenotypes, co-expression of markers, and rare cell-type detection. The different advantages and disadvantages related to the study of multiple markers on a single slide are summarized in the Table 1, showing the methodologies described above. The first component after the staining is the image acquisition which must provide images with high enough quality to perform the analysis on. Currently the image acquisition systems are software-driven, robotically–controlled microscope systems that provide high quality monochrome cameras with high-resolution and multi-band filter cubes set to have greater flexibility and to match with the samples. Image acquisition systems alone or with their own analysis platform are used in the different methodologies described above, such as the Olympus scanner, Nikon Eclipse Ci-E [8], the Hamamatsu Nanozoomer S60 scanner with a Fluorescence Imaging Module [23], Zeiss/confocal laser scanning microscopy [22], Olympus America/VS110, Akoya/PerkinElmer Vectra®-Polaris™ [30], Neo Genomics/MultiOmyx scanner [74], Ventana/Roche/iScan, Leica Biosystems/Aperio FL, 3Dhistech/Pannoramic/250 FLASH III [75], TissueGnostics/TissueFAXS [76], just to mention some. These have shown high versatility and quality imaging as well as the images generated by mass spectrometry techniques (Supplementary Table S1). Image acquisition systems for multiplexed immunofluorescence support multiple filters using mechanical switching or using tunable LED excitation, similar to the confocal microscope, to capture the fluorescence signals to assemble compose images [77] for analysis. The alignment of image acquired systems during successive rounds of staining is required for some staining techniques, such as MICSSS, SIMPLE, MELC, MultiOmyx™, t-CyCIF, and CODEX, where it is essential to retain the information from each image during registration to stitch together images from overlapping fields to allow a precise representation of co-localization from different markers by the cells. Although the alignment of images is not necessary in other multiplexed methodologies because the image is acquired at the end of all staining process, it is still impossible to accelerate the process of scanning, which can take min to several hours [78] depending the size of the area scanned (whole section or region-of-interest, ROI), the number of ROIs scanned, and the methodology used [79,80]. In fluorescence methodologies, image acquisition is performed using one filter at a time or by changing the filter at each capture to obtain the co-localized [80] expression of the markers. The multidimensional tissue image generated by mass spectrometry techniques from the metal-labeled antibodies, such as MALDI-TOF, MIBI and CyTOF, that are used to perform highly multiplexed analyses are very comparable with the bright field or fluorescent images generated by the systems described above [81] (Figure 1). Overall, important considerations for cost estimation are the scan time, image resolution, hardware robustness, slide holder capacity, image focusing and stitching algorithms, acquisition modes, the use of bright field versus fluorescence, the file compression method/format/size, and the application capacity for these different techniques that need to be addressed, understood and discussed with the different vendors of image acquisition systems. The next component after the image acquisition is the image analysis and for that, several types of software have demonstrated their overall capability with different detection modules, including tissue segmentation, cell segmentation, co-localization, and spatial distribution of cell phenotyping, which is critically important to allow the combination of image layers to delineate the structures of interest to study multiplex staining tissues. A wide variety of image analysis software is applicable and is being developed to make high-dimensional image-based data exploration feasible for researchers who lack computational skills and flexible for computer scientists who want to develop and add advanced new methods for image-based machine learning-based phenotype scoring (Table 2). The combination of image analysis systems with automated scanning, such as Vectra®-Polaris™/InForm Cell Analysis/Akoya/PerkinElmer [30], MultiOmyx/analysis software [74], Aperio FL/digital image analysis tools [82], is increasingly being employed to take advantage of multiplexed staining methodologies, all of which can scan slides affixed to whole tissue or tissue microarray slices prior to image analysis. Stand-alone image analysis software packages used to evaluate these virtual multiplex slides include Definiens TissueMap [83], HistoRx AQUA [84], SlidePath [85], Indica labs/HALO™ Image Analysis Software [86], and VISIOPHARM/Phenomap™ [87]. These are the most well-known software packages available in the market that offer high quality interpretation for multiplexed histological specimens. Open image analysis software, such as ImageJ/FIJI [88], QuPath [89], Icy [90] and Cell Profiler/Cell Analyst [91–93] are also available as open sources for multiplex image analysis with a high level of performance. In addition, it is important to mention that there are several companies that can provide different solutions for high content and/or high throughput scanning service and analytical algorithms, such as the TissueGnostics platform (https://www.news-medical.net/suppliers/TissueGnostics.aspx), Oncotopix® (https://www.visiopharm.com/solutions/oncotopix), 3DHISTECH Ltd. (https://www.3dhistech.com/quantcenter) and others such as Akoya/PerkinElmer (http://www.perkinelmer.com/corporate/what-we-do/markets/life-sciences/), Definiens (https://www.definiens.com/), Neogenomics (https://neogenomics.com/pharma-services/lab-services/multiomyx), and IONpath (https://www.ionpath.com/) include a multiplex staining process with customized panels, scanning service and data analysis, and different strategies. High resolution performance during the multiplexing analysis across the ROIs/whole section needs to be combined with the signals of the immune markers to enable further different cell subpopulations to be identified and localized using the image analysis software. However, there are several types of image analysis software involving fluorescence and non-fluorescence multiplexed staining, as mentioned above, and their basic characteristics, such as having an easy algorithm workflow creation, and especially, having manual interactive or automated segmentation, with high flexibility cell phenotyping are important criteria to consider when choosing the image analysis system [94]. The power of different image analysis systems is reflected in the identification of cell phenotypes and in the specific pattern of immune cell identification, based either on the spatial distribution (distance between different subpopulations and cancer cells) or the relationships between different cells, such as lymphocyte subclasses, with each other (e.g., cytotoxic/regulatory cells) that can be associated with pathology, clinical patient information, and prognoses to give us important information about the tumor behavior [95].

However, although multiplex techniques are a powerful and efficient tool that allows us to identify several markers in a single slide, each methodology has a plethora of parameters that have significant effects on the outcome of the results and these need to be carefully validated in the lab, including antibody validation, tissue processing (cases and controls), signal acquisition calibration to obtain reproducible, reliable, and high-quality staining, and analysis that will be applied to clinical biopsies to provide a basic characterization of immune infiltrates to guide clinical decisions in the era of immunotherapy.

Table 1. Multiplex staining methodologies and their advantages and disadvantages.

Multiplex Staining Method	Advantage	Disadvantage
	Non-fluorescence based platform	
Multiplexed immunohistochemical consecutive staining on a single slide	• Uses conventional chromogenic-immunohistochemistry (IHC) staining • Allows colocalization and detection of multiples proteins	• Relatively slow process • Request automatization • Allows 10 labeled antibodies per slide
Sequential immunoperoxidase labeling and erasing	• Use conventional chromogenic-IHC staining • Allows colocalization and detection of multiple proteins • Compatible with primary antibodies from same species	• Relatively slow process • Maximum of five antibody labels per section
	Fluorescence based platform	
	Bleaching techniques without signal amplification system	
Multi-epitope-ligand cartography	• Allows colocalization and detection of a large number of proteins • High functional resolution	• The multiprobe image is limited to a single microscopic medium-to-high power field • Longer sampling time • The method requires robotic staining integrated with an inverted fluorescence microscope (high cost)
MultiOmyx^{TM} staining or hyperplexed Immunofluorescence Assay	• Allows the analysis of up to 60 biomarkers in a single slide	• Cycles of two antibodies with a longer sampling scan time
Tissue-based cyclic immunofluorescence method	• Allows sequential immunostaining of around 30 markers	• Slow process of around 6–8 h
Co-detection by indexing or fluorescent immunohisto-PCR	• Eliminates autofluorescence • Allows the analysis of several markers	• Longer scan sampling time • Limited use in formalin-fixed, paraffin-embedded (FFPE) tissues
DNA exchange imaging	• Flexible for adaptation to diverse imaging platforms	• Longer scan sampling time • Small data analyzed
	Amplification of the epitope detection	
Hapten-based modified multiplex	• Fast staining around 2 h • Cocktails of markers	• Allows a maximum of 4 markers per slide • Not tested with an autostainer
Tyramide signal amplification	• Compatible with primary antibodies from the same species • Available for autostainer	• Allows a maximum of 7 labeled antibodies per slide
Nanocrystal quantum dots	• Eliminates autofluorescence	• Limited nanocrystals

Table 1. *Cont.*

Multiplex Staining Method	Advantage	Disadvantage
	Mass Spectrometry Imaging	
Secondary Ion Mass Spectrometry	• The most sensitive system	• The ionized particles destroy the region of interest (ROI) of analysis • A current limitation is the availability of antibodies (high cost)
Laser Desorption/Ionization	• Use of lasers (UV or IR) instead of ion beams • High sensitivity and quantitative abilities	• Low resolution
Matrix-assisted laser desorption/ionization	• Organic compound matrix used	• Sampling time and resolution • A current limitation is the availability of antibodies (high cost)
Multiplexed ion beam imaging	• Simultaneous labeling of up 40 antibodies with metals	• Sampling time and small area sampling • A current limitation is the availability of antibodies (high cost)
Imaging Mass Cytometry	• Eliminates sample autofluorescence • Preprocessing using routine immunohistochemistry protocols • The signals are plotted using coordinates of each single laser shot • No amplification step of the signal needed • No matrix needed	• Current limitations are the availability of antibodies (high cost), the sampling time, and the resolution • Laser tissue ablation

Table 2. Image analysis software packages for multiplex staining.

Vendor	Software Package	Capabilities	Data Visualization	Availability	Reference
Akoya/PerkinElmer	InForm	Color-Based Co-localization, Tissue Segmentation, Cell/Object Segmentation, Cell Phenotyping, Scoring and Automated Quantitation using Batch Analysis	Density Raw Data	Licensed	[6,96]
Neo Genomics	MultiOmyx Quantification Program	Epithelial tissue reconstruction, Cellular and Subcellular Segmentation, Cell Phenotyping, Quantification Algorithms	Density Raw Data	Licensed	[3,20]
Leica Biosystems	Aperio eSlide Manager Analysis	Pixel-Based Analysis, Cellular identification, Area Quantification and Positive Pixel Count IF Algorithm	Density Raw Data	Licensed	[82]
Definiens	Tissue Studio/Image Developer	Imaging Segmentation, Marker Intensity Measurement, Cell Quantification, Batch Analysis, Statistical Analysis, and Algorithm Creator.	Histograms and Profile Plots	Licensed	[83]
HistoRx	AQUAnalysis	Signal Intensity Quantification Per Unit Area and Per Layer	Density Raw Data	Licensed	[84]
SlidePath	SlidePath's Tissue Image Analysis	Membrane, Nuclear and Positive Pixel Quantification	Density Raw Data	Licensed	[85]
Indica Labs	HALO	Membrane, Co-localization, Immune Cell Proximity, Spatial Analysis, Batch Analysis	Spatial Plot, Histogram	Licensed	[86]
VISIOPHARM	Visimoph Tissuemorph	Signal Intensity, Area, Counting Objects, Spatial Analysis, Clustering Statistical Analysis, Batch Analysis and Algorithm Creator.	Phenotypic Matrix, t-SNE Plots	Licensed	[87]
Media Cybernetics	Image-Pro	Color-Based, Nuclear segmentation, Cell quantification, Macro-enabled Advanced Image Processing Solution	Density Raw Data	Licensed	[97]
CompuCyte	iCyte/iBroser/iNovator	Nucleus Segmentation or Phantom Contouring, Measures Associated Signals	Density Raw Data	Licensed	[98]
TissueGnostics	HistoQuest/ TissueQuest/StrataQuest	Nuclei-Based Segmentation of Tissues, Cell Phenotyping	Density Raw Data	Licensed	[99]
NIH	Image J	Color-Based, User Interactive Segmentation	Histograms and Profile Plots	Open	[88]
https://qupath.github.io	QuPath	View Measurements in Context by Color Coding Objects According to Their Features, Flexible Object Classification, Trainable Cell Classification and Quantification	Density Raw Data	Open	[89]
http://icy. bioimageanalysis.org	Icy	Based and Color Object Identification, Size, Shape, Color Intensity, Texture, Spatial Analysis.	Plots, Histogram	Open	[90]
https://cellprofiler.org/	Cell Profiler/Cell Analyst	Based and Color Object Identification, Size, Shape, Color Intensity, Texture, and Number Neighbor Quantification.	Density Plot, Histogram	Open	[91–93]

8. Clinical and Translational Use of Multiplexed Methodologies

Despite the evolution in previous years at different levels of cancer research concerning prevention, diagnosis, therapeutic options, and follow up methods, cancer still remains a major public health problem worldwide [100]. Immune contexture profiling is currently a powerful metric that can be used for tumor subclassification and the prediction of clinical outcomes [101]. A great variety of cancer research screening tools are applied to diagnose tumors, and these have been established for different tumors. Simultaneous quantification of more than one biomarker at the same time has become more and more interesting in cancer research using the technologies described previously [102]. Multiplexed methodologies can allow different biomarkers, representing different important systemic processes, such as inflammation, angiogenesis, or cell death, can be combined with established tumor markers in one single panel to potentially improve the study of cancer to aid in prevention, diagnostic accuracy, and treatment (Figure 4). Multiplex based immunoassays can offer important advantages, such as a high-throughput performance, low material requirement, a wide range of applications and cost- and time-effective multiplexing through the use of several parameters [23,96,103]. Several biomarkers could be cancer-specific, since malignant cells of different histologic types can produce different tumor-related patterns of proangiogenic factors, growth factors, and immune cells [68]. The study of biomarker panels can be used for early diagnosis and assessment of therapy responses [102]. The use of multiplexed methodologies to identify multiple biomarkers can be used to allow for the early detection of pre-neoplastic lesions, trying to identify basic microenvironment patterns on those cases to determine their progression to cancer [95] (Figure 5). Therefore, these new technology assays may represent an ideal method for developing personalized therapies if efficient multiplexing panels are created [4]. These technologies could help us to better understand the cancer microenvironment, highlighting the benefit for exploring immune evasion mechanisms and finding potential biomarkers that allow researchers to assess the mechanisms of action and predict and track responses [95].

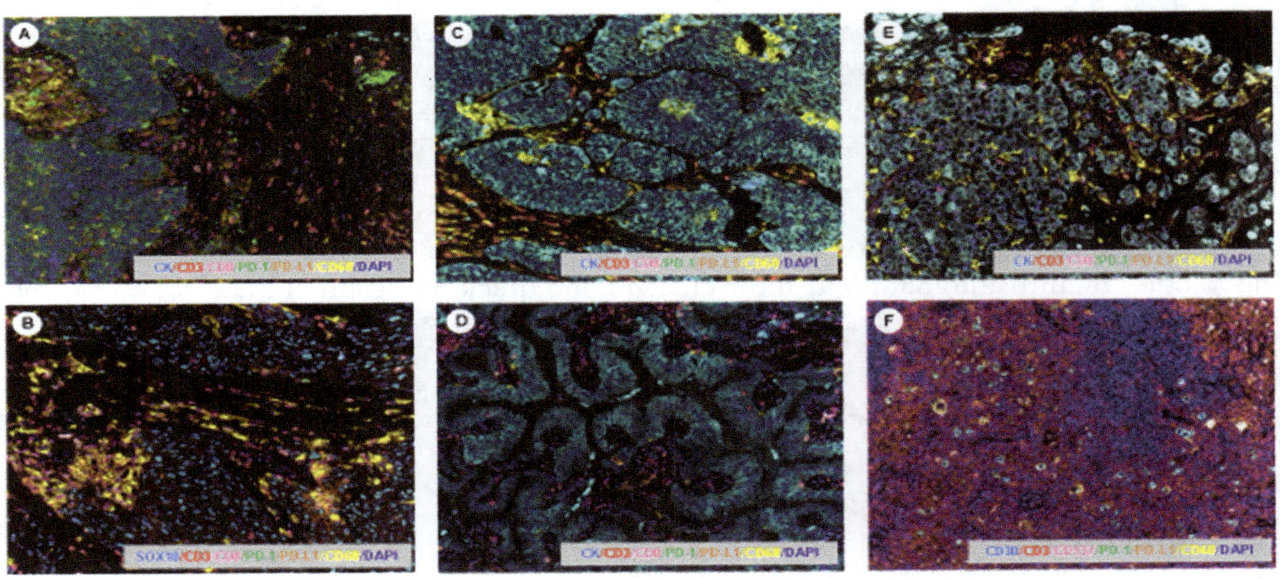

Figure 4. Multiplex immunoflorescencce microphotography. Images representing the immunoprofiling of different tumor types using the multiplexed tyramine signal amplification system: (**A**) esophageal squamous cell carcinoma, (**B**) malignant melanoma, (**C**) lung squamous cell carcinoma, (**D**) lung adenocarcinoma, (**E**) colorectal adenocarcinoma, (**F**) Hodgkin's lymphoma. Scale bar: 200× magnification.

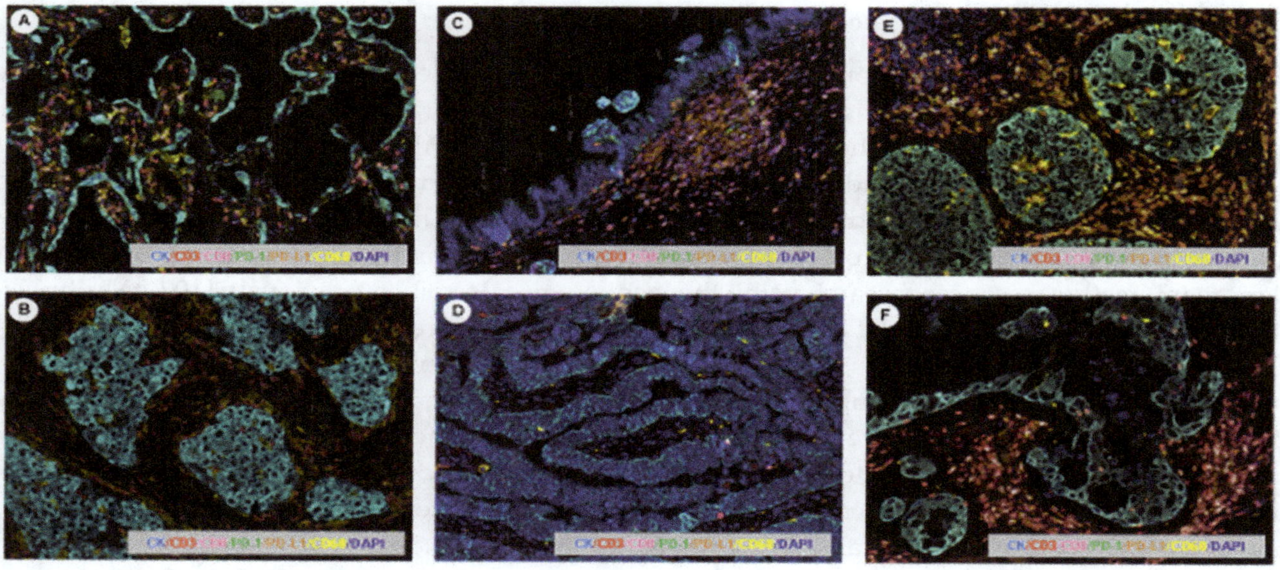

Figure 5. Multiplex immunofluorescence microphotography. Images representing the immunoprofiling of different stages of progression in lung, pancreas and breast cancer using the multiplexed tyramine signal amplification system: (**A**) pre-neoplastic lung lesion, (**B**) lung adenocarcinoma, (**C**) pre-neoplastic pancreatic lesion, (**D**) invasive pancreatic carcinoma, (**E**) non-invasive breast carcinoma, (**F**) invasive breast carcinoma. Scale bar: 200× magnification.

9. Conclusions

Multiplexed methods can provide an important and efficient way to study disease diagnosis, prevention, and to carry out translational research. These systems are showing more and more different capabilities, from research labs towards the clinic, increasing the opportunity to better understand tumor–immune interactions. Multiplexed methodologies and image analysis strategies can allow important information about immune cell co-expression and their spatial-pattern distribution in the tumor microenvironment. However, the development of these new methods requires a multidisciplinary team including pathologists, oncologists, immunologists, engineers, and/or computer scientists. In addition, for research pathologists to use highly-multiplexed methods, these methodologies require automation to allow efficient and quick provision of information as well as easy analysis.

Author Contributions: All authors were involved in drafting this review manuscript and revising it critically for important intellectual content, and all authors approved the final manuscript.

References

1. Steiner, C.; Ducret, A.; Tille, J.C.; Thomas, M.; McKee, T.A.; Rubbia-Brandt, L.; Scherl, A.; Lescuyer, P.; Cutler, P. Applications of mass spectrometry for quantitative protein analysis in formalin-fixed paraffin-embedded tissues. *Proteomics* **2014**, *14*, 441–451. [CrossRef] [PubMed]
2. Stauber, J.; MacAleese, L.; Franck, J.; Claude, E.; Snel, M.; Kaletas, B.K.; Wiel, I.M.; Wisztorski, M.; Fournier, I.; Heeren, R.M. On-tissue protein identification and imaging by MALDI-ion mobility mass spectrometry. *J. Am. Soc. Mass Spectrom.* **2010**, *21*, 338–347. [CrossRef] [PubMed]
3. Sood, A.; Miller, A.M.; Brogi, E.; Sui, Y.; Armenia, J.; McDonough, E.; Santamaria-Pang, A.; Carlin, S.; Stamper, A.; Campos, C.; et al. Multiplexed immunofluorescence delineates proteomic cancer cell states associated with metabolism. *JCI Insight* **2016**, *1*, e87030. [CrossRef] [PubMed]

4. Gorris, M.A.J.; Halilovic, A.; Rabold, K.; van Duffelen, A.; Wickramasinghe, I.N.; Verweij, D.; Wortel, I.M.N.; Textor, J.C.; de Vries, I.J.M.; Figdor, C.G. Eight-Color Multiplex Immunohistochemistry for Simultaneous Detection of Multiple Immune Checkpoint Molecules within the Tumor Microenvironment. *J. Immunol.* **2017**, *200*, 347–354. [CrossRef] [PubMed]
5. Rost, S.; Giltnane, J.; Bordeaux, J.M.; Hitzman, C.; Koeppen, H.; Liu, S.D. Multiplexed ion beam imaging analysis for quantitation of protein expresssion in cancer tissue sections. *Lab. Investig.* **2017**, *97*, 992–1003. [CrossRef] [PubMed]
6. Stack, E.C.; Wang, C.; Roman, K.A.; Hoyt, C.C. Multiplexed immunohistochemistry, imaging, and quantitation: A review, with an assessment of Tyramide signal amplification, multispectral imaging and multiplex analysis. *Methods* **2014**, *70*, 46–58. [CrossRef] [PubMed]
7. Dixon, A.R.; Bathany, C.; Tsuei, M.; White, J.; Barald, K.F.; Takayama, S. Recent developments in multiplexing techniques for immunohistochemistry. *Expert Rev. Mol. Diagn.* **2015**, *15*, 1171–1186. [CrossRef] [PubMed]
8. Remark, R.; Merghoub, T.; Grabe, N.; Litjens, G.; Damotte, D.; Wolchok, J.D.; Merad, M.; Gnjatic, S. In-depth tissue profiling using multiplexed immunohistochemical consecutive staining on single slide. *Sci. Immunol.* **2016**, *1*, aaf6925. [CrossRef] [PubMed]
9. Glass, G.; Papin, J.A.; Mandell, J.W. SIMPLE: A sequential immunoperoxidase labeling and erasing method. *J. Histochem. Cytochem.* **2009**, *57*, 899–905. [CrossRef] [PubMed]
10. Tsujikawa, T.; Kumar, S.; Borkar, R.N.; Azimi, V.; Thibault, G.; Chang, Y.H.; Balter, A.; Kawashima, R.; Choe, G.; Sauer, D.; et al. Quantitative Multiplex Immunohistochemistry Reveals Myeloid-Inflamed Tumor-Immune Complexity Associated with Poor Prognosis. *Cell Rep.* **2017**, *19*, 203–217. [CrossRef] [PubMed]
11. Schubert, W.; Bonnekoh, B.; Pommer, A.J.; Philipsen, L.; Bockelmann, R.; Malykh, Y.; Gollnick, H.; Friedenberger, M.; Bode, M.; Dress, A.W. Analyzing proteome topology and function by automated multidimensional fluorescence microscopy. *Nat. Biotechnol.* **2006**, *24*, 1270–1278. [CrossRef] [PubMed]
12. Friedenberger, M.; Bode, M.; Krusche, A.; Schubert, W. Fluorescence detection of protein clusters in individual cells and tissue sections by using toponome imaging system: Sample preparation and measuring procedures. *Nat. Protoc.* **2007**, *2*, 2285–2294. [CrossRef] [PubMed]
13. Herman, B.; Krishnan, R.V.; Centonze, V.E. Microscopic analysis of fluorescence resonance energy transfer (FRET). *Methods Mol. Biol.* **2004**, *261*, 351–370. [CrossRef] [PubMed]
14. Ostalecki, C.; Konrad, A.; Thurau, E.; Schuler, G.; Croner, R.S.; Pommer, A.J.; ael Sturzl, M. Combined multi-gene analysis at the RNA and protein levels in single FFPE tissue sections. *Exp. Mol. Pathol.* **2013**, *95*, 1–6. [CrossRef] [PubMed]
15. Philipsen, L.; Engels, T.; Schilling, K.; Gurbiel, S.; Fischer, K.D.; Tedford, K.; Schraven, B.; Gunzer, M.; Reichardt, P. Multimolecular analysis of stable immunological synapses reveals sustained recruitment and sequential assembly of signaling clusters. *Mol. Cell. Proteom.* **2013**, *12*, 2551–2567. [CrossRef] [PubMed]
16. Ostalecki, C.; Wittki, S.; Lee, J.H.; Geist, M.M.; Tibroni, N.; Harrer, T.; Schuler, G.; Fackler, O.T.; Baur, A.S. HIV Nef- and Notch1-dependent Endocytosis of ADAM17 Induces Vesicular TNF Secretion in Chronic HIV Infection. *EBioMedicine* **2016**, *13*, 294–304. [CrossRef] [PubMed]
17. Berndt, U.; Philipsen, L.; Bartsch, S.; Wiedenmann, B.; Baumgart, D.C.; Hammerle, M.; Sturm, A. Systematic high-content proteomic analysis reveals substantial immunologic changes in colorectal cancer. *Cancer Res.* **2008**, *68*, 880–888. [CrossRef] [PubMed]
18. Berndt, U.; Philipsen, L.; Bartsch, S.; Hu, Y.; Rocken, C.; Bertram, W.; Hammerle, M.; Rosch, T.; Sturm, A. Comparative Multi-Epitope-Ligand-Cartography reveals essential immunological alterations in Barrett's metaplasia and esophageal adenocarcinoma. *Mol. Cancer* **2010**, *9*, 177. [CrossRef]
19. Hollman-Hewgley, D.; Lazare, M.; Bordwell, A.; Zebadua, E.; Tripathi, P.; Ross, A.S.; Fisher, D.; Adams, A.; Bouman, D.; O'Malley, D.P.; et al. A single slide multiplex assay for the evaluation of classical Hodgkin lymphoma. *Am. J. Surg. Pathol.* **2014**, *38*, 1193–1202. [CrossRef]
20. Gerdes, M.J.; Sevinsky, C.J.; Sood, A.; Adak, S.; Bello, M.O.; Bordwell, A.; Can, A.; Corwin, A.; Dinn, S.; Filkins, R.J.; et al. Highly multiplexed single-cell analysis of formalin-fixed, paraffin-embedded cancer tissue. *Proc. Natl. Acad. Sci. USA* **2013**, *110*, 11982–11987. [CrossRef]

21. Li, C.; Ma, H.; Wang, Y.; Cao, Z.; Graves-Deal, R.; Powell, A.E.; Starchenko, A.; Ayers, G.D.; Washington, M.K.; Kamath, V.; et al. Excess PLAC8 promotes an unconventional ERK2-dependent EMT in colon cancer. *J. Clin. Investig.* **2014**, *124*, 2172–2187. [CrossRef]
22. Lin, J.R.; Izar, B.; Wang, S.; Yapp, C.; Mei, S.; Shah, P.M.; Santagata, S.; Sorger, P.K. Highly multiplexed immunofluorescence imaging of human tissues and tumors using t-CyCIF and conventional optical microscopes. *Elife* **2018**, *7*, e31657. [CrossRef] [PubMed]
23. Bolognesi, M.M.; Manzoni, M.; Scalia, C.R.; Zannella, S.; Bosisio, F.M.; Faretta, M.; Cattoretti, G. Multiplex Staining by Sequential Immunostaining and Antibody Removal on Routine Tissue Sections. *J. Histochem. Cytochem.* **2017**, *65*, 431–444. [CrossRef] [PubMed]
24. Goltsev, Y.; Samusik, N.; Kennedy-Darling, J.; Bhate, S.; Hale, M.; Vasquez, G.; Nolan, G. Deep profiling of mouse splenic architecture with CODEX multiplexed imaging. *Cell* **2018**, *174*, 968–981. [CrossRef] [PubMed]
25. Wang, Y.; Woehrstein, J.B.; Donoghue, N.; Dai, M.; Avendano, M.S.; Schackmann, R.C.J.; Zoeller, J.J.; Wang, S.S.H.; Tillberg, P.W.; Park, D.; et al. Rapid Sequential in Situ Multiplexing with DNA Exchange Imaging in Neuronal Cells and Tissues. *Nano Lett.* **2017**, *17*, 6131–6139. [CrossRef] [PubMed]
26. Jungmann, R.; Avendano, M.S.; Woehrstein, J.B.; Dai, M.; Shih, W.M.; Yin, P. Multiplexed 3D cellular super-resolution imaging with DNA-PAINT and Exchange-PAINT. *Nat. Methods* **2014**, *11*, 313–318. [CrossRef] [PubMed]
27. Levin, M.; Kron, S.J.; Schwartz, D.; Snyder, H. Rapid 5-marker multiplex phenotyping of breast cancer subtypes & tumor-infiltrating leukocytes "in situ" in FFPE sections. *Cancer Res.* **2016**, *76*. [CrossRef]
28. Bobrow, M.N.; Harris, T.D.; Shaughnessy, K.J.; Litt, G.J. Catalyzed reporter deposition, a novel method of signal amplification. Application to immunoassays. *J. Immunol. Methods* **1989**, *125*, 279–285. [CrossRef]
29. Bobrow, M.N.; Shaughnessy, K.J.; Litt, G.J. Catalyzed reporter deposition, a novel method of signal amplification. II. Application to membrane immunoassays. *J. Immunol. Methods* **1991**, *137*, 103–112. [CrossRef]
30. Parra, E.R.; Uraoka, N.; Jiang, M.; Cook, P.; Gibbons, D.; Forget, M.A.; Bernatchez, C.; Haymaker, C.; Wistuba, I.I.; Rodriguez-Canales, J. Validation of multiplex immunofluorescence panels using multispectral microscopy for immune-profiling of formalin-fixed and paraffin-embedded human tumor tissues. *Sci. Rep.* **2017**, *7*, 13380. [CrossRef]
31. Faget, L.; Hnasko, T.S. Tyramide Signal Amplification for Immunofluorescent Enhancement. *Methods Mol. Biol.* **2015**, *1318*, 161–172. [CrossRef] [PubMed]
32. Ju, X.; Shen, R.; Huang, P.; Zhai, J.; Qian, X.; Wang, Q.; Chen, M. Predictive relevance of PD-L1 expression with pre-existing TILs in gastric cancer. *Oncotarget* **2017**, *8*, 99372–99381. [CrossRef] [PubMed]
33. Carey, C.D.; Gusenleitner, D.; Lipschitz, M.; Roemer, M.G.M.; Stack, E.C.; Gjini, E.; Hu, X.; Redd, R.; Freeman, G.J.; Neuberg, D.; et al. Topological analysis reveals a PD-L1-associated microenvironmental niche for Reed-Sternberg cells in Hodgkin lymphoma. *Blood* **2017**, *130*, 2420–2430. [CrossRef] [PubMed]
34. Edwards, J.; Wilmott, J.S.; Madore, J.; Gide, T.N.; Quek, C.; Tasker, A.; Ferguson, A.L.; Chen, J.; Hewavisenti, R.; Hersey, P.; et al. CD103+ tumor-resident CD8+ T cells are associated with improved survival in immunotherapy naive melanoma patients and expand significantly during anti-PD1 treatment. *Clin. Cancer Res.* **2018**, *24*, 3036–3045. [CrossRef] [PubMed]
35. Buisseret, L.; Pommey, S.; Allard, B.; Garaud, S.; Bergeron, M.; Cousineau, I.; Ameye, L.; Bareche, Y.; Paesmans, M.; Crown, J.P.A.; et al. Clinical significance of CD73 in triple-negative breast cancer: Multiplex analysis of a phase III clinical trial. *Ann. Oncol.* **2018**, *29*, 1056–1062. [CrossRef] [PubMed]
36. Fang, M.; Peng, C.W.; Pang, D.W.; Li, Y. Quantum dots for cancer research: Current status, remaining issues, and future perspectives. *Cancer Biol. Med.* **2012**, *9*, 151–163. [CrossRef] [PubMed]
37. Bostick, R.M.; Kong, K.Y.; Ahearn, T.U.; Chaudry, Q.; Cohen, V.; Wang, M.D. Detecting and quantifying biomarkers of risk for colorectal cancer using quantum dots and novel image analysis algorithms. *Conf. Proc. IEEE Eng. Med. Biol. Soc.* **2006**, *1*, 3313–3316. [CrossRef] [PubMed]
38. Kairdolf, B.A.; Smith, A.M.; Stokes, T.H.; Wang, M.D.; Young, A.N.; Nie, S. Semiconductor quantum dots for bioimaging and biodiagnostic applications. *Annu. Rev. Anal. Chem.* **2013**, *6*, 143–162. [CrossRef] [PubMed]

39. Peng, C.W.; Liu, X.L.; Chen, C.; Liu, X.; Yang, X.Q.; Pang, D.W.; Zhu, X.B.; Li, Y. Patterns of cancer invasion revealed by QDs-based quantitative multiplexed imaging of tumor microenvironment. *Biomaterials* **2011**, *32*, 2907–2917. [CrossRef] [PubMed]
40. Liu, J.; Lau, S.K.; Varma, V.A.; Moffitt, R.A.; Caldwell, M.; Liu, T.; Young, A.N.; Petros, J.A.; Osunkoya, A.O.; Krogstad, T.; et al. Molecular mapping of tumor heterogeneity on clinical tissue specimens with multiplexed quantum dots. *ACS Nano* **2010**, *4*, 2755–2765. [CrossRef] [PubMed]
41. Mansfield, J.R.; Gossage, K.W.; Hoyt, C.C.; Levenson, R.M. Autofluorescence removal, multiplexing, and automated analysis methods for in-vivo fluorescence imaging. *J. Biomed. Opt.* **2005**, *10*, 41207. [CrossRef] [PubMed]
42. Zrazhevskiy, P.; True, L.D.; Gao, X. Multicolor multicycle molecular profiling with quantum dots for single-cell analysis. *Nat. Protoc.* **2013**, *8*, 1852–1869. [CrossRef] [PubMed]
43. Zhang, Y.; Wang, T.H. Quantum dot enabled molecular sensing and diagnostics. *Theranostics* **2012**, *2*, 631–654. [CrossRef] [PubMed]
44. Perez-Trevino, P.; la Cerda, H.H.; Perez-Trevino, J.; Fajardo-Ramirez, O.R.; Garcia, N.; Altamirano, J. 3D Imaging Detection of HER2 Based in the Use of Novel Affibody-Quantum Dots Probes and Ratiometric Analysis. *Transl. Oncol.* **2018**, *11*, 672–685. [CrossRef] [PubMed]
45. Matros, A.; Mock, H.P. Mass spectrometry based imaging techniques for spatially resolved analysis of molecules. *Front. Plant Sci.* **2013**, *4*, 89. [CrossRef] [PubMed]
46. Reyzer, M.L.; Caprioli, R.M. The Development of Imaging Mass Spectrometry. *Encycl. Mass Spectrom.* **2016**, *9*, 285–304.
47. Dong, Y.; Li, B.; Malitsky, S.; Rogachev, I.; Aharoni, A.; Kaftan, F.; Svatos, A.; Franceschi, P. Sample Preparation for Mass Spectrometry Imaging of Plant Tissues: A Review. *Front. Plant Sci.* **2016**, *7*, 60. [CrossRef]
48. Pohl, L.; Kolbl, A.; Werner, F.; Mueller, C.W.; Hoschen, C.; Hausler, W.; Kogel-Knabner, I. Imaging of Al/Fe ratios in synthetic Al-goethite revealed by nanoscale secondary ion mass spectrometry. *Rapid Commun. Mass Spectrom.* **2018**, *32*, 619–628. [CrossRef]
49. Andersen, C.A.; Hinthorne, J.R. Ion microprobe mass analyzer. *Science* **1972**, *175*, 853–860. [CrossRef]
50. Liebl, H. SIMS Instrumentation and Imaging Techniques. *Scanning* **1980**, *3*, 79–89. [CrossRef]
51. Morrison, G.H.; Slodzian, G. Ion Microscopy. *Anal. Chem.* **1975**, *47*, 932A–943A. [CrossRef]
52. Liebl, H. Ion Microprobe Mass Analyzer. *J. Appl. Phys.* **1967**, *38*, 5277–5283. [CrossRef]
53. Baker, M.J.; Brown, M.D.; Gazi, E.; Clarke, N.W.; Vickerman, J.C.; Lockyer, N.P. Discrimination of prostate cancer cells and non-malignant cells using secondary ion mass spectrometry. *Analyst* **2008**, *133*, 175–179. [CrossRef] [PubMed]
54. Gostek, J.; Awsiuk, K.; Pabijan, J.; Rysz, J.; Budkowski, A.; Lekka, M. Differentiation between single bladder cancer cells using principal component analysis of time-of-flight secondary ion mass spectrometry. *Anal. Chem.* **2015**, *87*, 3195–3201. [CrossRef] [PubMed]
55. Kulp, K.S.; Berman, E.S.; Knize, M.G.; Shattuck, D.L.; Nelson, E.J.; Wu, L.; Montgomery, J.L.; Felton, J.S.; Wu, K.J. Chemical and biological differentiation of three human breast cancer cell types using time-of-flight secondary ion mass spectrometry. *Anal. Chem.* **2006**, *78*, 3651–3658. [CrossRef] [PubMed]
56. Theiner, S.; Van Malderen, S.J.M.; Van Acker, T.; Legin, A.; Keppler, B.K.; Vanhaecke, F.; Koellensperger, G. Fast High-Resolution Laser Ablation-Inductively Coupled Plasma Mass Spectrometry Imaging of the Distribution of Platinum-Based Anticancer Compounds in Multicellular Tumor Spheroids. *Anal. Chem.* **2017**, *89*, 12641–12645. [CrossRef] [PubMed]
57. Yalcin, E.B.; de la Monte, S.M. Review of matrix-assisted laser desorption ionization-imaging mass spectrometry for lipid biochemical histopathology. *J. Histochem. Cytochem.* **2015**, *63*, 762–771. [CrossRef]
58. Di Girolamo, F.; Lante, I.; Muraca, M.; Putignani, L. The Role of Mass Spectrometry in the "Omics" Era. *Curr. Org. Chem.* **2013**, *17*, 2891–2905. [CrossRef]
59. Chan, T.W.; Duan, L.; Sze, T.P. Accurate mass measurements for peptide and protein mixtures by using matrix-assisted laser desorption/ionization Fourier transform mass spectrometry. *Anal. Chem.* **2002**, *74*, 5282–5289. [CrossRef]
60. Sauer, S.; Kliem, M. Mass spectrometry tools for the classification and identification of bacteria. *Nat. Rev. Microbiol.* **2010**, *8*, 74–82. [CrossRef]
61. Gao, X.; Tan, B.H.; Sugrue, R.J.; Tang, K. MALDI mass spectrometry for nucleic acid analysis. *Top. Curr. Chem.* **2013**, *331*, 55–77. [CrossRef] [PubMed]

62. Vogel, N.; Schiebel, K.; Humeny, A. Technologies in the Whole-Genome Age: MALDI-TOF-Based Genotyping. *Transfus. Med. Hemother.* **2009**, *36*, 253–262. [CrossRef] [PubMed]
63. Yanagisawa, K.; Shyr, Y.; Xu, B.J.; Massion, P.P.; Larsen, P.H.; White, B.C.; Roberts, J.R.; Edgerton, M.; Gonzalez, A.; Nadaf, S.; et al. Proteomic patterns of tumour subsets in non-small-cell lung cancer. *Lancet* **2003**, *362*, 433–439. [CrossRef]
64. Steinhauser, M.L.; Bailey, A.P.; Senyo, S.E.; Guillermier, C.; Perlstein, T.S.; Gould, A.P.; Lee, R.T.; Lechene, C.P. Multi-isotope imaging mass spectrometry quantifies stem cell division and metabolism. *Nature* **2012**, *481*, 516–519. [CrossRef] [PubMed]
65. Angelo, M.; Bendall, S.C.; Finck, R.; Hale, M.B.; Hitzman, C.; Borowsky, A.D.; Levenson, R.M.; Lowe, J.B.; Liu, S.D.; Zhao, S.; et al. Multiplexed ion beam imaging of human breast tumors. *Nat. Med.* **2014**, *20*, 436–442. [CrossRef] [PubMed]
66. Bandura, D.R.; Baranov, V.I.; Ornatsky, O.I.; Antonov, A.; Kinach, R.; Lou, X.; Pavlov, S.; Vorobiev, S.; Dick, J.E.; Tanner, S.D. Mass cytometry: Technique for real time single cell multitarget immunoassay based on inductively coupled plasma time-of-flight mass spectrometry. *Anal. Chem.* **2009**, *81*, 6813–6822. [CrossRef] [PubMed]
67. Rimm, D.L. What brown cannot do for you. *Nat. Biotechnol.* **2006**, *24*, 914–916. [CrossRef] [PubMed]
68. Keren, L.; Bosse, M.; Marquez, D.; Angoshtari, R.; Jain, S.; Varma, S.; Yang, S.R.; Kurian, A.; Van Valen, D.; West, R.; et al. A Structured Tumor-Immune Microenvironment in Triple Negative Breast Cancer Revealed by Multiplexed Ion Beam Imaging. *Cell* **2018**, *174*, 1373–1387. [CrossRef]
69. Di Palma, S.; Bodenmiller, B. Unraveling cell populations in tumors by single-cell mass cytometry. *Curr. Opin. Biotechnol.* **2015**, *31*, 122–129. [CrossRef]
70. Dempsey, L.A. CyTOF analysis of anti-tumor responses. *Nat. Immunol.* **2017**, *18*, 254. [CrossRef]
71. Bendall, S.C.; Simonds, E.F.; Qiu, P.; Amir el, A.D.; Krutzik, P.O.; Finck, R.; Bruggner, R.V.; Melamed, R.; Trejo, A.; Ornatsky, O.I.; et al. Single-cell mass cytometry of differential immune and drug responses across a human hematopoietic continuum. *Science* **2011**, *332*, 687–696. [CrossRef] [PubMed]
72. Giesen, C.; Wang, H.A.; Schapiro, D.; Zivanovic, N.; Jacobs, A.; Hattendorf, B.; Schuffler, P.J.; Grolimund, D.; Buhmann, J.M.; Brandt, S.; et al. Highly multiplexed imaging of tumor tissues with subcellular resolution by mass cytometry. *Nat. Methods* **2014**, *11*, 417–422. [CrossRef] [PubMed]
73. Schulz, D.; Zanotelli, V.R.T.; Fischer, J.R.; Schapiro, D.; Engler, S.; Lun, X.K.; Jackson, H.W.; Bodenmiller, B. Simultaneous Multiplexed Imaging of mRNA and Proteins with Subcellular Resolution in Breast Cancer Tissue Samples by Mass Cytometry. *Cell Syst.* **2018**, *6*, 531. [CrossRef] [PubMed]
74. Ribas, A.; Dummer, R.; Puzanov, I.; VanderWalde, A.; Andtbacka, R.H.I.; Michielin, O.; Olszanski, A.J.; Malvehy, J.; Cebon, J.; Fernandez, E.; et al. Oncolytic Virotherapy Promotes Intratumoral T Cell Infiltration and Improves Anti-PD-1 Immunotherapy. *Cell* **2017**, *170*, 1109–1119. [CrossRef] [PubMed]
75. Zheng, P.P.; van der Weiden, M.; Kros, J.M. Fast tracking of co-localization of multiple markers by using the nanozoomer slide scanner and NDPViewer. *J. Cell. Physiol.* **2014**, *229*, 967–973. [CrossRef] [PubMed]
76. Saylor, J.; Ma, Z.; Goodridge, H.S.; Huang, F.; Cress, A.E.; Pandol, S.J.; Shiao, S.L.; Vidal, A.C.; Wu, L.; Nickols, N.G.; et al. Spatial Mapping of Myeloid Cells and Macrophages by Multiplexed Tissue Staining. *Front. Immunol.* **2018**, *9*, 2925. [CrossRef]
77. Sanderson, M.J.; Smith, I.; Parker, I.; Bootman, M.D. Fluorescence microscopy. *Cold Spring Harb. Protoc.* **2014**, *2014*, pdb.top071795. [CrossRef]
78. Spindel, S.; Sapsford, K.E. Evaluation of optical detection platforms for multiplexed detection of proteins and the need for point-of-care biosensors for clinical use. *Sensors* **2014**, *14*, 22313–22341. [CrossRef]
79. Blom, S.; Paavolainen, L.; Bychkov, D.; Turkki, R.; Maki-Teeri, P.; Hemmes, A.; Valimaki, K.; Lundin, J.; Kallioniemi, O.; Pellinen, T. Systems pathology by multiplexed immunohistochemistry and whole-slide digital image analysis. *Sci. Rep.* **2017**, *7*, 15580. [CrossRef]
80. Isse, K.; Lesniak, A.; Grama, K.; Roysam, B.; Minervini, M.I.; Demetris, A.J. Digital transplantation pathology: Combining whole slide imaging, multiplex staining and automated image analysis. *Am. J. Transplant.* **2012**, *12*, 27–37. [CrossRef]
81. Bodenmiller, B. Multiplexed Epitope-Based Tissue Imaging for Discovery and Healthcare Applications. *Cell Syst.* **2016**, *2*, 225–238. [CrossRef] [PubMed]

82. Lyons, C.; Lawler, D. Aperio Cellular IF Algorithm Validation. *Pathologist* **2016**. [CrossRef]
83. Harder, N.; Athelogou, M.; Hessel, H.; Brieu, N.; Yigitsoy, M.; Zimmermann, J.; Baatz, M.; Buchner, A.; Stief, C.G.; Kirchner, T.; et al. Tissue Phenomics for prognostic biomarker discovery in low- and intermediate-risk prostate cancer. *Sci. Rep.* **2018**, *8*, 4470. [CrossRef] [PubMed]
84. Klimowicz, A.C.; Bose, P.; Petrillo, S.K.; Magliocco, A.M.; Dort, J.C.; Brockton, N.T. The prognostic impact of a combined carbonic anhydrase IX and Ki67 signature in oral squamous cell carcinoma. *Br. J. Cancer* **2013**, *109*, 1859–1866. [CrossRef] [PubMed]
85. Rojo, M.G.; Bueno, G.; Slodkowska, J. Review of imaging solutions for integrated quantitative immunohistochemistry in the Pathology daily practice. *Folia Histochem. Cytobiol.* **2009**, *47*, 349–354. [CrossRef] [PubMed]
86. Ma, Z.; Shiao, S.L.; Yoshida, E.J.; Swartwood, S.; Huang, F.; Doche, M.E.; Chung, A.P.; Knudsen, B.S.; Gertych, A. Data integration from pathology slides for quantitative imaging of multiple cell types within the tumor immune cell infiltrate. *Diagn. Pathol.* **2017**, *12*, 69. [CrossRef] [PubMed]
87. Sideras, K.; Galjart, B.; Vasaturo, A.; Pedroza-Gonzalez, A.; Biermann, K.; Mancham, S.; Nigg, A.L.; Hansen, B.E.; Stoop, H.A.; Zhou, G.; et al. Prognostic value of intra-tumoral CD8(+) /FoxP3(+) lymphocyte ratio in patients with resected colorectal cancer liver metastasis. *J. Surg. Oncol.* **2018**, *118*, 68–76. [CrossRef]
88. Schneider, C.A.; Rasband, W.S.; Eliceiri, K.W. NIH Image to ImageJ: 25 years of image analysis. *Nat. Methods* **2012**, *9*, 671–675. [CrossRef]
89. Bankhead, P.; Loughrey, M.B.; Fernandez, J.A.; Dombrowski, Y.; McArt, D.G.; Dunne, P.D.; McQuaid, S.; Gray, R.T.; Murray, L.J.; Coleman, H.G.; et al. QuPath: Open source software for digital pathology image analysis. *Sci. Rep.* **2017**, *7*, 16878. [CrossRef]
90. De Chaumont, F.; Dallongeville, S.; Chenouard, N.; Herve, N.; Pop, S.; Provoost, T.; Meas-Yedid, V.; Pankajakshan, P.; Lecomte, T.; Le Montagner, Y.; et al. Icy: An open bioimage informatics platform for extended reproducible research. *Nat. Methods* **2012**, *9*, 690–696. [CrossRef]
91. Jones, T.R.; Kang, I.H.; Wheeler, D.B.; Lindquist, R.A.; Papallo, A.; Sabatini, D.M.; Golland, P.; Carpenter, A.E. CellProfiler Analyst: Data exploration and analysis software for complex image-based screens. *BMC Bioinform.* **2008**, *9*, 482. [CrossRef] [PubMed]
92. Lamprecht, M.R.; Sabatini, D.M.; Carpenter, A.E. CellProfiler: Free, versatile software for automated biological image analysis. *Biotechniques* **2007**, *42*, 71–75. [CrossRef] [PubMed]
93. McQuin, C.; Goodman, A.; Chernyshev, V.; Kamentsky, L.; Cimini, B.A.; Karhohs, K.W.; Doan, M.; Ding, L.; Rafelski, S.M.; Thirstrup, D.; et al. CellProfiler 3.0: Next-generation image processing for biology. *PLoS Biol.* **2018**, *16*, e2005970. [CrossRef] [PubMed]
94. Wiesmann, V.; Franz, D.; Held, C.; Munzenmayer, C.; Palmisano, R.; Wittenberg, T. Review of free software tools for image analysis of fluorescence cell micrographs. *J. Microsc.* **2015**, *257*, 39–53. [CrossRef] [PubMed]
95. Barua, S.; Fang, P.; Sharma, A.; Fujimoto, J.; Wistuba, I.; Rao, A.U.K.; Lin, S.H. Spatial interaction of tumor cells and regulatory T cells correlates with survival in non-small cell lung cancer. *Lung Cancer* **2018**, *117*, 73–79. [CrossRef]
96. Stack, E.C.; Foukas, P.G.; Lee, P.P. Multiplexed tissue biomarker imaging. *J. Immunother. Cancer* **2016**, *4*, 9. [CrossRef]
97. Johansson, A.C.; Visse, E.; Widegren, B.; Sjogren, H.O.; Siesjo, P. Computerized image analysis as a tool to quantify infiltrating leukocytes: A comparison between high- and low-magnification images. *J. Histochem. Cytochem.* **2001**, *49*, 1073–1079. [CrossRef]
98. Henriksen, M. Quantitative imaging cytometry: Instrumentation of choice for automated cellular and tissue analysis. *Nat. Methods* **2010**, *7*, 330. [CrossRef]
99. Miller, A.; Nagy, C.; Knapp, B.; Laengle, J.; Ponweiser, E.; Groeger, M.; Starkl, P.; Bergmann, M.; Wagner, O.; Haschemi, A. Exploring Metabolic Configurations of Single Cells within Complex Tissue Microenvironments. *Cell Metab.* **2017**, *26*, 788–800. [CrossRef]
100. Siegel, R.L.; Miller, K.D.; Jemal, A. Cancer Statistics, 2017. *CA Cancer J. Clin.* **2017**, *67*, 7–30. [CrossRef]
101. Parra, E.R.; Villalobos, P.; Behrens, C.; Jiang, M.; Pataer, A.; Swisher, S.G.; William, W.N., Jr.; Zhang, J.; Lee, J.; Cascone, T.; et al. Effect of neoadjuvant chemotherapy on the immune microenvironment in non-small cell lung carcinomas as determined by multiplex immunofluorescence and image analysis approaches. *J. Immunother. Cancer* **2018**, *6*, 48. [CrossRef] [PubMed]

102. Parra, E.R. Novel Technology to Assess Programmed Death-Ligand 1 Expression by Multiplex Immunofluorescence and Image Analysis. *Appl. Immunohistochem. Mol. Morphol.* **2018**, *26*, e22–e24. [CrossRef] [PubMed]
103. Parra, E.R. Novel Platforms of Multiplexed Immunofluorescence for Study of Paraffin Tumor Tissues. *J. Cancer Treat. Diagn.* **2018**, *2*, 43–53. [CrossRef]

13

Systematic Review and Network Meta-Analysis of Immune Checkpoint Inhibitors in Combination with Chemotherapy as a First-Line Therapy for Extensive-Stage Small Cell Carcinoma

Hsiao-Ling Chen [1], Yu-Kang Tu [2,3], Hsiu-Mei Chang [1], Tai-Huang Lee [4], Kuan-Li Wu [5], Yu-Chen Tsai [5], Mei-Hsuan Lee [5,*], Chih-Jen Yang [5,6,7,8,*], Jen-Yu Hung [4,5,7] and Inn-Wen Chong [6,7,8,9]

1 Department of Pharmacy, Kaohsiung Municipal Ta-Tung Hospital, Kaohsiung 80145, Taiwan; hlchen369@gmail.com (H.-L.C.); 880504@kmhk.org.tw (H.-M.C.)

2 Institute of Epidemiology and Preventive Medicine, National Taiwan University, Taipei 100225, Taiwan; yukangtu@ntu.edu.tw

3 Department of Medical Research, National Taiwan University Hospital, Taipei 100225, Taiwan

4 Department of Internal Medicine Kaohsiung Municipal Ta-Tung Hospital, Kaohsiung Medical University, Kaohsiung 88145, Taiwan; weatlee@gmail.com (T.-H.L.); jenyuhung@gmail.com (J.-Y.H.)

5 Division of Pulmonary and Critical Care Medicine, Department of Internal Medicine, Kaohsiung Medical University Hospital, Kaohsiung Medical University, Kaohsiung 88708, Taiwan; 980448kmuh@gmail.com (K.-L.W.); 1010362kmuh@gmail.com (Y.-C.T.)

6 Department of General Medicine, Kaohsiung Medical University Hospital, Kaohsiung Medical University, Kaohsiung 88708, Taiwan; chong@kmu.edu.tw

7 Faculty of Medicine, College of Medicine, Kaohsiung Medical University, Kaohsiung 88708, Taiwan

8 Respiratory Therapy, College of Medicine, Kaohsiung Medical University, Kaohsiung 88708, Taiwan

9 Department of Biological Science & Technology, National Chiao Tung University, Hsinchu 300, Taiwan

* Correspondence: mhsuan99@gmail.com (M.-H.L.); chjeya@cc.kmu.edu.tw (C.-J.Y.)

Simple Summary: Patients with extensive-stage small cell lung cancer (ED-SCLC) have a very short survival time even if they receive standard chemotherapy. Currently, the combination of chemotherapy plus immune checkpoint inhibitors (ICIs) as the first line treatment had superior survival than chemotherapy alone in randomized control trials. However, there is a lack of head-to-head comparisons for these combination regimens. We conducted a systematic review and network meta-analysis to provide a treatment ranking of ICIs for ED-SCLC. In summary, the probability of nivolumab was associated with the best ranking for overall survival, followed by atezolizumab, durvalumab, pembrolizumab, and ipilimumab. The ranking of progression free survival from the best to the worst was as follows: nivolumab, pembrolizumab, atezolizumab, durvalumab, and ipilimumab. However, nivolumab had the highest probability of grade 3–4 adverse events in our study. Further head-to head large-scale phase III randomized controlled studies are needed to verify our conclusions.

Abstract: Patients with extensive-stage small cell lung cancer (ED-SCLC) have a very short survival time even if they receive standard cytotoxic chemotherapy with etoposide and platinum (EP). Several randomized controlled trials have shown that patients with ED-SCLC who received a combination of EP plus immune checkpoint inhibitors (ICIs) had superior survival compared with those who received EP alone. We conducted a systematic review and network meta-analysis to provide a ranking of ICIs for our primary endpoints in terms of overall survival (OS), progression free survival (PFS), and objective response rate (ORR), as well as our secondary endpoint in terms of adverse events. The fractional polynomial model was used to evaluate the adjusted hazard ratios for the survival indicators (OS and PFS). Treatment rank was estimated using the surface under the cumulative ranking curve (SUCRA), as well as the probability of being best (Prbest) reference. EP plus nivolumab, atezolizumab or durvalumab had significant benefits compared with EP alone in terms of OS (Hazard Ratio HR = 0.67, 95% Confidence Interval CI = 0.46–0.98 for nivolumab, HR = 0.70, 95% CI = 0.54–0.91 for atezolizumab, HR = 0.73, 95% CI = 0.59–0.90 for durvalumab) but no significant differences were observed for pembrolizumab or ipilimumab. The probability of nivolumab being ranked first among all treatment arms was highest (SCURA = 78.7%, Prbest = 46.7%). All EP plus ICI combinations had a longer PFS compared with EP alone (HR = 0.65, 95% CI = 0.46–0.92 for nivolumab, HR = 0.77, 95% CI = 0.61–0.96 for atezolizumab, HR = 0.78, 95% CI = 0.65–0.94 for durvalumab, HR = 0.75, 95% CI = 0.61–0.92 for pembrolizumab), and nivolumab was ranked first in terms of PFS (SCURA = 85.0%, Prbest = 66.8%). In addition, nivolumab had the highest probability of grade 3–4 adverse events (SUCRA = 84.8%) in our study. We found that nivolumab had the best PFS and OS in all combinations of ICIs and EP, but nivolumab also had the highest probability of grade 3–4 adverse events in our network meta-analysis. Further head-to head large-scale phase III randomized controlled studies are needed to verify our conclusions.

Keywords: immune checkpoint inhibitors; extensive-stage small cell lung cancer; nivolumab; ipilimumab; pembrolizumab; atezolizumab; durvalumab; chemotherapy

---

1. Introduction

Small cell lung cancer (SCLC) accounts for 10–15% of all lung cancer cases and is known for its aggressive behavior, rapid doubling time, growth, and early spread to distant sites. The most common risk factor for SCLC is smoking tobacco, and up to 98% of patients with SCLC have a history of smoking. SCLC is characterized by multiple genetic alterations, reflecting its genomic instability [1,2]. The majority of SCLCs express alterations in chromosome 3p and mutations in *RB1, TP53, RASSF1, MYC, FGFR1,* and *PTEN* [3,4]. In addition to these genomic alterations, there are also malfunctions in specific regulatory pathways. Long term exposure to tobacco smoke causes an increase in the tumor mutation burden (TMB) and SCLC is associated with a higher expression of DNA damage response (DDR) pathway mediators [5]. Early detection of SCLC is very challenging due to the lack of specific symptoms and the rapid tumor growth, making current approaches to screening ineffective for diagnosing patients at early disease stages [6–8]. Around 70% of cases present with extensive-stage SCLC at diagnosis (ED-SCLC); the remaining 30% of patients have limited-stage SCLC (LD-SCLC) [8]. First-line standard chemotherapy is a combination of etoposide with platinum (EP) [6,7]. In ED-SCLC, chemotherapy is the mainstay treatment in the first-line setting. The median overall survival (OS) rates range from 15 to 20 months for LS-SCLC and 8 to 13 months for ED-SCLC. The five-year survival rate is 20% to 25% for LS-SCLC, but only about 2% for ED-SCLC, and there is an average OS period of only two to four months for untreated ED-SCLC patients [6]. SCLC is usually sensitive to the initial chemotherapy treatment; however, most patients develop recurrent disease, often with metastasis to additional sites after the initial treatment. Currently, radiation therapy to the chest and prophylactic cranial irradiation are applied to destroy undetectable cancer cells and decrease the risk of recurrence. Topotecan is a standard second-line treatment choice but its efficacy is very limited [6]. There is no standard of care beyond second-line therapy. Systemic therapy for SCLC patients has not changed substantially in several decades [2,6]. Consequently, there is an urgent medical need to bring new treatment options to SCLC patients.

SCLC is a tumor with one of the highest rates of somatic mutations and this characteristic can result in a higher likelihood of identifying tumor-specific neoantigens that may ultimately trigger an adaptive immune response that is capable of detecting and eradicating tumor cells [1,2]. Preclinical data has demonstrated that treatment with antibodies specific for anti-cytotoxic T lymphocyte associated antigen 4 (CTLA-4) can restore an immune response through the increased accumulation and survival of memory T cells and depletion of regulatory T cells (Tregs). The use of monoclonal antibodies (mAbs) to block either programmed cell death 1 (PD-1) or anti-programmed cell death ligand 1 (PD-L1) prevents the downregulation of T cell effector function, allowing T cells to mediate tumor cell death. Several phase III trials reported that immune checkpoint inhibitors (ICIs) in combination with chemotherapy had clinical benefit in terms of progression free survival (PFS) and OS when used as a salvage therapy for advanced non-small cell lung cancer compared with those patients who received chemotherapy alone [9–12]. Since then, several trials have been designed to combine chemotherapy with ICIs, including anti-CTLA4, anti-PD-1 or anti-PD-L1, as a first line therapy for ED-SCLC [13–18]. Except for anti-CTLA4, ICIs plus chemotherapy provided a better survival benefit for newly diagnosed ED-SCLC. However, there is a lack of head-to-head comparisons for these combination regimens in the treatment of ED-SCLC. As ICIs are very expensive and ED-SCLC patients have a short survival time, we urgently need to know which ICI plus EP is most effective and reliable. Therefore, we used PFS, OS, objective response rate (ORR) and grade 3–4 adverse drug reactions as the major outcomes in a network meta-analysis of current randomized phase II and phase III trials which reported on ICI plus EP treatment to evaluate their clinical efficacy.

2. Results

2.1. Literature Search

A total of 393 studies were identified following electronic searches, and eight studies were identified from American Society of Clinical Oncology (ASCO) and European Medical Oncology (ESMO). After the exclusion of duplicate studies, 211 papers underwent title/abstract screening. Of those, 82 were excluded due to being incomplete randomized controlled trials (RCTs)and 93 were excluded on the basis of the title/abstract review, leaving 36 studies that underwent a full text review. At the end of the review process, six met the inclusion criteria and underwent qualitative synthesis and quantitative meta-analysis. A Preferred Reporting Items for Systematic Reviews and Meta-Analyses (PRISMA) flow diagram is presented in Figure 1 and the reasons for exclusion are provided in Table S1.

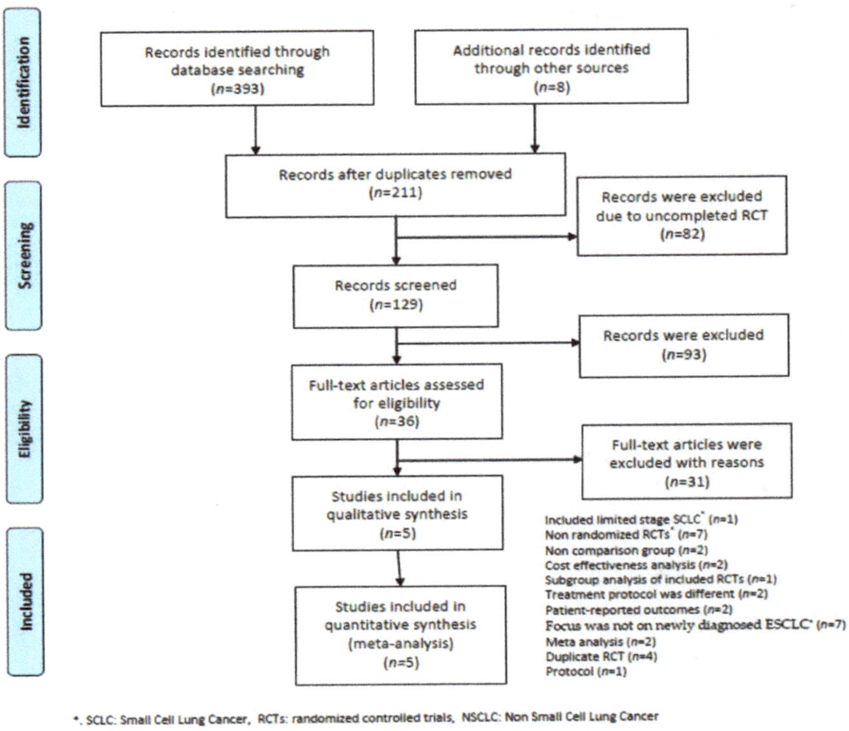

Figure 1. PRIMSA flow diagram.

Study Characteristics and Quality Evaluation

The characteristics of the included studies are provided in Table 1. All six trials were phase II or III and were completed between 2013 and 2020 for newly diagnosed ED-SCLC patients who had not received previous treatment. Except for CA184-041 [16], the control group of all included trials was chemotherapy with etoposide plus platinum (EP) agents. There were two study arms in four of the trials which compared chemotherapy plus ICIs, such as ipilimumab [17], nivolumab [14], pembrolizumab [18], or atezolizumab [13], to chemotherapy alone, while there were three study arms in the CASPIAN [15] and CA184-041 trials. However, the groups with durvalumab, tremelimumab and EP in the CASPIAN trial did not meet the predefined statistical significance threshold at the time of the interim analysis and therefore the result was not presented in the final report. Besides, the group with the concurrent regimen in CA184-041 [16], a phase II trial for ipilimumab, was not regarded as a treatment arm in CA184-156 [17], a phase III trial for ipilimumab, due to there being no improvement in efficacy. The percentage of patients aged ≥ 65 years across the trials ranged from 23.1% to 52.3%, and the percentage of males ranged from 44.4% to 78.4%. The percentage of brain or CNS metastases ranged from 8.68% to 12.14% across all included trials. Response evaluation criteria in solid tumors version 1.1 (RECIST) was used to assess tumor shrinkage (objective response) and disease progression in four of the trials. The other two trials for ipilimumab (CA184-041 and CA184-156) assessed the tumor burden using the modified World Health Organization (mWHO) criteria, as well as the immune-related (IR) response criteria. In conclusion, CA-184-041 [16] was excluded from our analysis due to heterogeneity in the chemotherapy regimen. Furthermore, data from CA184-156 was not included in the network comparisons for PFS and ORR because different criteria were used for cancer progression and treatment response.

The results of the quality assessment are presented in Figure S1. Detailed information about EA5161 was determined from the protocol in ClinicalTrials.gov because limited data was provided in the report from the 2020 annual meeting of the American Society of Clinical Oncology. Both CASPIAN and EA5161 were open label studies; therefore, a high risk of bias was declared for blinding. Besides, unclear assessments were presented and resulted from a lack of detailed information about the random sequence generation and allocation process.

Table 1. Characteristics of the included studies.

Trial Name	ICI-Based Treatment	Year	Phase	Age ≥ 65 (%)	Males (%)	Brain or CNS * Meta (%)	Experimental Arm 1 (Number)	Experimental Arm 2 (Number)	Control Arm (Number)	Criteria for Progression or Response	Criteria for AE *
PD-1 inhibitors											
Keynote-604	pembrolizumab	2020	3	52.3%	64.9%	12.14%	($n = 228$)		($n = 225$)	RECIST *	CTCAE *
[18]							Induction: 4 × 21 days cycle		EP alone	version 1.1	
							Pembrolizumab + EP *		4 × 21 days cycle		
							maintenance *				
							pembrolizumab every 3 weeks				
EA5161	nivolumab	2020	2	unknown	44.4%	11.25%	($n = 80$)		($n = 80$)	RECIST	CTCAE
[14]				median			induction: 4 × 21 days cycle		EP alone	version 1.1	
				Age = 65			Nivolumab + EP		4 × 21 days cycle		
							maintenance *				
							nivolumab every 2 weeks				
PD-L1 inhibitors											
IMpower133	atezolizumab	2018	3	46.2%	64.8%	8.68%	($n = 201$)		($n = 202$)	RECIST	CTCAE
[13]							induction: 4 × 21 days cycle		EP alone	version 1.1	
							atezolizumab + EP		4×21 days cycle		
							maintenance *				
							atezolizumab every 3 weeks				
CASPIAN	durvalumab	2019	3	39.7%	69.6%	10.24%	($n = 268$)	($n = 268$)	($n = 269$)	RECIST	CTCAE
[15]							induction: 4 × 21 days cycle	induction: 4 × 21 days cycle	EP alone	version 1.1	
							durvalumab + EP	durvalumab + EP + tremelimumab	4 × 21 days cycle		
							Maintenance *	Maintenance *			
							durvalumab every 4 weeks	durvalumab every 4 weeks			
CTLA4 inhibitors											
CA184-041	ipilimumab	2013	2	23.1%	78.4%	unknown	($n = 42$)	($n = 42$)	($n = 45$)	1. mWHO *	CTCAE

Table 1. *Cont.*

Trial Name	ICI-Based Treatment	Year	Phase	Age ≥ 65 (%)	Males (%)	Brain or CNS * Meta (%)	Experimental Arm 1 (Number)	Experimental Arm 2 (Number)	Control Arm (Number)	Criteria for Progression or Response	Criteria for AE *
[16]							phase regman 6 × 21 days cycle	concurrent regman 6 × 21 days cycle	paclitaxel + carboplatin 4 × 21 days cycle		
							paclitaxel + carboplatin at cycle 1–2	ipilimumab +paclitaxel +		2. irRC *	
							ipilimumab +paclitaxel + carboplatin at cycle 3–6	carboplatin at cycle 1–4			
								paclitaxel + carboplatin at cycle 5–6			
							maintenance *	maintenance *			
							ipilimumab every 12 weeks	ipilimumab every 12 weeks			
CA184-156	ipilimumab	2016	3	39.6%	56.9%	10.48%	(n = 478)		(n = 476)	1. mWHO	CTCAE
[17]							phase regman: 6 × 21 days cycle		EP alone 4 × 21 days cycle		
							EP at cycle 1–2			2. irRC	
							ipilimumab + EP at cycle 3–6				
							maintenance *				
							Ipilimumab every 12 weeks				

* CNS: central nervous system, EP: etoposide and platinum, AE: adverse event, RECIST: Response evaluation criteria in solid tumors version, CTCAE: Common Terminology Criteria for Adverse Events, mWHO: modified World Health Organization criteria, irRC: immune-related response criteria.

2.2. *Pooled Results for ICIs and Their Effect on Efficacy and Safety*

Pooled results for the effect of different ICIs on OS, PFS and ORR as well as grade 3–4 adverse events are provided in Figures S2 and S3. Compared to chemotherapy alone, ICI plus chemotherapy significantly increased the OS and PFS but no significant effect was observed for ORR. On the other hand, ICI plus chemotherapy slightly increased the risk of grade 3–4 adverse events. With regards to the blockade of ICIs, anti-PD-1 agents (nivolumab and pembrolizumab) were associated with significant benefits in OS and PFS. A noticeable OS benefit was seen in the patients who received anti-PD-L1 agents (atezolizumab and durvalumab), but there were no significant effects in PFS and ORR. Only one RCT evaluated the efficacy of an anti-CTLA4 agent (ipilimumab), but there was no improvement in OS between the patients who received ipilimumab plus chemotherapy and those who received chemotherapy alone. In terms of safety, no statistical risks were reported among the patients who received ICIs plus chemotherapy, regardless of the subgroup of ICIs.

Efficacy and Safety Evaluation from the Network Meta-Analysis

The network constructions are presented in Figure 2. For OS and grade 3–4 adverse events, five ICIs plus chemotherapy and chemotherapy alone were included in the network meta-analysis. In terms of PFS and ORR, four ICIs plus chemotherapy and chemotherapy alone were included in the network meta-analysis. The effect sizes of the pairwise comparisons are summarized in Figure 3 and the surface under cumulative ranking curve (SUCRA) rankings are detailed in Figure 4. The probability of being the best treatment is shown in Figure 5 for all efficacy and safety indicators.

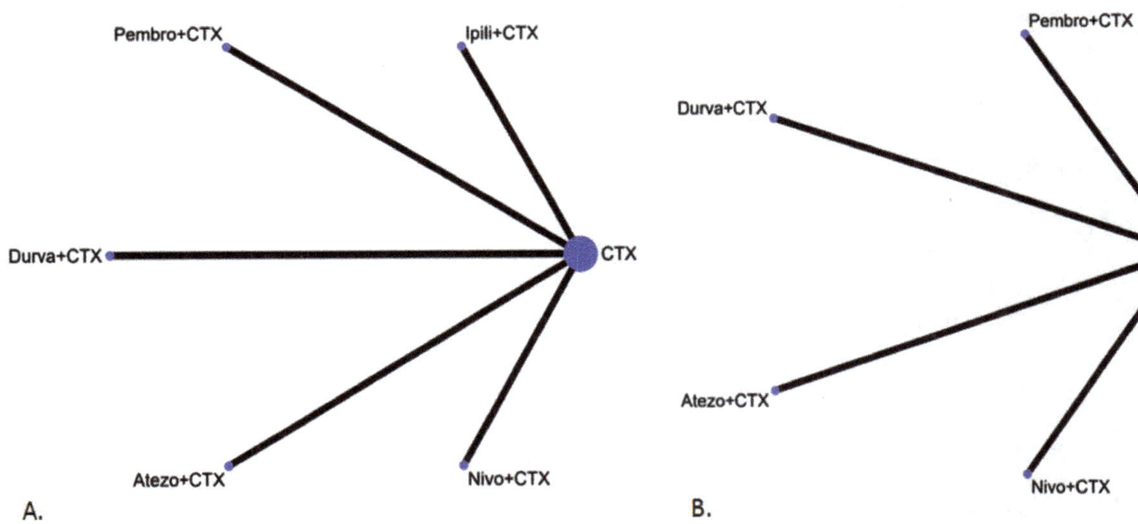

Figure 2. Network construction. (**A**) Network constructions for comparison in overall survival and grade 3–4 adverse events; (**B**) Network constructions for comparison in progression free survival and objective response ratio.

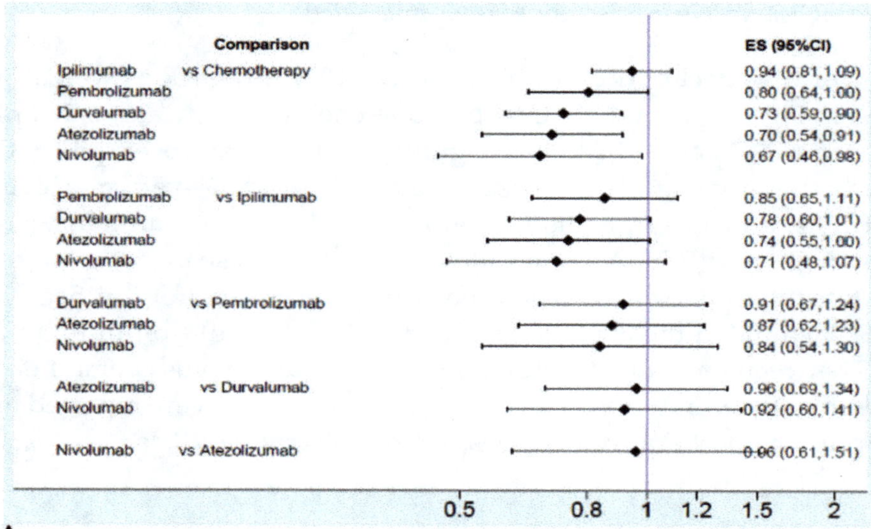

A.

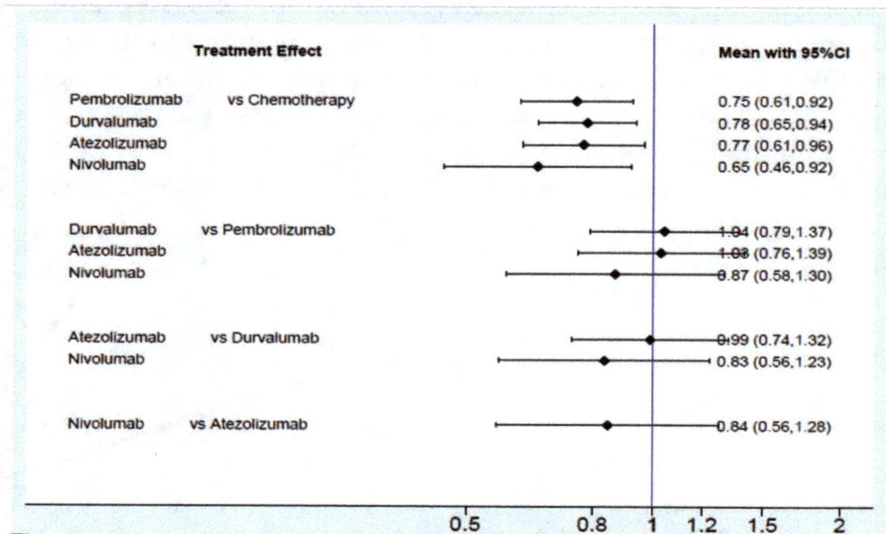

B.

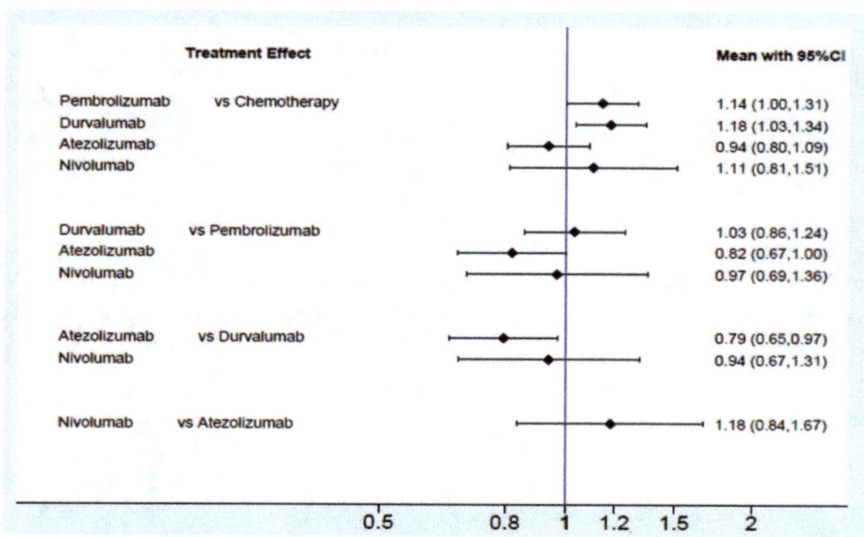

C.

Figure 3. *Cont.*

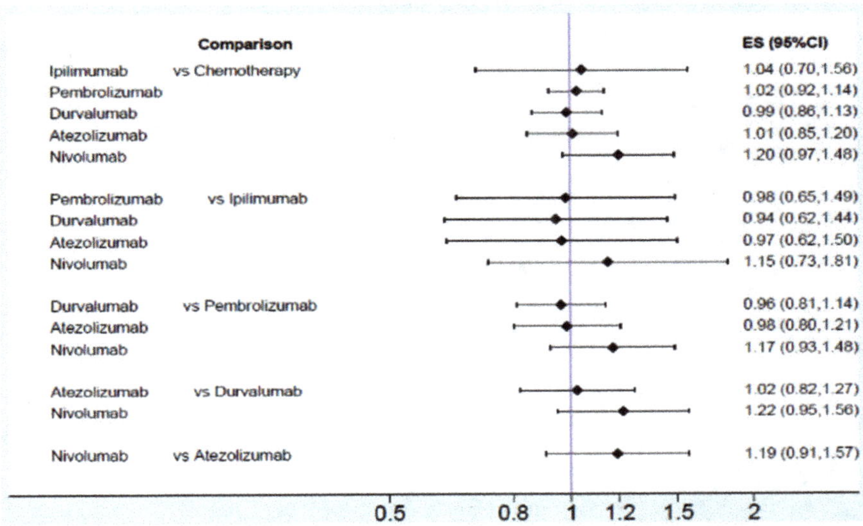

D.

Figure 3. Summary of effect sizes from pairwise comparisons. (**A**) Hazard Ratio for overall survival; (**B**) Hazard Ratio for progression free survival; (**C**) Response Ratio for objective response rate; (**D**) Risk Ratio for grade 3–4 adverse events.

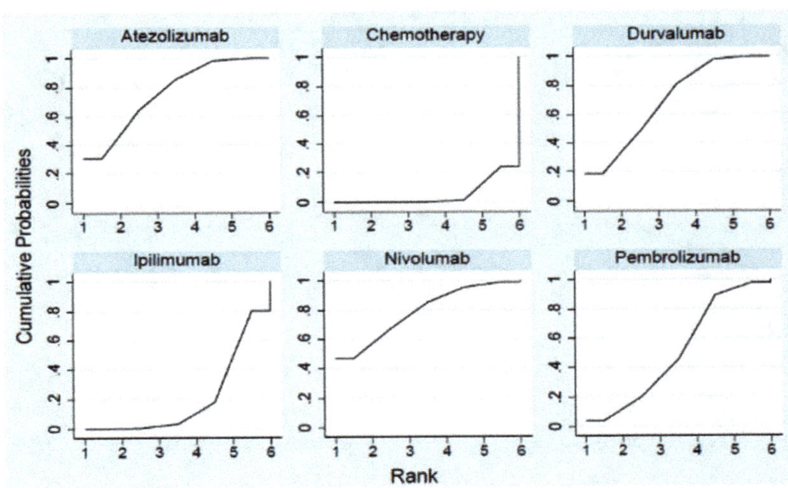

A.

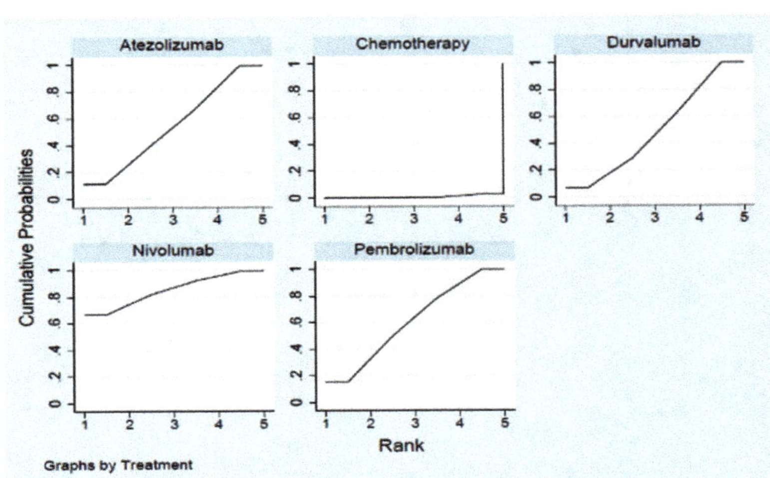

B.

Figure 4. *Cont.*

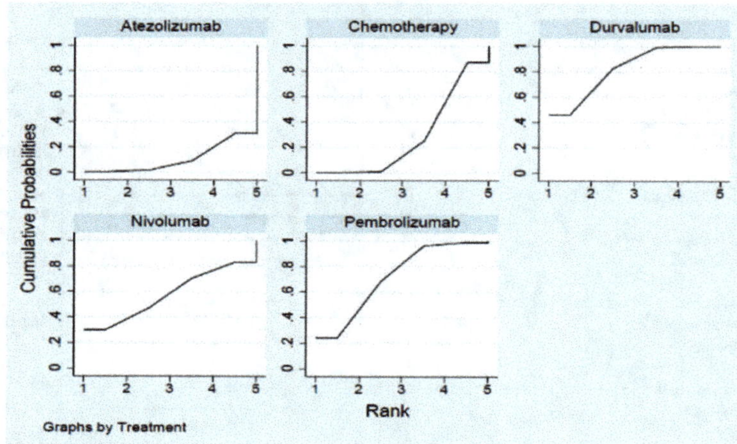

C.

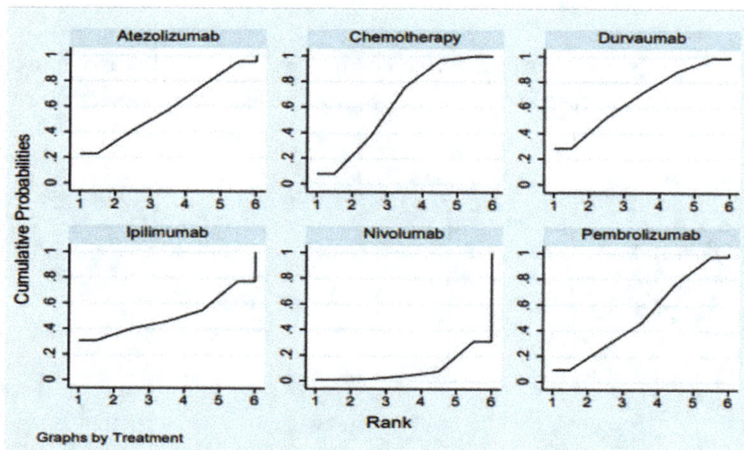

D.

Figure 4. Cumulative ranking probability for different treatments. (**A**) Overall survival; (**B**) Progression free survival; (**C**) Objective response rate; (**D**) Grade 3–4 adverse events.

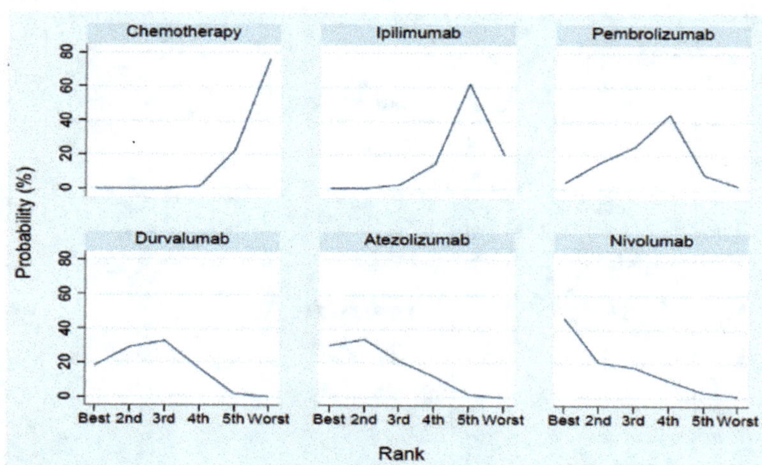

A.

Figure 5. *Cont.*

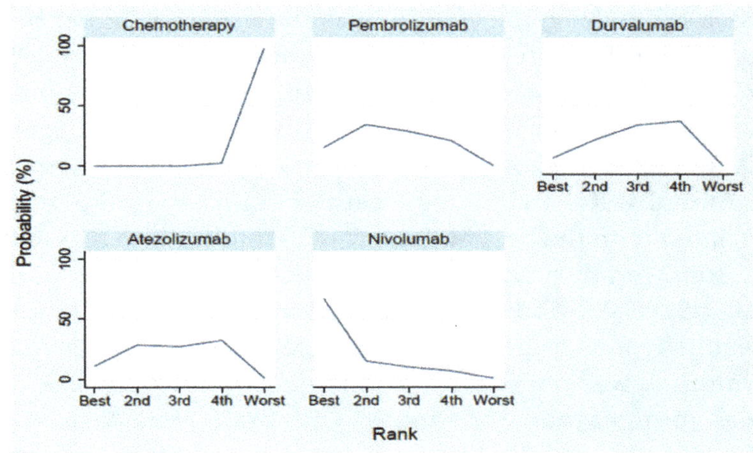

B.

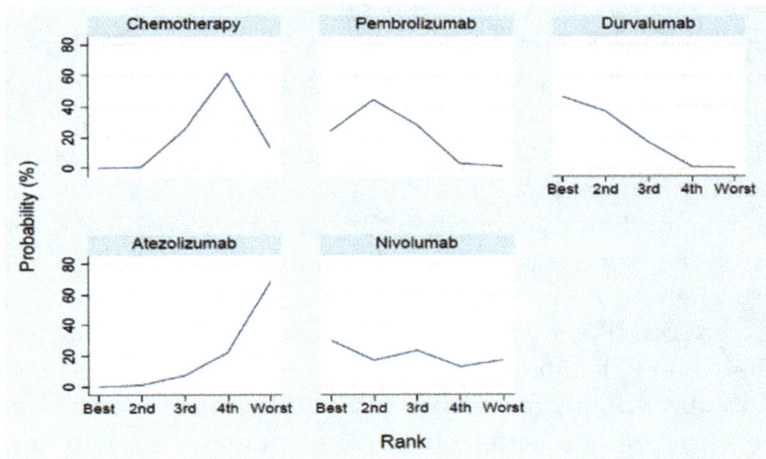

C.

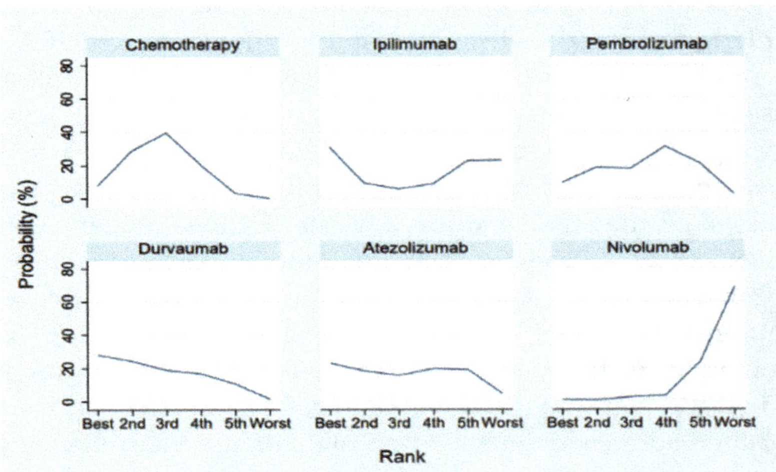

D.

Figure 5. Probability to be the best treatment for different treatments. (**A**) Overall survival; (**B**) Progression free survival; (**C**) Objective response rate; (**D**) Grade 3–4 adverse events.

2.3. Efficacy and Safety Evaluation

In terms of pairwise comparisons for OS (Figure 3A), chemotherapy plus nivolumab, atezolizumab or durvalumab gave a significantly improved benefit compared with chemotherapy alone (HR = 0.67, 95% CI = 0.46–0.98 for nivolumab, HR = 0.70, 95% CI = 0.54–0.91 for atezolizumab, HR = 0.73, 95% CI

= 0.59–0.90 for durvalumab). However, the efficacy was shown to be similar between pembrolizumab or ipilimumab plus chemotherapy and chemotherapy alone (HR = 0.80, 95% CI = 0.64–1.00 for pembrolizumab, HR = 0.92, 95% CI = 0.80–1.09 for ipilimumab). Although no superior effects were indicated in pairwise comparisons between different ICIs, anti-PD-1 agents (pembrolizumab or nivolumab) and anti-PD-L1 agents (atezolizumab or durvalumab) had lower HRs compared with the anti-CTLA4 agent (ipilimumab). Regarding the treatment efficacy ranking, the probability showed that nivolumab was associated with the best ranking for OS (highest SCURA and Prbest value; SCURA = 78.6%, Prbest = 46.7%), followed by atezolizumab (SCURA = 75.7%), durvalumab (SCURA = 68.9%), pembrolizumab (SCURA = 51.3%), ipilimumab (SCURA = 20.4%) and chemotherapy alone (SCURA = 5.0%). Based on the results from subgroup analysis (Figure S4), ranking was similar to the overall subjects. Although durvalumab was not regarded as being a better ICI in OS, it was recommended as the best choice for females younger than 65 years old with brain metastasis at baseline.

In terms of PFS (Figure 3B), all ICIs included in our analysis improved PFS compared with chemotherapy alone (HR = 0.65, 95% CI = 0.46–0.92 for nivolumab, HR = 0.77, 95% CI = 0.61–0.96 for atezolizumab, HR = 0.78, 95% CI = 0.65–0.94 for durvalumab, HR = 0.75, 95% CI = 0.61–0.92 for pembrolizumab). Even though the different ICIs had a similar effect on PFS, treatment with nivolumab had a lower HR than the others. Additionally, the probability showed that nivolumab was associated with the best ranking for PFS (highest SUCRA and Prbest; SCURA = 85.0%, Prbest = 66.8%). As for the blockade of ICIs, anti-PD-1 agents (SCURA = 85.0% for nivolumab and 60.8% for pembrolizumab) were associated with better rankings than anti-PD-L1 agents (SCURA = 54.2% for atezolizumab and 49.5% for durvalumab). Chemotherapy alone had the lowest score (SCURA = 0.6%).

In terms of the objective response rate (Figure 3C), durvalumab was associated with a superior ranking compared with chemotherapy alone (response ratio = 1.18, 95% CI = 1.03–1.34) but no significant differences were observed between the other ICIs and chemotherapy alone. Based on pairwise comparisons between ICIs, no significant difference was observed between any comparable ICIs except for durvalumab, which produced a noticeable benefit over atezolizumab. Moreover, durvalumab was regarded to have a better objective response rate. Durvalumab had the highest SUCRA and Prbest scores (SCURA = 82.1%, Prbest = 46.2%), followed by pembrolizumab (SCURA = 71.8%) and nivolumab (SCURA = 57.4%). However, adding atezolizumab to chemotherapy treatment did not give a better ranking compared with chemotherapy alone, as the SCURA value of atezolizumab was the lowest (SUCRA = 28.3% for chemotherapy alone and SCURA = 10.4% for atezolizumab).

In terms of pairwise comparisons for grade 3–4 adverse events (Figure 3D), we found no significant differences in the risk of grade 3–4 adverse events between any two treatment arms. Although a higher risk was observed among nivolumab users, the risk ratios were close to one and there were no statistical differences. Based on the SUCRA value, a larger SUCRA value indicated a higher treatment risk. Nivolumab (SUCRA = 86.9%, Prbest = 61.3%) had the highest probability of grade 3–4 adverse events, followed by ipilimumab (SUCRA = 51.3%), pembrolizumab (SUCRA = 49.4%), atezolizumab (SUCRA = 42.3%), chemotherapy alone (SUCRA = 37.4%) and durvalumab (SUCRA = 32.7%). Finally, death events for the included RCTs are summarized in Table S2. Due to the limited data that was provided in the published RCTs, it was not possible to classify death events into any events leading to death, immune-mediated adverse events leading to death, or chemotherapy leading to death, so we did not conduct network meta-analyses for death events. The ranking of specific toxicities was similar to the ranking of overall adverse events, except for ipilimumab (Figure S5). Ipilimumab had a lower risk for anemia (ranking = five of six), neutropenia (ranking = six of six) and thrombocytopenia (ranking = six of six); however, ipilimumab had worse safety data for overall adverse events (ranking = two of six).

3. Discussion

ICI plus chemotherapy has been shown to be superior to traditional chemotherapy in both OS and PFS for patients with treatment naïve ED-SCLC in several trials [13–15,18]. Our network meta-analysis firstly proposed a ranking for PFS, OS, ORR and grade 3–4 adverse events for different combinations of ICI and chemotherapy for ED-SCLC treatment.

Add-on ICIs are a feasible way of improving the very short survival time of ED-SCLC patients who receive the standard EP regimen [13–15,18]. Although a response rate of 50% to 80% is achieved in first-line treatment with EP chemotherapy, progression occurs rapidly and there is only a 15–20% response to secondary topotecan chemotherapy [6,8]. Since SCLC has a very short survival time, new treatment strategies are urgently needed. The clinical efficacy of immunotherapies has been observed in patients with refractory or metastatic SCLC [12,19–23]. The phase II KEYNOTE-158 study [21] showed that the PFS of pembrolizumab for relapsed SCLC was 2.0 months, the median OS was 9.1 months, and the one-year PFS and OS were 16.8% and 40.2%, respectively. In a non-randomized cohort of patients with advanced SCLC treated in the CheckMate 032 study [19], the estimated two-year OS rate was 14% with nivolumab monotherapy and 26% with nivolumab plus ipilimumab. Nivolumab plus ipilimumab appeared to provide a greater clinical benefit than nivolumab monotherapy in SCLC patients with a high tumor mutation burden [5]. Furthermore, several trials were designed as a first line therapy for ED-SCLC.

A randomized phase II study (CA184-041) led by Reck et al. was designed to compare paclitaxel with carboplatin plus ipilimumab and paclitaxel with carboplatin alone, but the results did not reveal a significant difference in the ORR, PFS or OS between the treatments [16]. A randomized phase III trial (CA184-156) was further designed to compared ipilimumab and EP with EP alone, and the study showed a minimal increase in median PFS, but there was no significant change in median OS [17]. Recently, several phase II and III trials have been designed to evaluate the addition of PD-1 and PD-L1 inhibitors to EP, and they have demonstrated positive results [13–15,18]. Some traditional meta-analyses of the efficacy of ICIs plus EP have shown that a combination of EP plus ICIs gives superior PFS and OS compared with EP alone for the treatment of ED-SCLC [24,25]. However, the current network meta-analysis proposed not only the efficacies, but also showed the ranking of these ICIs plus chemotherapy combinations on PFS, OS, ORR and grade 3–4 adverse events in different combinations. Firstly, our study showed that all ICIs with EP combination regimens had superior PFS compared with EP treatment alone. All combinations of ICIs with EP enrolled in our network meta-analysis improved the PFS compared with chemotherapy alone. Among all ICI plus EP combinations, nivolumab plus EP had the lowest HR, and nivolumab plus EP ranked first in the treatment of ED-SCLC for PFS and could be regarded as the most reliable combination among all evaluated regimens. In addition, anti-PD-1 agents plus EP ranked better than anti-PD-L1 agents plus EP and EP alone in our analysis.

EP plus nivolumab, atezolizumab or durvalumab all had a significantly better ranking for OS compared with EP alone, but no significant benefits were observed for pembrolizumab or ipilimumab plus EP. Anti-PD-1 agents and anti-PD-L1 agents had lower HRs compared with the anti-CTLA4 agent. In fact, ipilimumab plus paclitaxel and carboplatin failed to demonstrate the efficacy of paclitaxel and carboplatin alone in a phase II trial and it also failed in a phase III study when compared with ipilimumab plus EP [16,17]. Furthermore, nivolumab was ranked as the most optimal ICI among all ICIs plus EP in the treatment arms, followed by atezolizumab, durvalumab, pembrolizumab, ipilimumab and EP alone.

Some previous trial results indicated that ICIs plus chemotherapy were better than chemotherapy alone in terms of ORR and disease control rate (DCR) [15,18]. However, some showed that there was no significant difference in the ORR and DCR between ICIs plus chemotherapy and chemotherapy alone [13,14]. In our analysis, ICIs with EP were compared with EP alone in terms of ORR and DCR. Durvalumab was determined to be the optimal treatment regimen with a better objective response rate, but no significant differences were presented between other ICIs and chemotherapy alone in our network meta-analysis. Interestingly, there was a discrepancy between the ranking of ORR benefit and OS/PFS benefit. This discrepancy may have been caused by measurement bias due to how tumor measurements were taken (in the setting of the subjectivity of RECIST) and also when these measurements were made [26].

Clinically, grade 3–4 adverse events always limit the application of effective combinations of ICIs and EP and grade 3–4 adverse events become the main concern [9,16]. Some previous analyses of these trials indicated that there were fewer serious hematology-related toxicities for the ICI plus chemotherapy group compared with the chemotherapy alone group, however, serious non-hematology-related toxicities were more common in patients receiving an ICI combined with chemotherapy, and there were significant increases in fatigue, rashes, diarrhea, and elevated aminotransferase enzymes [16,27]. In the current study, we found non-significant differences in the risk of grade 3–4 adverse events between any two treatment arms, but nivolumab plus EP had the highest risk. Among all ICIs, nivolumab plus EP had the highest probability of grade 3–4 adverse events as determined by the SUCRA ranking method.

Our meta-analysis had some limitations. First, heterogeneity was present among these included RCTs, such as the regimen for chemotherapy and criteria for treatment response or progression. Therefore, the CA184-041 phase II RCT was excluded from the quantitative synthesis. In addition, the EA5161 study is a small sample phase II trial assessing the effect of nivolumab on ED-SCLC. Although narrow Cls provided strong evidence in EA5161, further RCTs with large sample sizes are needed to confirm our findings. Therefore, our results only serve as a platform for future trials that attempt to introduce nivolumab as a first-line therapy for ES-SCLC in a large phase III RCT, not as direct evidence to promote nivolumab-based therapy as a frontline option at present.

4. Methods

This study was conducted in accordance with the Preferred Reporting Items for Systematic Reviews and Meta-Analyses (PRISMA) guidelines. A prospective protocol was created in advance and registered on the International Prospective Register of Systematic Reviews PROSPERO website (registration number: CRD42020215762) [27].

4.1. Search Strategy and Study Selection

A comprehensive literature search was performed of PubMed, Embase, Cochrane library ClinicalTrials.gov, the database of the American Society of Clinical Oncology (ASCO) and the dataset of European Medical Oncology (ESMO) from their conception until 30 September 2020 without a language limitation. Full details of the search strategy are presented in Tables S3 and S4 and the search keywords were as follows: small cell lung cancer (SCLC or small cell lung carcinoma), immune checkpoint inhibitors (ICIs) anti-CTLA4, anti-PD-1 or anti-PD-L1, and the specific names of drugs (ipilimumab, nivolumab, durvalumab, pembrolizumab, atezolizumab, lambrolizumab, avelumab or tremelimumab). In order to include more relevant studies, controlled vocabulary search terms for PubMed (MeSH) and Embase (Emtree) were used and additional references were sought from the reference lists of the retrieved studies. The inclusion criteria were as follows: (1) completed phase II–III randomized control trials (RCTs) involving adults with ED-SCLC; (2) the RCTs involved newly diagnosed untreated patients with ED-SCLC; (3) the RCTs investigated and compared the efficacy and safety of an ICI combined with chemotherapy with chemotherapy alone.

4.2. Data Extraction and Quality Assessment

Two independent reviewers (H.L. Chen and C.J. Yang) performed the data extraction and quality assessment. Any unresolved discrepancies in the data extraction or appraisal of the results were resolved by discussion with a third reviewer (M.S. Lee). The extracted information included trial details, such as trial name, year published, phase of trial, baseline characteristics, regimen and patient number, primary endpoints, secondary endpoints, and criteria for treatment response. Only grade 3–4 adverse events as defined by the Common Terminology Criteria for Adverse Events (CTCAE) were included for the safety analysis [28]. Quality assessment was performed using the Cochrane

Collaboration's Risk of Bias tool. Quality assessment was performed using Review Manager version 5.1 [29].

4.3. Data Synthesis and Statistical Analysis

Treatment efficacies were evaluated in terms of OS, PFS and ORR. The safety outcomes focused on grade 3–4 adverse events as determined by the CTCAE. A fractional polynomial model was used to evaluate the adjusted hazard ratios (HRs) for the survival indicators (OS and PFS). In terms of binomial indicators, response ratio was regarded as the effect size for the objective response rate and risk ratio was used for adverse events along with 95% confidence intervals (CIs).

We first generated the network graphs for different outcomes separately to determine which treatments were directly or indirectly comparable. After that, we performed a frequentist network meta-analysis to estimate the comparative effect of each pair of treatments included in the constructed network. Fixed-effect models were used, since in most cases the treatment of interest was evaluated in one trial and the number of included trials per comparison was too small to estimate between-study heterogeneity. Finally, treatment rank was estimated by a surface under cumulative ranking curve (SUCRA), as well as the probability of being best (Prbest). SUCRA was computed for a more precise estimation of the ranking probabilities and the larger the SUCRA value, the better the intervention. The Prbest value indicated that the treatment was the best choice in the top rank. All statistical analyses and network graph generation were performed using Stata 11.2 [30].

5. Conclusions

In summary, our network meta-analysis showed that EP plus all ICIs have longer PFS compared with chemotherapy alone, while nivolumab ranked first in the SUCRA ranking analysis. Furthermore, EP plus nivolumab, atezolizumab or durvalumab all provided significant improvements for OS compared with EP alone, and nivolumab also ranked first among all treatment arms. In addition, durvalumab plus EP showed a better objective response rate than the other ICIs plus EP. Finally, nivolumab had the highest probability of grade 3–4 adverse events according to the SUCRA ranking. Given the limited number of studies included in the meta-analysis, additional large-scale phase III RCT studies are needed to verify these conclusions.

Author Contributions: H.-L.C., C.-J.Y. and M.-H.L.: protocol development, data analysis, and manuscript writing. Y.-K.T.: data analysis. H.-M.C., T.-H.L., K.-L.W. and I.-W.C.: data interpretation. Y.-C.T. and J.-Y.H.: data extraction. All authors have read and agreed to the published version of the manuscript.

References

1. Sabari, J.K.; Lok, B.H.; Laird, J.H.; Poirier, J.T.; Rudin, C.M. Unravelling the biology of sclc: Implications for therapy. *Nat. Rev. Clin. Oncol.* **2017**, *14*, 549–561. [CrossRef] [PubMed]
2. Subbiah, S.; Nam, A.; Garg, N.; Behal, A.; Kulkarni, P.; Salgia, R. Small cell lung cancer from traditional to innovative therapeutics: Building a comprehensive network to optimize clinical and translational research. *J. Clin. Med.* **2020**, *9*, 2433. [CrossRef] [PubMed]
3. George, J.; Lim, J.S.; Jang, S.J.; Cun, Y.; Ozretic, L.; Kong, G.; Leenders, F.; Lu, X.; Fernandez-Cuesta, L.; Bosco, G.; et al. Comprehensive genomic profiles of small cell lung cancer. *Nature* **2015**, *524*, 47–53. [CrossRef] [PubMed]
4. Peifer, M.; Fernandez-Cuesta, L.; Sos, M.L.; George, J.; Seidel, D.; Kasper, L.H.; Plenker, D.; Leenders, F.; Sun, R.; Zander, T.; et al. Integrative genome analyses identify key somatic driver mutations of small-cell lung cancer. *Nat. Genet.* **2012**, *44*, 1104–1110. [CrossRef]

5. Dong, Z.; Bing, X.; Yong, Y.; Peng, Y.; Sheng-Nan, L.; Qiang, L. Progress in immunotherapy for small cell lung cancer. *World J. Clin. Oncol.* **2020**, *11*, 370–377.
6. Oze, I.; Hotta, K.; Kiura, K.; Ochi, N.; Takigawa, N.; Fujiwara, Y.; Tabata, M.; Tanimoto, M. Twenty-seven years of phase iii trials for patients with extensive disease small-cell lung cancer: Disappointing results. *PLoS ONE* **2009**, *4*, e7835. [CrossRef]
7. Rudin, C.M.; Ismaila, N.; Hann, C.L.; Malhotra, N.; Movsas, B.; Norris, K.; Pietanza, M.C.; Ramalingam, S.S.; Turrisi, A.T., 3rd; Giaccone, G. Treatment of small-cell lung cancer: American society of clinical oncology endorsement of the american college of chest physicians guideline. *J. Clin. Oncol.* **2015**, *33*, 4106–4111. [CrossRef]
8. Nicholson, A.G.; Chansky, K.; Crowley, J.; Beyruti, R.; Kubota, K.; Turrisi, A.; Eberhardt, W.E.; van Meerbeeck, J.; Rami-Porta, R.; Goldstraw, P.; et al. The international association for the study of lung cancer lung cancer staging project: Proposals for the revision of the clinical and pathologic staging of small cell lung cancer in the forthcoming eighth edition of the tnm classification for lung cancer. *J. Thorac. Oncol.* **2016**, *11*, 300–311. [CrossRef]
9. Almutairi, A.R.; Alkhatib, N.; Martin, J.; Babiker, H.M.; Garland, L.L.; McBride, A.; Abraham, I. Comparative efficacy and safety of immunotherapies targeting the pd-1/pd-l1 pathway for previously treated advanced non-small cell lung cancer: A bayesian network meta-analysis. *Crit. Rev. Oncol. Hematol.* **2019**, *142*, 16–25. [CrossRef]
10. Ando, K.; Kishino, Y.; Homma, T.; Kusumoto, S.; Yamaoka, T.; Tanaka, A.; Ohmori, T.; Ohnishi, T.; Sagara, H. Nivolumab plus ipilimumab versus existing immunotherapies in patients with pd-l1-positive advanced non-small cell lung cancer: A systematic review and network meta-analysis. *Cancers* **2020**, *12*, 1905. [CrossRef]
11. Franek, J.; Cappelleri, J.C.; Larkin-Kaiser, K.A.; Wilner, K.D.; Sandin, R. Systematic review and network meta-analysis of first-line therapy for advanced egfr-positive non-small-cell lung cancer. *Future Oncol.* **2019**, *15*, 2857–2871. [CrossRef] [PubMed]
12. Calles, A.; Aguado, G.; Sandoval, C.; Alvarez, R. The role of immunotherapy in small cell lung cancer. *Clin. Transl. Oncol.* **2019**, *21*, 961–976. [CrossRef] [PubMed]
13. Horn, L.; Mansfield, A.S.; Szczesna, A.; Havel, L.; Krzakowski, M.; Hochmair, M.J.; Huemer, F.; Losonczy, G.; Johnson, M.L.; Nishio, M.; et al. First-line atezolizumab plus chemotherapy in extensive-stage small-cell lung cancer. *N. Engl. J. Med.* **2018**, *379*, 2220–2229. [CrossRef] [PubMed]
14. Leal, T.; Wang, Y.; Dowlati, A.; Chen, Y.; Ramesh, A.; Razaq, M.; Liu, J.; Joseph, C.; King, D.M.; Ahuja, H.G.; et al. Randomized phase II clinical trial of cisplatin/carboplatin and etoposide (CE) alone or in combination with nivolumab as frontline therapy for extensivestage small cell lung cancer (ESSCLC): ECOG-ACRIN EA5161. *J. Clin. Oncol.* **2020**, *38*, 9000. [CrossRef]
15. Paz-Ares, L.; Dvorkin, M.; Chen, Y.; Reinmuth, N.; Hotta, K.; Trukhin, D.; Statsenko, G.; Hochmair, M.J.; Ozguroglu, M.; Ji, J.H.; et al. Durvalumab plus platinum-etoposide versus platinum-etoposide in first-line treatment of extensive-stage small-cell lung cancer (caspian): A randomised, controlled, open-label, phase 3 trial. *Lancet* **2019**, *394*, 1929–1939. [CrossRef]
16. Reck, M.; Bondarenko, I.; Luft, A.; Serwatowski, P.; Barlesi, F.; Chacko, R.; Sebastian, M.; Lu, H.; Cuillerot, J.M.; Lynch, T.J. Ipilimumab in combination with paclitaxel and carboplatin as first-line therapy in extensive-disease-small-cell lung cancer: Results from a randomized, double-blind, multicenter phase 2 trial. *Ann. Oncol.* **2013**, *24*, 75–83. [CrossRef]
17. Reck, M.; Luft, A.; Szczesna, A.; Havel, L.; Kim, S.W.; Akerley, W.; Pietanza, M.C.; Wu, Y.L.; Zielinski, C.; Thomas, M.; et al. Phase iii randomized trial of ipilimumab plus etoposide and platinum versus placebo plus etoposide and platinum in extensive-stage small-cell lung cancer. *J. Clin. Oncol.* **2016**, *34*, 3740–3748. [CrossRef]
18. Rudin, C.M.; Awad, M.M.; Navarro, A.; Gottfried, M.; Peters, S.; Csoszi, T.; Cheema, P.K.; Rodriguez-Abreu, D.; Wollner, M.; Yang, J.C.; et al. Pembrolizumab or placebo plus etoposide and platinum as first-line therapy for extensive-stage small-cell lung cancer: Randomized, double-blind, phase iii keynote-604 study. *J. Clin. Oncol.* **2020**, *38*, 2369–2379. [CrossRef]
19. Antonia, S.J.; Lopez-Martin, J.A.; Bendell, J.; Ott, P.A.; Taylor, M.; Eder, J.P.; Jager, D.; Pietanza, M.C.; Le, D.T.; de Braud, F.; et al. Nivolumab alone and nivolumab plus ipilimumab in recurrent small-cell lung cancer (checkmate 032): A multicentre, open-label, phase 1/2 trial. *Lancet Oncol.* **2016**, *17*, 883–895. [CrossRef]

20. Iams, W.T.; Porter, J.; Horn, L. Immunotherapeutic approaches for small-cell lung cancer. *Nat. Rev. Clin. Oncol.* **2020**, *17*, 300–312. [CrossRef]
21. Chung, H.C.; Piha-Paul, S.A.; Lopez-Martin, J.; Schellens, J.H.M.; Kao, S.; Miller, W.H., Jr.; Delord, J.P.; Gao, B.; Planchard, D.; Gottfried, M.; et al. Pembrolizumab after two or more lines of previous therapy in patients with recurrent or metastatic sclc: Results from the keynote-028 and keynote-158 studies. *J. Thorac. Oncol.* **2020**, *15*, 618–627. [CrossRef] [PubMed]
22. Ma, X.; Wang, S.; Zhang, Y.; Wei, H.; Yu, J. Efficacy and safety of immune checkpoint inhibitors (icis) in extensive-stage small cell lung cancer (sclc). *J. Cancer Res. Clin. Oncol.* **2020**. [CrossRef] [PubMed]
23. Jones, G.S.; Elimian, K.; Baldwin, D.R.; Hubbard, R.B.; McKeever, T.M. A systematic review of survival following anti-cancer treatment for small cell lung cancer. *Lung Cancer* **2020**, *141*, 44–55. [CrossRef] [PubMed]
24. Facchinetti, F.; Di Maio, M.; Tiseo, M. Adding pd-1/pd-l1 inhibitors to chemotherapy for the first-line treatment of extensive stage small cell lung cancer (sclc): A meta-analysis of randomized trials. *Cancers* **2020**, *12*, 2645. [CrossRef]
25. Landre, T.; Chouahnia, A.K.; Des Guetz, G.; Assié, J.B.; Chouaid, C. 1799P Immune checkpoint inhibitor plus chemotherapy versus chemotherapy alone as first-line for extensive stage small cell lung cancer: A meta-analysis. *Ann. Oncol.* **2020**, *31* (Suppl. S4), S1041. [CrossRef]
26. Villaruz, L.C.; Socinski, M.A. The Clinical Viewpoint: Definitions, Limitations of RECIST, Practical Considerations of Measurement. *Clin. Cancer Res.* **2013**, *19*, 2629–2636. [CrossRef]
27. Systematic Review and Network Meta-Analysis of First-Line Therapy Combination of Immune Checkpoint Inhibitors and Chemotherapy for Extensive-Stage Small Cell Carcinoma (ID: CRD42020215762). Available online: https://www.crd.york.ac.uk/prospero/ (accessed on 26 November 2020).
28. U.S. Department of Health and Human Services. Common Terminology Criteria for Adverse Events (CTCAE) Version 5.0. Available online: https://ctep.cancer.gov/protocolDevelopment/electronicapplications/docs/ (accessed on 9 October 2020).
29. The Nordic Cochrane Centre, The Cochrane Collaboration. *Review Manager (RevMan)*; Version 5.3; The Nordic Cochrane Centre, The Cochrane Collaboration: Copenhagen, Denmark, 2014.
30. Stata Corp. *Stata Statistical Software: Release 12, Version*; StataCorp LP: College Station, TX, USA, 2011.

14

The OncoAge Consortium: Linking Aging and Oncology from Bench to Bedside and Back Again

Paul Hofman [1,2,*], Nicholas Ayache [3], Pascal Barbry [4], Michel Barlaud [5], Audrey Bel [6], Philippe Blancou [4], Frédéric Checler [4], Sylvie Chevillard [7], Gael Cristofari [2], Mathilde Demory [8], Vincent Esnault [9], Claire Falandry [10,11], Eric Gilson [2], Olivier Guérin [12], Nicolas Glaichenhaus [4], Joel Guigay [13], Marius Ilié [1,2], Bernard Mari [4], Charles-Hugo Marquette [14], Véronique Paquis-Flucklinger [2], Frédéric Prate [12], Pierre Saintigny [15], Barbara Seitz-Polsky [4,16], Taycir Skhiri [6], Ellen Van Obberghen-Schilling [17], Emmanuel Van Obberghen [18] and Laurent Yvan-Charvet [19]

1 Laboratory of Clinical and Experimental Pathology/Biobank 0033-00025, CHU Nice, FHU OncoAge, Université Côte d'Azur, 06001 Nice, France; Ilie.m@chu-nice.fr

2 Inserm U1081, CNRS UMR7284, Institut de Recherche sur le Cancer et le Vieillissement (IRCAN), FHU OncoAge, Université Côte d'Azur, 06107 Nice, France; gael.cristofari@unice.fr (G.C.); eric.gilson@unice.fr (E.G.); veronique.paquis@unice.fr (V.P.-F.)

3 Epione Team, Inria, FHU OncoAge, Université Côte d'Azur, 06902 Sophia Antipolis, France; Nicholas.ayache@inria.fr

4 CNRS UMR7275, Institut de Pharmacologie Cellulaire et Moléculaire, FHU OncoAge, Université Côte d'Azur, 06560 Valbonne, France; pascal.barbry@unice.fr (P.B.); philippe.blancou@unice.fr (P.B.); frederic.checler@unice.fr (F.C.); nicolas.glaichenhaus@unice.fr (N.G.); bernard.mari@unice.fr (B.M.); Seitz-polski.b@chu-nice.fr (B.S.-P.)

5 i3S Sophia Antipolis, FHU OncoAge, Université Côte d'Azur, 06560 Sophia Antipolis, France; michel.barlaud@unice.fr

6 Centre d'Innovation et d'Usages en Santé (CIUS), FHU OncoAge, Université Côte d'Azur, 06000 Nice, France; audrey.bel@ciusante.org (A.B.); Skhiri.t@chu-nice.fr (T.S.)

7 Laboratoire de Cancérologie Expérimentale, Institut François Jacob, CEA Direction de la Recherche Fondamentale, FHU OncoAge, Université Côte d'Azur, 92265 Fontenay-aux-Roses, France; sylvie.chevillard@cea.fr

8 Ville de Nice, Mairie de Nice, FHU OncoAge, Université Côte d'Azur, 06364 Nice, France; mathilde.demory@ville-nice.fr

9 Nephrology Department, CHU Nice, FHU OncoAge, Université Côte d'Azur, 06001 Nice, France; esnault.v@chu-nice.fr

10 Geriatric Unit, Centre Hospitalier Lyon Sud, Hospices Civils de Lyon, FHU OncoAge, Université Claude Bernard Lyon 1, 69310 Pierre-Benite, France; Claire.falandry@chu-lyon.fr

11 Laboratoire CarMeN, Inserm U1060, INRA U139, INSA Lyon, Ecole de Médecine Charles Mérieux, Université Claude Bernard Lyon 1, 69921 Oullins, France

12 Geriatric Coordination Unit for Geriatric Oncology (UCOG) PACA Est, CHU Nice, FHU OncoAge, Université Côte d'Azur, 06000 Nice, France; guerin.o@chu-nice.fr (O.G.); prate.f@chu-nice.fr (F.P.)

13 Oncology Department, Centre Antoine Lacassagne, FHU OncoAge, Université Côté d'Azur, 06189 Nice, France; joel.guigay@nice.unicancer.fr

14 Department of Pulmonary Medicine and Oncology, CHU Nice, FHU OncoAge, Université Côte d'Azur, 06000 Nice, France; marquette.c@chu-nice.fr

15 Département de Médecine, INSERM 1052, CNRS 5286, Centre de recherche en cancérologie de Lyon, Centre Léon Bérard, FHU OncoAge, Université Claude Bernard Lyon 1, 69008 Lyon, France; pierre.saintigny@lyon.unicancer.fr

16 Laboratory of Immunology, CHU Nice, FHU OncoAge, Université Côte d'Azur, 06200 Nice, France

17 CNRS, Inserm, iBV, Centre Antoine Lacassagne, FHU OncoAge, Université Côte d'Azur, 06108 Nice, France; ellen.van-obberghen@unice.fr

18 CNRS, LP2M, FHU OncoAge, Université Côte d'Azur, 06107 Nice, France; emmanuel.Van-obberghen@unice.fr

19 Inserm U1065, Centre Méditerranéen de Médecine Moléculaire (C3M), FHU OncoAge, Université Côte d'Azur, 06200 Nice, France; laurent.yvan-charvet@unice.fr

* Correspondence: hofman.p@chu-nice.fr

Abstract: It is generally accepted that carcinogenesis and aging are two biological processes, which are known to be associated. Notably, the frequency of certain cancers (including lung cancer), increases significantly with the age of patients and there is now a wealth of data showing that multiple mechanisms leading to malignant transformation and to aging are interconnected, defining the so-called common biology of aging and cancer. OncoAge, a consortium launched in 2015, brings together the multidisciplinary expertise of leading public hospital services and academic laboratories to foster the transfer of scientific knowledge rapidly acquired in the fields of cancer biology and aging into innovative medical practice and silver economy development. This is achieved through the development of shared technical platforms (for research on genome stability, (epi)genetics, biobanking, immunology, metabolism, and artificial intelligence), clinical research projects, clinical trials, and education. OncoAge focuses mainly on two pilot pathologies, which benefit from the expertise of several members, namely lung and head and neck cancers. This review outlines the broad strategic directions and key advances of OncoAge and summarizes some of the issues faced by this consortium, as well as the short- and long-term perspectives.

Keywords: aging; cancer; optimization; research; education; elderly; well-being

1. Introduction

Chronological age is the most important single risk factor for the development of a variety of cancers and chronic diseases that account for the majority of societal morbidity, mortality, and public health costs. Recent findings suggest that changes in certain basic biological processes are shared in physiological aging, cancer, and degenerative pathologies [1,2]. Importantly, similar processes can be altered in diseases as diverse as cancer, neurodegeneration, cardiovascular disorders, chronic obstructive pulmonary disease (COPD), osteoarthritis, and diabetes, to name a few. For instance, at the cellular level, the accumulation in tissues of senescent cells (permanent cell cycle arrest in response to various types of stress or tissue remodeling) emerges as an important contributor to aging and age-related pathologies, through both cell autonomous and non-autonomous mechanisms driving inflammation, immunosenescence, and tissue degeneration [3,4]. Therefore, a key challenge now is to rapidly improve our knowledge on the biological processes in common that lead to malignant transformation and degenerative pathologies [1,5–7]. From a cellular standpoint, the mechanisms that drive degenerative diseases and cancer are shared at an initial phase (e.g., during the accumulation of senescent cells), before adopting a particular direction and specific genetic and epigenetic modifications that orient cells toward distinct fates (e.g., escape of cellular checkpoints for cancer cells) [1,5–8]. Thus, schematically, degenerative aging and cancer can be considered as two sides of the same coin, involving many common fundamental biological mechanisms (Figure 1).

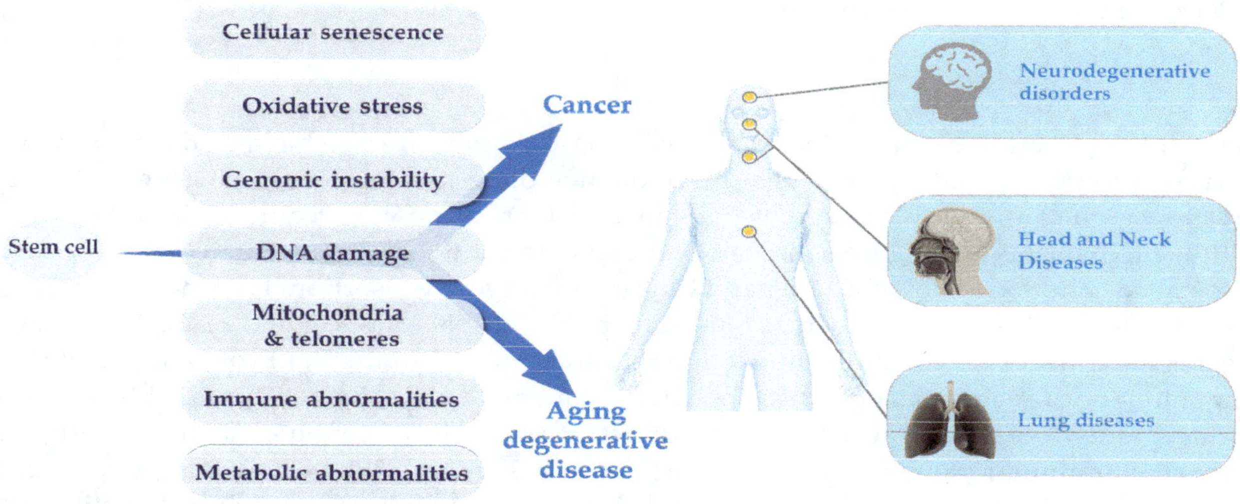

Figure 1. Common mechanisms that drive degenerative diseases and cancer. OncoAge is dedicated to three major pathologies: thoracic diseases (tumoral or non-tumoral), head and neck and thyroid pathologies, and neuromuscular degenerative disorders.

Hence, the progressive degeneration of tissues can lead to transformation into cancer after activation of chronic inflammation and immunosenescence [9–12]. Finally, from an epidemiological standpoint, the risk of emergence and incidence of most cancers increase with the age of the population [13–15].

Although cancer and aging biology are closely related, they are often investigated separately. Thus, whereas a number of fundamental and translational research centers or institutes worldwide have oriented their research in the direction of aging, only a few of them have really focused their studies on the links between aging and cancer. This is the case for the Institute for Research on Cancer and Aging, Nice (IRCAN) in France, which bases its overarching strategy on combining the research developed by scientists and physicians on cancer and aging mechanisms (https://www.ircan.org). It is within this context that the OncoAge consortium was launched in Nice to facilitate the transfer of this growing knowledge on cancer and aging to medical innovation and current medical practice. This consortium was certified and recognized in 2015 as a Hospital-University Federation (HUF) by AVIESAN (https://www.aviesan.fr; https://www.oncoage.org). The global aim of the HUF program in France is to develop excellence within the university hospitals by targeting medical topics optimizing care, research, and education in these subject areas (https://www.aviesan.fr). In short, OncoAge is a HUF based on the expertise of medical and scientific teams oriented toward cancer pathologies associated with aging. The key aim of OncoAge is to improve the care of elderly patients, in particular those with cancer, to set up research projects, and develop training and educational programs in this domain (https://www.oncoage.org). These efforts should not only deepen our understanding of the mechanisms underlying cancer and aging, but also improve the daily well-being of the patients.

The aging of the world's populations has progressively modified the profile of the most frequent diseases [13]. While infectious and cardiovascular disorders have until recently been the most frequent, and resulted in the highest number of deaths around the globe, considerable progression towards an increase in the number of certain cancers and diseases linked to aging has been observed in recent years. According to epidemiological predictions, these diseases will be among the most common in 2030, in both industrialized and non-industrialized countries. Among them, lung cancer will be the fifth cause of death in 2030, whereas according to the Global Burden of Disease (GBD), COPD is already now the third leading cause of death worldwide, a progression WHO had not predicted to occur until 2030 [16,17].

In this context, it is crucial to rapidly advance the molecular understanding of genetic and epigenetic mechanisms, as well as immune and metabolic abnormalities leading to the development of cancers associated with age, and to improve the care and well-being of patients with cancers that have become chronic and often invalidating. This has generated an urgent need to address many new challenges in translational projects in this field [18].

Importantly, elderly patients with lung cancer and head and neck cancer (HNC) are rarely enrolled in clinical trials, particularly in phase 1, and even less so in dedicated trials in curative or palliative settings. As an example, no standards of treatment exist for these populations, and frail elderly lung and HNC patients may be over-treated with a risk of increased toxicity while fit patients may be proposed for suboptimal treatment. It is, therefore, crucial to develop and evaluate appropriate treatments by enrolling elderly patients with cancer in a higher number of therapeutic trials. Beyond research-related concerns, OncoAge faces epidemiologic and environmental issues such as the procurement of well-controlled demographic data and the means of measuring air pollutants according to geolocalization of the patients in the Alpes-Maritimes area. Moreover, questions concerning costs (obtaining funding from public and private sources) and organization (steering multicenter efforts in the same direction) must be anticipated and managed to assure the sustainability of the consortium in the near years.

The genesis and objectives of the OncoAge consortium since its creation in 2015 at the Côte d'Azur University (Nice, France), its first accomplishments, and its future perspectives are described below.

2. OncoAge: The Origin of the Project

OncoAge was established in France after acceptance and certification by AVIESAN, subsequent to a national tender for HUF proposals (https://www.aviesan.fr). The application called for unique and original projects covering an aspect of health for which a program optimizing the healthcare of patients, research, and teaching in the specified domain could be addressed. The HUF OncoAge project was submitted in 2015 and selected by AVIESAN after the representatives of the project were examined by an international committee.

3. OncoAge at the Côte d'Azur University: Why?

The choice of setting up a HUF within the Nice Hospital of the University Côte d'Azur was motivated by several aspects, in particular, based on epidemiological arguments (Figure 2).

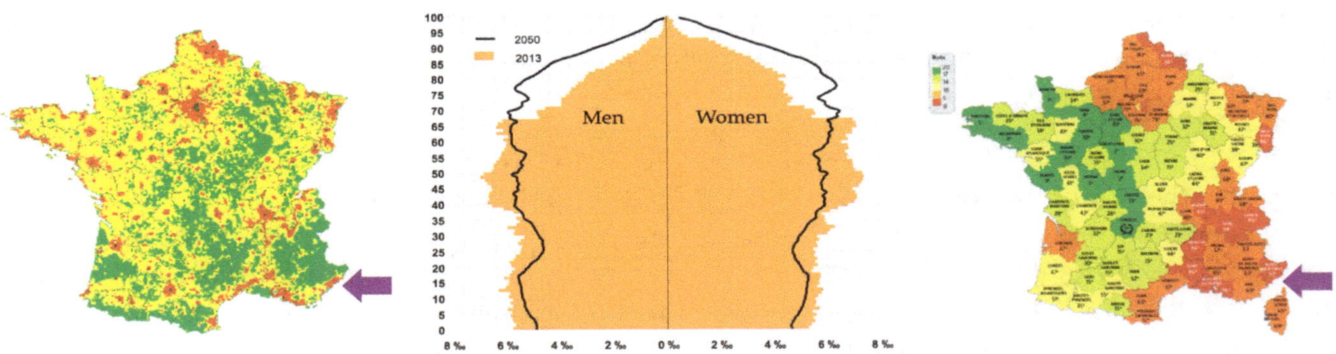

(a) (b) (c)

Figure 2. (**a**) High population density within the Alpes-Maritimes area (purple arrow) (INSEE data). (**b**) Age pyramid within the Alpes-Maritimes area in 2013 and pre-visions for 2050 (INSEE data). (**c**) Air pollution levels (in red, very high air pollution) within the Alpes-Maritimes area (purple arrow; www.prevair.org).

According to the data from the National Institute of Statistics and Economic studies ("INSEE"), in contrast to other regions in France, the population of the Alpes-Maritimes region, where the HUF is located, is populated by a high number of elderly people (>65 years old) (https://www.insee.fr).

This region has a population density above the average in France, and which is increasing yearly (https://www.insee.fr). Indeed, the Nice University Hospital already treats many patients above 65 years of age, and this number is expected to increase. In this context, due to the global aging of the world population, it is estimated that the number of elderly patients admitted to this healthcare center today is similar to that which will be observed in most hospitals in the world in 2030. The high incidence of lung cancer and the above average level of atmospheric pollution in the Alpes-Maritimes region, as compared to national levels, were among the other reasons that motivated the decision to develop the OncoAge project (Figure 2). Moreover, no other HUF in France has focused on aging and cancer. Therefore, we felt that this important issue should be developed within this geographical area. Finally, the presence of IRCAN, a research center focusing on the mechanisms linking cancer and aging, provides a unique opportunity to associate the most recent biological discoveries with the health-oriented aims of OncoAge.

4. OncoAge at the Côte d'Azur University: How?

OncoAge efforts are based, for the greater part, on a limited number of "pilot" pathologies that were selected within the Nice Hospital, taking into consideration the following parameters: (i) optimal organization of the hospital sectors in the concerned domains and the potential recruitment of patients, (ii) activities of the university (publications and teaching) of the hospital departments, (iii) the organized clinical and/or biological databases, (iv) clinical and translational research performed in collaboration with scientists of the teams studying fundamental research in the specified subjects. For this, three major pathologies were initially chosen to set up the foundations of OncoAge: thoracic diseases (tumoral or non-tumoral), head and neck and thyroid pathologies, and neuromuscular degenerative disorders. Transversal studies were initiated to reinforce the fundamental knowledge on these medical questions, combining various (epi)genomics, immunology, metabolism, and artificial intelligence (AI) approaches since these topics are particularly important for aging and cancer [1,19–27]. Actions that support common structures have been established, such as innovative programs and connection to the silver economy (https://www.france-silvereco.fr/notre-observatoire/tableau-de-bord-de-la-filiere), technological platforms (including geriatric screening tools to identify elderly cancer patients who could benefit from comprehensive geriatric assessment), and new biorepository space, training and education, dissemination of knowledge and information [28–33]. The participants working on these different aspects (work package leaders) interact in concert with the unique aim of building a dynamic, collaborative network.

In addition to several departments of the Nice University Hospital, the OncoAge consortium brings together a number of institutes of the Côte d'Azur University (UCA), such as the Antoine Lacassagne Comprehensive Cancer Center (CAL), the Etablissement de Santé Privé d'Intérêt Collectif (ESPIC) Hôpitaux Pédiatriques de Nice Centre Hospitalier Universitaire Fondation Lenval, and many teams of different research centers (Institut of Research and Aging, Nice (IRCAN), Centre Méditerranéen de Médecine Moléculaire (C3M), Institut de Biologie Valrose (iBV), Institut de Pharmacologie Cellulaire et Moléculaire (IPMC), Laboratoire de PhysioMédecine Moléculaire (LP2M), and Institut National de Recherche en Informatique et en Automatique (Inria)). OncoAge is not only composed of different stakeholders belonging to the Côte d'Azur University but also of teams of the Lyon University (Lyon University Hospital; Hospices Civils de Lyon; HCL; and Leon Bérard Comprehensive Cancer Center (CLB) and of the International Agency for Research on Cancer (IARC, Lyon, France), the Centre d'Energie Atomique (CEA; Fontenay aux Roses, France), and the Gustave Roussy Institute (IGR; Villejuif, France) (Figure 3).

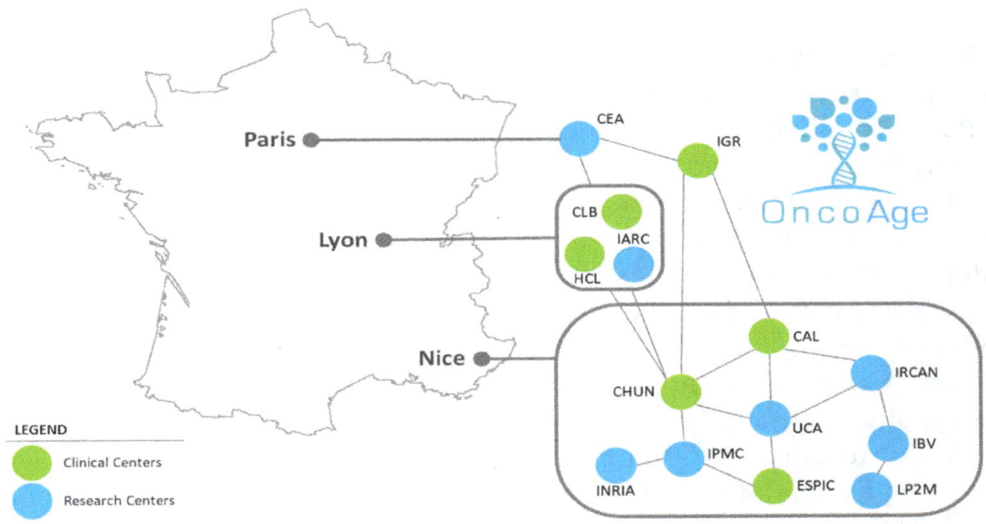

Figure 3. The OncoAge consortium members. CEA: Centre d'Energie Atomique; IGR: Gustave Roussy Institute; CLB: Léon Bérard Comprehensive Cancer Center; IARC: International Agency for Resarch on Cancer; HCL: Hospices Civils de Lyon; CAL: Antoine Lacassagne Comprehensive Cancer Center; CHUN: Centre Hospitalier Universitaire de Nice; UCA: Université Côte d'Azur; IRCAN: Institut of Research and Aging, Nice; IBV: Institut de Biologie Valrose; LP2M: Laboratoire de PhysioMédecine Moléculaire; ESPIC: Etablissement de Santé Privé d'Intérêt Collectif Hôpitaux Pédiatriques de Nice Centre Hospitalier Universitaire Fondation Lenval; IPMC: Institut de Pharmacologie Cellulaire et Moléculaire; INRIA: Institut National de Recherche en Informatique et en Automatique.

The governance of OncoAge is provided by a strategic committee and a scientific council (https://www.oncoage.org). To ensure proper functioning and to benefit from expert advice, an international scientific advisory board (SAB) composed of medical and scientific opinion leaders in the field of cancer and aging has been set up (https://www.oncoage.org).

5. OncoAge: Main Objectives

The overarching objective of OncoAge is to create and foster a network of expertise, and to develop collaborations and projects to improve the healthcare of elderly patients with cancer. To attain these objectives, a number of initiatives have been undertaken: (i) definition of different indicators of tracking (using publications), (ii) development of clinical and translational research projects funded by regional, national, and international bodies, (iii) introduction into the university lectures of themes developed by OncoAge, (iv) organization of workshops and conferences, and (v) communication of information to the general public and the creation of a dedicated website. These different initiatives put forward by OncoAge were first evaluated by the SAB of OncoAge in 2015, and found to be highly appropriate.

6. OncoAge: Main Results After Three Years of Existence (2015–2018)

Several key accomplishments both at the level of clinical and translational research projects and at the level of the structuring and dissemination of information were achieved. The clinical expertise in HNC within OncoAge is highlighted by the ELAN (ELderly Head and Neck cancer) program. These clinical studies on curative or palliative personalized treatment of elderly head and neck cancer patients after geriatric assessment (Elan Geriatric Evaluation, EGE) currently represent the only multi-center therapeutic trials dedicated to this group of patients worldwide [34–36]. Studies were completed in 2018 and results will be presented in 2019. Moreover, an early phase clinical trial unit was set up in the Comprehensive Cancer Center Antoine Lacassagne to favor the emergence of therapeutic innovations.

Since 2015, OncoAge has been associated with the publication of 86 scientific articles referenced in NCBI PubMed (the "FHU OncoAge" was listed with the author's affiliation). For example, some publications are related to epidemiological, clinical, and translational research projects made in lung cancer and COPD, such as lung cancer screening and assessment of biomarkers [37–46]. Recently, a new project was accomplished by physicians from the Nice University Hospital and researchers belonging to the "Institut National de Recherche en Informatique et en Automatique" (Inria) who aimed to develop a lung cancer screening program based on the integration of three signatures: clinical data (leading to better risk factor assessment), chest low dose CT scan (by using computer-aided diagnosis), and biological blood signatures [47]. Since the HUF OncoAge was established, a strong partnership between oncologists and geriatricians belonging to the consortium was set up in order to optimize the care of the elderly cancer population. In this context, a large comprehensive geriatric assessment program using a multidimensional interdisciplinary diagnostic process was rapidly developed [48].

Other specific studies concern the head and neck pilot pathology [49,50]. Several scientific projects managed by leaders of OncoAge were financed by different organizations, including the Institut National du Cancer (the French NCI), l'Agence Nationale de la Recherche, la Fondation de l'Association de la Recherche contre le Cancer, le Cancéropôle Provence Alpes Côte d'Azur" (PACA), and the Infrastructure en Biologie Santé et Agronomie" (IBiSA). A master's program on "Biobanks and Complex Data Management" was set up through the association of the Côte d'Azur University and the Nice Hospital (https://MScbiobanks-complex-data) [51]. The Laboratory of Clinical and Experimental Pathology within OncoAge has been selected by the European Society of Pathology to serve as an advanced training center for molecular pathology with an emphasis on liquid biopsy. Since 2015, the master's program has enrolled students from all around the world and so far, three classes of students have been trained.

This master's is supported by the biobank of the Nice University Hospital (BB-0033-0025), which has benefited since 2015 from new infrastructures and developments (http://univ-cotedazur.fr/en/education/informations-utiles/les-informations-utiles/biobanks-complex-data/#.XGlsb7jjJ4E) [51].

This biobank has integrated the technological platform of OncoAge and the biological specimens associated with the clinical data and is available to the teams of OncoAge after a material transfer agreement has been signed. The visibility of OncoAge has been ensured through the creation of a website and the organization of several symposiums, including the first joint meeting on lung cancer associating the MD Anderson Cancer Center and the HUF OncoAge (https://www.oncoage.org/news-and-events-2/3/). Moreover, recently, on behalf of the HUF OncoAge, different actors of the consortium have had the opportunity to participate in the writing of a next Encyclopedia of Aging and Population Aging, edited by Springer, which will be available at the end of 2019. The HUF OncoAge will lead the "Cancer and Treatment" section of this encyclopedia.

The different actions accomplished by OncoAge were favorably evaluated by the SAB of OncoAge at the end of 2018.

7. OncoAge: Current Developments and Perspectives

A number of perspectives have been envisioned for the short term (2020). First, broadening the pathologies that OncoAge intends to investigate, in particular, skin cancers (including melanoma), will be integrated in 2019. New clinical–biological collections will be built, either as a complement to existing collections or from a new population of patients. Concerning the complementary collections (from patients with lung cancer and chronic obstructive pulmonary disease), the samples will include urine, total blood, and peripheral blood mononuclear cells (PBMCs). A new collection of blood (plasma, PBMCs, and total blood) obtained from healthy individuals older than 80 years and residents of the Alpes-Maritimes region will be assembled. Finally, a collection of bronchial and transthoracic biopsies (tissues fixed and paraffin embedded) obtained from lung cancer patients will be set up for future translational research projects.

Several other objectives have been defined. Amongst these, an international master's degree on aging, dedicated to researching questions concerning aging and associated diseases, should be created. Further, a national project implicating private–public partners targeting innovation in the domain of aging should initiate several national and international collaborations (http://www.agence-nationale-recherche.fr/). Finally, new clinical trials, all with translational studies (including mechanisms of resistance to immunotherapy), have been launched or are in advanced phases of discussion with academic institutional groups and pharmacological companies. Indeed, immunotherapy in elderly patients has become a promising treatment alternative and put in the limelight [52–56]. In this context, the development and assessment of biomarkers of senescence will be associated with clinical trials thanks to the biobank (BB-0033-00025) and the OncoAge research teams [57,58]. These studies will benefit from the acquisition by OncoAge of technical platforms of state-of-the-art equipment and AI-based software (HALO AI^{TM}, Indica Labs, London, UK) for high-speed whole slide imaging and quantitative multiplexing.

8. Conclusions

The most prominent feature of aging is a gradual deterioration/loss of cells that is associated with organ dysfunction and the rise of age-related chronic pathologies. Amongst these, cancer stands out as its occurrence significantly increases with age and has a devastating human and public health cost. Deciphering the clinical features, the biological markers, and the lifestyle and environmental factors that are shared between common chronic age-related pathologies and cancer should lead to the development of new clinical approaches, including the validation of surrogate biomarkers of frailty and predisposition. A deeper understanding of the common mechanisms involved both in aging and cancer is expected to considerably improve our knowledge on how to prevent age-related pathologies and how to optimize the care of elderly patients. In this context, OncoAge is a unique consortium composed of more than 1000 participants and actors located in Nice, Lyon, and Paris with the exclusive ambition of working together on clinical–biological and medical–scientific projects that aim to improve the care of elderly patients with cancer. This consortium has actively developed translational and clinical projects and has created innovation in the domain of geriatric oncology. The increase in the age of the world's populations has created new urgent demands on healthcare, as well as major strategic and economic issues. Improving the autonomy of elderly patients with cancer, avoiding repeated and long hospitalizations, performing early screening for certain cancers, and predicting, as well as preventing complications, are all objectives set out by OncoAge. Moreover, understanding the relationships between the aging phenomenon and cancer is a timely and multifaceted challenge where high-level research efforts in medicine, genomics, and biology have to be combined with societal approaches focused on individuals. In this context, OncoAge has designed and made operational an original holistic approach combining genotype and phenotype analyses of the aging and cancer processes.

To conclude, our expert multipronged approach is consolidated by the enthusiasm of the many physicians and scientists of several leading hospitals and strong research centers and warrants the future of OncoAge.

Author Contributions: Conceptualization, P.H.; methodology, P.H., N.A., P.B. (Pascal Barbry), M.B., A.B., P.B. (Philippe Blancou), F.C., S.C., G.C., M.D., V.E., C.F., E.G., O.G., N.G., J.G., M.I., B.M., C.-H.M., V.P.-F., F.P., P.S., B.S.-P., T.S., E.V.-O.-S., E.V.-O., L.Y.-C.; software, N.A.; validation, P.H., M.I., E.O., E.G., E.V.-S.; formal analysis, P.H.; investigation, P.H.; resources, P.H.; data curation, P.H.; writing—original draft preparation, P.H., M.I., E.V.-O., E.G., E.V.-O.-S.; writing—review and editing, P.H., M.I., E.O., E.G., E.V.-S.; visualization, P.H., M.I., E.V.-O., E.G., E.V.-O.-S.; supervision, P.H.; project administration, P.H.; funding acquisition, P.H.

Acknowledgments: Frédéric Checler is supported by the Laboratory of Excellence DistALZ.

References

1. Falandry, C.; Bonnefoy, M.; Freyer, G.; Gilson, E. Biology of cancer and aging: A complex association with cellular senescence. *J. Clin. Oncol.* **2014**, *32*, 2604–2610. [CrossRef] [PubMed]
2. Kennedy, B.K.; Berger, S.L.; Brunet, A.; Campisi, J.; Cuervo, A.M.; Epel, E.S.; Franceschi, C.; Lithgow, G.J.; Morimoto, R.I.; Pessin, J.E.; et al. Geroscience: Linking aging to chronic disease. *Cell* **2014**, *159*, 709–713. [CrossRef] [PubMed]
3. Grimes, A.; Chandra, S.B. Significance of cellular senescence in aging and cancer. *Cancer Res. Treat* **2009**, *41*, 187–195. [CrossRef]
4. Lopez-Otin, C.; Blasco, M.A.; Partridge, L.; Serrano, M.; Kroemer, G. The hallmarks of aging. *Cell* **2013**, *153*, 1194–1217. [CrossRef] [PubMed]
5. Aunan, J.R.; Cho, W.C.; Soreide, K. The Biology of Aging and Cancer: A Brief Overview of Shared and Divergent Molecular Hallmarks. *Aging Dis.* **2017**, *8*, 628–642. [CrossRef] [PubMed]
6. Rozhok, A.I.; DeGregori, J. The evolution of lifespan and age-dependent cancer risk. *Trends Cancer* **2016**, *2*, 552–560. [CrossRef] [PubMed]
7. Shay, J.W. Role of Telomeres and Telomerase in Aging and Cancer. *Cancer Discov.* **2016**, *6*, 584–593. [CrossRef]
8. Pawelec, G. Immunosenescence and cancer. *Biogerontology* **2017**, *18*, 717–721. [CrossRef] [PubMed]
9. Barreiro, E.; Bustamante, V.; Curull, V.; Gea, J.; Lopez-Campos, J.L.; Munoz, X. Relationships between chronic obstructive pulmonary disease and lung cancer: Biological insights. *J. Thorac. Dis.* **2016**, *8*, E1122–E1135. [CrossRef]
10. Biswas, A.; Mehta, H.J.; Folch, E.E. Chronic obstructive pulmonary disease and lung cancer: Inter-relationships. *Curr. Opin. Pulm. Med.* **2018**, *24*, 152–160. [CrossRef] [PubMed]
11. Murata, M. Inflammation and cancer. *Environ. Health Prev. Med.* **2018**, *23*, e50. [CrossRef] [PubMed]
12. Serrano, M. Unraveling the links between cancer and aging. *Carcinogenesis* **2016**, *37*, 107. [CrossRef] [PubMed]
13. Fitzmaurice, C.; Akinyemiju, T.F.; Al Lami, F.H.; Alam, T.; Alizadeh-Navaei, R.; Allen, C.; Alsharif, U.; Alvis-Guzman, N.; Amini, E.; Anderson, B.O.; et al. Global, Regional, and National Cancer Incidence, Mortality, Years of Life Lost, Years Lived With Disability, and Disability-Adjusted Life-Years for 29 Cancer Groups, 1990 to 2016: A Systematic Analysis for the Global Burden of Disease Study. *JAMA Oncol.* **2018**, *4*, 1553–1568. [CrossRef] [PubMed]
14. Micheli, A.; Mugno, E.; Krogh, V.; Quinn, M.J.; Coleman, M.; Hakulinen, T.; Gatta, G.; Berrino, F.; Capocaccia, R. Cancer prevalence in European registry areas. *Ann. Oncol.* **2002**, *13*, 840–865. [CrossRef] [PubMed]
15. Yancik, R. Population aging and cancer: A cross-national concern. *Cancer J.* **2005**, *11*, 437–441. [CrossRef] [PubMed]
16. Lozano, R.; Naghavi, M.; Foreman, K.; Lim, S.; Shibuya, K.; Aboyans, V.; Abraham, J.; Adair, T.; Aggarwal, R.; Ahn, S.Y.; et al. Global and regional mortality from 235 causes of death for 20 age groups in 1990 and 2010: A systematic analysis for the Global Burden of Disease Study 2010. *Lancet* **2012**, *380*, 2095–2128. [CrossRef]
17. Quaderi, S.A.; Hurst, J.R. The unmet global burden of COPD. *Glob. Health Epidemiol. Genom.* **2018**, *3*, e4. [CrossRef]
18. Partridge, L.; Deelen, J.; Slagboom, P.E. Facing up to the global challenges of ageing. *Nature* **2018**, *561*, 45–56. [CrossRef]
19. Benz, C.C.; Yau, C. Ageing, oxidative stress and cancer: Paradigms in parallax. *Nat. Rev. Cancer* **2008**, *8*, 875–879. [CrossRef]
20. Bernardes de Jesus, B.; Blasco, M.A. Telomerase at the intersection of cancer and aging. *Trends Genet.* **2013**, *29*, 513–520. [CrossRef]
21. Birch, J.; Anderson, R.K.; Correia-Melo, C.; Jurk, D.; Hewitt, G.; Marques, F.M.; Green, N.J.; Moisey, E.; Birrell, M.A.; Belvisi, M.G.; et al. DNA damage response at telomeres contributes to lung aging and chronic obstructive pulmonary disease. *Am. J. Physiol. Lung Cell Mol. Physiol.* **2015**, *309*, L1124–L1137. [CrossRef] [PubMed]
22. Bottazzi, B.; Riboli, E.; Mantovani, A. Aging, inflammation and cancer. *Semin. Immunol.* **2018**, *40*, 74–82. [CrossRef] [PubMed]
23. Caron, A.; Briscoe, D.M.; Richard, D.; Laplante, M. DEPTOR at the Nexus of Cancer, Metabolism, and Immunity. *Physiol. Rev.* **2018**, *98*, 1765–1803. [CrossRef] [PubMed]

24. Lawrence, R.E.; Zoncu, R. The lysosome as a cellular centre for signalling, metabolism and quality control. *Nat. Cell Biol.* **2019**. [CrossRef] [PubMed]
25. Ovadya, Y.; Landsberger, T.; Leins, H.; Vadai, E.; Gal, H.; Biran, A.; Yosef, R.; Sagiv, A.; Agrawal, A.; Shapira, A.; et al. Impaired immune surveillance accelerates accumulation of senescent cells and aging. *Nat. Commun.* **2018**, *9*, 5435. [CrossRef] [PubMed]
26. Raffaghello, L.; Longo, V. Metabolic Alterations at the Crossroad of Aging and Oncogenesis. *Int. Rev. Cell Mol. Biol.* **2017**, *332*, 1–42. [PubMed]
27. Zhavoronkov, A.; Mamoshina, P.; Vanhaelen, Q.; Scheibye-Knudsen, M.; Moskalev, A.; Aliper, A. Artificial intelligence for aging and longevity research: Recent advances and perspectives. *Ageing Res. Rev.* **2019**, *49*, 49–66. [CrossRef] [PubMed]
28. Bellera, C.A.; Rainfray, M.; Mathoulin-Pelissier, S.; Mertens, C.; Delva, F.; Fonck, M.; Soubeyran, P.L. Screening older cancer patients: First evaluation of the G-8 geriatric screening tool. *Ann. Oncol.* **2012**, *23*, 2166–2172. [CrossRef] [PubMed]
29. Bellera, C.A.; Artaud, F.; Rainfray, M.; Soubeyran, P.L.; Mathoulin-Pelissier, S. Modeling individual and relative accuracy of screening tools in geriatric oncology. *Ann. Oncol.* **2017**, *28*, 1152–1157. [CrossRef]
30. Kenis, C.; Bron, D.; Libert, Y.; Decoster, L.; Van Puyvelde, K.; Scalliet, P.; Cornette, P.; Pepersack, T.; Luce, S.; Langenaeken, C.; et al. Relevance of a systematic geriatric screening and assessment in older patients with cancer: Results of a prospective multicentric study. *Ann. Oncol.* **2013**, *24*, 1306–1312. [CrossRef]
31. Kenis, C.; Decoster, L.; Flamaing, J.; Debruyne, P.R.; De Groof, I.; Focan, C.; Cornelis, F.; Verschaeve, V.; Bachmann, C.; Bron, D.; et al. Adherence to geriatric assessment-based recommendations in older patients with cancer: A multicenter prospective cohort study in Belgium. *Ann. Oncol.* **2018**, *29*, 1987–1994. [CrossRef] [PubMed]
32. Magnuson, A.; Allore, H.; Cohen, H.J.; Mohile, S.G.; Williams, G.R.; Chapman, A.; Extermann, M.; Olin, R.L.; Targia, V.; Mackenzie, A.; et al. Geriatric assessment with management in cancer care: Current evidence and potential mechanisms for future research. *J. Geriatr. Oncol.* **2016**, *7*, 242–248. [CrossRef] [PubMed]
33. Mohile, S.G.; Dale, W.; Somerfield, M.R.; Hurria, A. Practical Assessment and Management of Vulnerabilities in Older Patients Receiving Chemotherapy: ASCO Guideline for Geriatric Oncology Summary. *J. Oncol. Pract.* **2018**, *14*, 442–446. [CrossRef] [PubMed]
34. Guigay, J.; Mertens, C.; Le Caer, H.; Michel, C.; Ortholan, C.; Auperin, A. A French multicenter research program for a personalized treatment of elderly head and neck cancer patient. *Bull. Cancer* **2017**, *104*, 816–819. [CrossRef] [PubMed]
35. Guigay, J.; Le Caer, H.; Ortholan, C.; Aupérin, A.; Michele, C.; Mertens, C. Treatment of inoperable elderly Head and Neck cancer patients. *Curr. Opin. Oncol.* **2019**, in press.
36. Mertens, C.; Le Caer, H.; Ortholan, C.; Blot, E.; Even, C.; Rousselot, H.; Peyrade, F.; Sire, C.; Cupissol, D.; Pointreau, Y.; et al. The ELAN-ONCOVAL (ELderly heAd and Neck cancer-Oncology eValuation) study: Evaluation of the feasibility of a suited geriatric assessment for use by oncologists to classify patients as fit or unfit. In Proceedings of the ESMO 2017 Congress, Madrid, Spain, 8–12 September 2017.
37. Boulahssass, R.; Gonfrier, S.; Ferrero, J.M.; Sanchez, M.; Mari, V.; Moranne, O.; Rambaud, C.; Auben, F.; Hannoun Levi, J.M.; Bereder, J.M.; et al. Predicting early death in older adults with cancer. *Eur. J. Cancer* **2018**, *100*, 65–74. [CrossRef] [PubMed]
38. Heeke, S.; Hofman, V.; Long-Mira, E.; Lespinet, V.; Lalvee, S.; Bordone, O.; Ribeyre, C.; Tanga, V.; Benzaquen, J.; Leroy, S.; et al. Use of the Ion PGM and the GeneReader NGS Systems in Daily Routine Practice for Advanced Lung Adenocarcinoma Patients: A Practical Point of View Reporting a Comparative Study and Assessment of 90 Patients. *Cancers* **2018**, *10*, 88. [CrossRef]
39. Ilie, M.; Beaulande, M.; Ben Hadj, S.; Chamorey, E.; Schiappa, R.; Long-Mira, E.; Lassalle, S.; Butori, C.; Cohen, C.; Leroy, S.; et al. Chromogenic Multiplex Immunohistochemistry Reveals Modulation of the Immune Microenvironment Associated with Survival in Elderly Patients with Lung Adenocarcinoma. *Cancers* **2018**, *9*, 326. [CrossRef]
40. Leroy, S.; Benzaquen, J.; Mazzetta, A.; Marchand-Adam, S.; Padovani, B.; Israel-Biet, D.; Pison, C.; Chanez, P.; Cadranel, J.; Mazieres, J.; et al. Circulating tumour cells as a potential screening tool for lung cancer (the AIR study): Protocol of a prospective multicentre cohort study in France. *BMJ Open* **2017**, *7*, e018884. [CrossRef]
41. Washetine, K.; Heeke, S.; Bonnetaud, C.; Kara-Borni, M.; Ilie, M.; Lassalle, S.; Butori, C.; Long-Mira, E.; Marquette, C.H.; Cohen, C.; et al. Establishing a Dedicated Lung Cancer Biobank at the University Center Hospital of Nice (France). Why and How? *Cancers* **2018**, *10*, 220. [CrossRef]

42. Giovannini-Chami, L.; Paquet, A.; Sanfiorenzo, C.; Pons, N.; Cazareth, J.; Magnone, V.; Lebrigand, K.; Chevalier, B.; Vallauri, A.; Julia, V.; et al. The "one airway, one disease" concept in light of Th2 inflammation. *Eur. Respir. J.* **2018**, *52*, e1800437. [CrossRef] [PubMed]
43. Falk, A.T.; Yazbeck, N.; Guibert, N.; Chamorey, E.; Paquet, A.; Ribeyre, L.; Bence, C.; Zahaf, K.; Leroy, S.; Marquette, C.H.; et al. Effect of mutant variants of the KRAS gene on PD-L1 expression and on the immune microenvironment and association with clinical outcome in lung adenocarcinoma patients. *Lung Cancer* **2018**, *121*, 70–75. [CrossRef] [PubMed]
44. Ilie, M.; Szafer-Glusman, E.; Hofman, V.; Chamorey, E.; Lalvee, S.; Selva, E.; Leroy, S.; Marquette, C.H.; Kowanetz, M.; Hedge, P.; et al. Detection of PD-L1 in circulating tumor cells and white blood cells from patients with advanced non-small-cell lung cancer. *Ann. Oncol.* **2018**, *29*, 193–199. [CrossRef] [PubMed]
45. Kemp, S.V.; Slebos, D.J.; Kirk, A.; Kornaszewska, M.; Carron, K.; Ek, L.; Broman, G.; Hillerdal, G.; Mal, H.; Pison, C.; et al. A Multicenter Randomized Controlled Trial of Zephyr Endobronchial Valve Treatment in Heterogeneous Emphysema (TRANSFORM). *Am. J. Respir. Crit. Care Med.* **2017**, *196*, 1535–1543. [CrossRef] [PubMed]
46. Revinski, D.R.; Zaragosi, L.E.; Boutin, C.; Ruiz-Garcia, S.; Deprez, M.; Thome, V.; Rosnet, O.; Gay, A.S.; Mercey, O.; Paquet, A.; et al. CDC20B is required for deuterosome-mediated centriole production in multiciliated cells. *Nat. Commun.* **2018**, *9*, e4668. [CrossRef] [PubMed]
47. Benzaquen, J.; Boutros, J.; Marquette, C.; Delingette, H.; Hofman, P. Lung Cancer Screening, Towards a Multidimensional Approach: Why and How? *Cancers* **2019**, *11*, 212. [CrossRef] [PubMed]
48. Boulahssass, R.; Gonfrier, S.; Champigny, N.; Lassalle, S.; Francois, E.; Hofman, P.; Guerin, O. The Desire to Better Understand Older Adults with Solid Tumors to Improve Management: Assessment and Guided Interventions-The French PACA EST Cohort Experience. *Cancers* **2019**, *11*, 192. [CrossRef] [PubMed]
49. Harrington, K.J.; Ferris, R.L.; Blumenschein, G., Jr.; Colevas, A.D.; Fayette, J.; Licitra, L.; Kasper, S.; Even, C.; Vokes, E.E.; Worden, F.; et al. Nivolumab versus standard, single-agent therapy of investigator's choice in recurrent or metastatic squamous cell carcinoma of the head and neck (CheckMate 141): Health-related quality-of-life results from a randomised, phase 3 trial. *Lancet Oncol.* **2017**, *18*, 1104–1115. [CrossRef]
50. Bozec, A.; Zangari, J.; Butori-Pepino, M.; Ilie, M.; Lalvee, S.; Juhel, T.; Butori, C.; Brest, P.; Hofman, P.; Vouret-Craviari, V. MiR-223-3p inhibits angiogenesis and promotes resistance to cetuximab in head and neck squamous cell carcinoma. *Oncotarget* **2017**, *8*, 57174–57186. [CrossRef]
51. Ilie, M.; Arrighi, N.; Hofman, P. Fueling the sustainability of Next Generation Biobanks by training. A New Master "Biobanks and Complex Data Management" at the Nice Côte d'Azur University, Nice, France. In Proceedings of the Global Biobank Week, Stockholm, Sweden, 13–15 September 2017.
52. Casaluce, F.; Sgambato, A.; Maione, P.; Spagnuolo, A.; Gridelli, C. Lung cancer, elderly and immune checkpoint inhibitors. *J. Thorac. Dis.* **2018**, *10*, S1474–S1481. [CrossRef]
53. Daste, A.; Domblides, C.; Gross-Goupil, M.; Chakiba, C.; Quivy, A.; Cochin, V.; de Mones, E.; Larmonier, N.; Soubeyran, P.; Ravaud, A. Immune checkpoint inhibitors and elderly people: A review. *Eur. J. Cancer* **2017**, *82*, 155–166. [CrossRef] [PubMed]
54. Elias, R.; Hartshorn, K.; Rahma, O.; Lin, N.; Snyder-Cappione, J.E. Aging, immune senescence, and immunotherapy: A comprehensive review. *Semin. Oncol.* **2018**, *45*, 187–200. [CrossRef] [PubMed]
55. Helissey, C.; Vicier, C.; Champiat, S. The development of immunotherapy in older adults: New treatments, new toxicities? *J. Geriatr. Oncol.* **2016**, *7*, 325–333. [CrossRef] [PubMed]
56. Kanesvaran, R.; Cordoba, R.; Maggiore, R. Immunotherapy in Older Adults With Advanced Cancers: Implications for Clinical Decision-Making and Future Research. *Am. Soc. Clin. Oncol. Educ. Book* **2018**, 400–414. [CrossRef] [PubMed]
57. Falandry, C.; Gilson, E.; Rudolph, K.L. Are aging biomarkers clinically relevant in oncogeriatrics? *Crit. Rev. Oncol. Hematol.* **2013**, *85*, 257–265. [CrossRef] [PubMed]
58. Ferrara, R.; Mezquita, L.; Auclin, E.; Chaput, N.; Besse, B. Immunosenescence and immunecheckpoint inhibitors in non-small cell lung cancer patients: Does age really matter? *Cancer Treat. Rev.* **2017**, *60*, 60–68. [CrossRef] [PubMed]

15

Ntrk1 Promotes Resistance to PD-1 Checkpoint Blockade in Mesenchymal Kras/p53 Mutant Lung Cancer

Jessica M. Konen [1], B. Leticia Rodriguez [1], Jared J. Fradette [1], Laura Gibson [1], Denali Davis [2], Rosalba Minelli [3], Michael D. Peoples [4], Jeffrey Kovacs [4], Alessandro Carugo [5], Christopher Bristow [4], Timothy Heffernan [5] and Don L. Gibbons [1,6,*]

1 Department of Thoracic/Head & Neck Medical Oncology, University of Texas MD Anderson Cancer Center, 1515 Holcombe Blvd, Houston, TX 77030, USA; jmkonen@mdanderson.org (J.M.K.); BLRodriguez@mdanderson.org (B.L.R.); jjfradette@mdanderson.org (J.J.F.); lagibson@mdanderson.org (L.G.)

2 Department of Chemistry, Indiana University of Pennsylvania, 1011 South Drive, Indiana, PA 15705, USA; denalihdavis@gmail.com

3 Department of Genomic Medicine, University of Texas MD Anderson Cancer Center, 1515 Holcombe Blvd, Houston, TX 77030, USA; RMinelli@mdanderson.org

4 Center for Co-Clinical Trials, University of Texas MD Anderson Cancer Center, 1515 Holcombe Blvd, Houston, TX 77030, USA; mdpeoples@mdanderson.org (M.D.P.); jjkovacs@mdanderson.org (J.K.); cabristow@mdanderson.org (C.B.)

5 Institute for Applied Cancer Science, University of Texas MD Anderson Cancer Center, 1515 Holcombe Blvd, Houston, TX 77030, USA; acarugo@mdanderson.org (A.C.); tpheffernan@mdanderson.org (T.H.)

6 Department of Molecular and Cellular Oncology, University of Texas MD Anderson Cancer Center, 1515 Holcombe Blvd, Houston, TX 77030, USA

* Correspondence: dlgibbon@mdanderson.org

Abstract: The implementation of cancer immunotherapeutics for solid tumors including lung cancers has improved clinical outcomes in a small percentage of patients. However, the majority of patients show little to no response or acquire resistance during treatment with checkpoint inhibitors delivered as a monotherapy. Therefore, identifying resistance mechanisms and novel combination therapy approaches is imperative to improve responses to immune checkpoint inhibitors. To address this, we performed an in vivo shRNA dropout screen that focused on genes encoding for FDA-approved drug targets (FDAome). We implanted epithelial and mesenchymal Kras/p53 (KP) mutant murine lung cancer cells expressing the FDAome shRNA library into syngeneic mice treated with an anti-PD-1 antibody. Sequencing for the barcoded shRNAs revealed *Ntrk1* was significantly depleted from mesenchymal tumors challenged with PD-1 blockade, suggesting it provides a survival advantage to tumor cells when under immune system pressure. Our data confirmed Ntrk1 transcript levels are upregulated in tumors treated with PD-1 inhibitors. Additionally, analysis of tumor-infiltrating T cell populations revealed that Ntrk1 can promote CD8+ T cell exhaustion. Lastly, we found that Ntrk1 regulates Jak/Stat signaling to promote expression of PD-L1 on tumor cells. Together, these data suggest that Ntrk1 activates Jak/Stat signaling to regulate expression of immunosuppressive molecules including PD-L1, promoting exhaustion within the tumor microenvironment.

Keywords: non-small cell lung cancer; immunotherapy; PD-1/PD-L1 checkpoint blockade

---

1. Introduction

Lung cancer is the leading cause of cancer-related deaths, killing more people in the U.S. than the next three most prevalent cancer types combined [1,2]. The five-year survival rate for all lung cancer patients is about 18%, which has improved marginally over the past several decades even with the improvement of genomic profiling and rational implementation of targeted therapies. Thus, a better understanding of the complexities of lung cancer progression, the contributing microenvironmental factors and how to target them would benefit patient outcomes.

Research focusing on systemic and tumor-infiltrating immune cell populations and their impact on shaping cancer progression in solid tumor types has provided compelling evidence for immune escape as a crucial survival mechanism. These studies have revealed that tumors avoid immune detection through a variety of complex mechanisms. For example, tumors can recruit immunosuppressive populations of cells such as myeloid derived suppressor cells or CD4+ T regulatory cells, which secrete suppressive cytokines that interfere with the cytotoxic functions of CD8+ T cells [3–5]. Additionally, tumors upregulate expression of PD-L1, which can occur de novo through oncogenic signaling or as a consequence of IFNγ-stimulation due to immune cell activation. PD-L1 binds to the PD-1 molecule on CD8+ T cells and blocks the full activation necessary for the cytotoxicity [6,7], thus representing an avenue of therapeutic intervention to promote cytotoxic activity of T cells.

The implementation of immunotherapies to release immune system braking mechanisms like those described above has been paradigm-shifting for cancer therapeutics. Clinical studies in lung cancer have revealed that inhibiting the PD-L1/PD-1 axis results in a significantly improved clinical outcome in ~15–20% of patients with lung cancer when compared to standard of care chemotherapy [8–10] and thus shows promise in improving patient prognosis. While some patients do show clinical benefit to checkpoint inhibitors when administered as single agents, the majority of patients either show no response or develop resistance to single agent checkpoint inhibition [9–15]; thus, discovering mechanisms of resistance and tumor cell dependencies in the face of immune-related pressure is imperative in furthering the potential for immunotherapy in treating lung tumors.

Several factors have been identified as impacting response to immune checkpoint inhibitors. For example, tumor mutational burden significantly correlates with response to immunotherapy, likely due to the creation of neoantigens that activate the immune response. Additional work has focused on oncogenic drivers of lung cancer. Kirsten rat sarcoma (KRAS) mutations occur in about 30% of lung adenocarcinomas, and unlike other common oncogenic drivers (such as epidermal growth factor receptor (EGFR) and anaplastic lymphoma kinase (ALK)), effective targeted therapeutic strategies for KRAS mutant lung cancer have been limited [16]. Interestingly, KRAS mutant lung tumors and their degree of immune system engagement and infiltration vary based upon the co-occurring mutations found within the tumor. Patients that present with a p53 mutation concurrently with oncogenic Kras (KP) exhibit higher expression of PD-L1 and other inflammatory markers when compared to other commonly co-occurring mutations such as STK11/LKB1 or CDKN2A [17], and these patients respond better to PD-1/PD-L1 axis blockade [18]. However, the mechanisms of tumor-regulated immunosuppression and the potential avenues of resistance in KP mutant lung cancer are vastly unknown, and the understanding of these factors is necessary for intelligent use of immunotherapies for maximum benefit to patients.

Previous work in our laboratory has focused on understanding the biology of KP mutant lung tumors through cancer cell intrinsic properties as well as extrinsic factors influencing cancer progression that are present within the tumor microenvironment. We have previously derived murine lung cancer cell lines from the primary or metastatic lesions of the $Kras^{LA1/+}/p53^{R172H\Delta g/+}$ genetically engineered mouse model of lung cancer [19,20]. These cells demonstrate heterogeneity in their epigenetic state and propensity to metastasize when re-implanted syngeneically into wildtype mice. Specifically, the KP murine cell lines that have undergone an epithelial-to-mesenchymal transition (EMT) are not only more metastatic and aggressive, but they also have lower CD8+ T cell infiltration and an increase in an exhaustive signature when compared to cells in an epithelial state [21]. This heterogeneity also translates to a response to PD-1 blockade, with mesenchymal cells responding initially to the anti-PD-1 antibody but ultimately acquiring resistance [22]. Thus, our in vivo models closely mimic patient disease progression and immune checkpoint inhibitor response, providing the opportunity to discover novel mechanisms regulating tumor response to immune checkpoint blockade in KP mutant lung cancer.

To identify novel mechanisms of KP lung cancer cell resistance to PD-1 checkpoint inhibition, we performed a clinically relevant and powerful in vivo dropout screen. KP murine mouse cell lines stably expressing the FDAome, a library of barcoded shRNAs specific to genes that encode for clinically actionable targets, were implanted into wildtype mice and treated with an anti-PD-1 antibody. Tumors were sequenced and analyzed for depleted shRNA sequences when mice were treated with an anti-PD-1 antibody, thus revealing genes essential for tumor survival in the face of PD-1 blockade. From this screen, neurotrophic receptor tyrosine kinase 1 (Ntrk1) was identified as a top lead candidate as it dropped out significantly in anti-PD-1 treated tumors. Our data indicate that Ntrk1 regulates KP cell biology including cell growth and invasion in vitro while also impacting the tumor-infiltrating immune populations and their functionality with a consistent promotion of an exhausted microenvironment. Thus, we determined that Ntrk1 is a novel regulator of immune functionality in KP lung cancer, and combinatory treatment strategies could circumvent PD-1 blockade resistance.

2. Results

2.1. An In Vivo Functional Genomics Screen to Identify Novel Tumor Cell Vulnerabilities in the Face of Immune Checkpoint Blockade

To explore novel avenues of therapeutic combinations with immune checkpoint blocking antibodies, we performed a powerful and clinically relevant in vivo dropout screen in combination with PD-1 checkpoint blockade treatment (Figure 1A). The screen library contained short hairpin RNAs (shRNAs) designed against ~200 genes, each of which encoded for a clinically actionable target, termed the FDAome. To ensure robustness and prevent false hits due to shRNA off-target effects, each gene was targeted with 10 unique shRNA sequences. Lentiviral particles expressing the shRNAs were used to transduce two murine Kras/p53 (KP) mutant lung cancer cells. The 393P epithelial cells are a non-metastatic line, whereas the 344P mesenchymal line is an aggressive and metastatic cell line, and each were originally derived from $Kras^{G12D/+}/p53^{R172H\Delta g}$ primary lung tumors as previously described by our laboratory [19]. The 393P and 344P cells stably expressing the FDAome library were implanted subcutaneously into 129/sv wildtype mice (3 mice/treatment group) (Figure 1B). Once tumors reached 150–200 mm^3, they were then treated with either an isotype control antibody or a PD-1 blocking antibody. 344P tumors, which responded to PD-1 treatment initially but eventually demonstrated resistance (Supplementary Figure S1), were collected at two time points of anti-PD-1 treatment to identify genes that synergize to prevent the development of resistance. After tumor collection and deep sequencing, quality control measures were completed to ensure sufficient barcode coverage across the library was maintained in vivo (Figure 1C). Importantly, strong separation of hairpins targeting positive controls (Psma1 and Rpl30) and hairpins targeting Luc was observed (Figure 1D, Supplementary Table S1). Furthermore, an additional positive control, the proteasomal gene Psmb1, ranks in the top 10 percent of the most significantly depleted genes across all conditions, thus strengthening the validity of the screen hits (Supplementary Table S2). To prioritize hits from the screen, a redundant shRNA activity (RSA) score method was used to assign significance of shRNA dropout, then assigning a rank from 1 to 192 for most significant to least significant dropout in each condition.

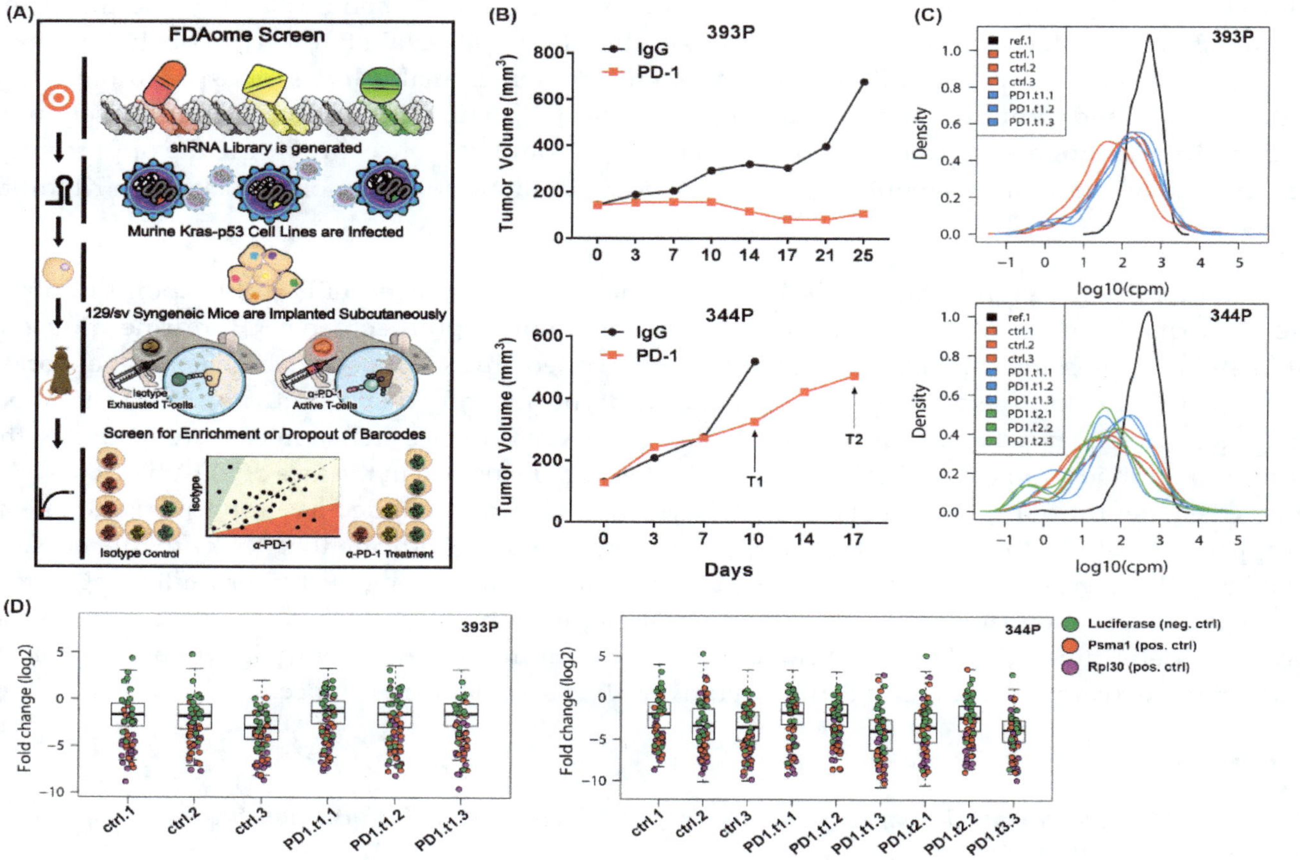

Figure 1. An in vivo functional genomics screen to identify novel tumor survival vulnerabilities when treated with PD-1 blocking antibody. (**A**) Schematic illustrating the workflow of the FDAome short hairpin RNA (shRNA) dropout screen. Briefly, a library of lentiviral particles expressing 10 different barcoded shRNAs for each of 192 genes was transduced into murine Kras/p53 mutant lung cancer cells. Genes included in the library have FDA-approved drugs that target the gene product. These cells were implanted into syngeneic 129/Sv and tumors were treated with PD-1 blocking antibody or IgG control. Tumors were sequenced for barcoded shRNAs and compared to reference cells for enriched or depleted shRNAs between isotype and PD-1 treated tumors. (**B**) 393P epithelial cells and 344P mesenchymal cells used in the FDAome screen were implanted subcutaneously and tumor growth was measured via calipers. T1 indicates time point 1 of tumor collection with PD-1 treatment in the 344P tumors, and T2 indicates time point 2. (**C**) Viral integration distribution of reference population and tumors determined through barcode sequencing (cmp counts per million). Ctrl.1-3 indicate 3 independent IgG treated tumors, and PD1.t1.1-3 label triplicates of anti-PD-1 treated tumors collected at the early time point. PD1.t2.1-3 indicate 344P tumors which were collected 1 week later at time point 2. (**D**) Fold change distribution (log2) of individual tumors relative to the initial transduction references with individual barcodes for positive controls Psma1 (red)/Rpl30 (purple), and the negative control Luc (green). Individual tumor samples per each group (ctrl, PD1.t1, PD1.t2) are shown.

2.2. Short Hairpin RNAs Targeting Ntrk1 Dropped out Significantly from 344P Mesenchymal Tumors Treated with PD-1 Blocking Antibody

The results of the FDAome screen revealed several shRNAs that dropped out from tumors treated with anti-PD-1 treatment, suggesting these genes to be vital for the survival of tumor cells when challenged with immune-related pressure through PD-1 treatment. We compared the differential in RSA value between isotype treated and anti-PD-1 treated tumors to compare nonessential to essential changes in the gene dropout score. Using this metric, we identified Ntrk1 as being one of the hits with the largest differential in RSA value between vehicle and PD-1 treated 344P tumors at both time points of treatment (Figure 2A, Supplementary Table S2). This was unique to the mesenchymal 344P tumors, as the epithelial 393P tumors do not show Ntrk1 shRNA dropout in anti-PD-1 treated tumors (Supplementary Figure S2). A similar screen using the same FDAome library but completed in vitro and in immunocompromised mice did not show significant dropout of Ntrk1 shRNAs [23]. These data suggest that Ntrk1 is nonessential for the survival of tumor cells in normal in vitro and in vivo conditions. However, when challenged with a PD-1 blocking antibody and therefore under immune system pressure, Ntrk1 then becomes essential for tumor cell survival. Importantly, Ntrk1 is a top hit across both time points of tumor collection and sequencing, suggesting the validity of this gene as a positive hit from the screen that is more likely to play a role in PD-1 treatment resistance in the face of long-term treatments.

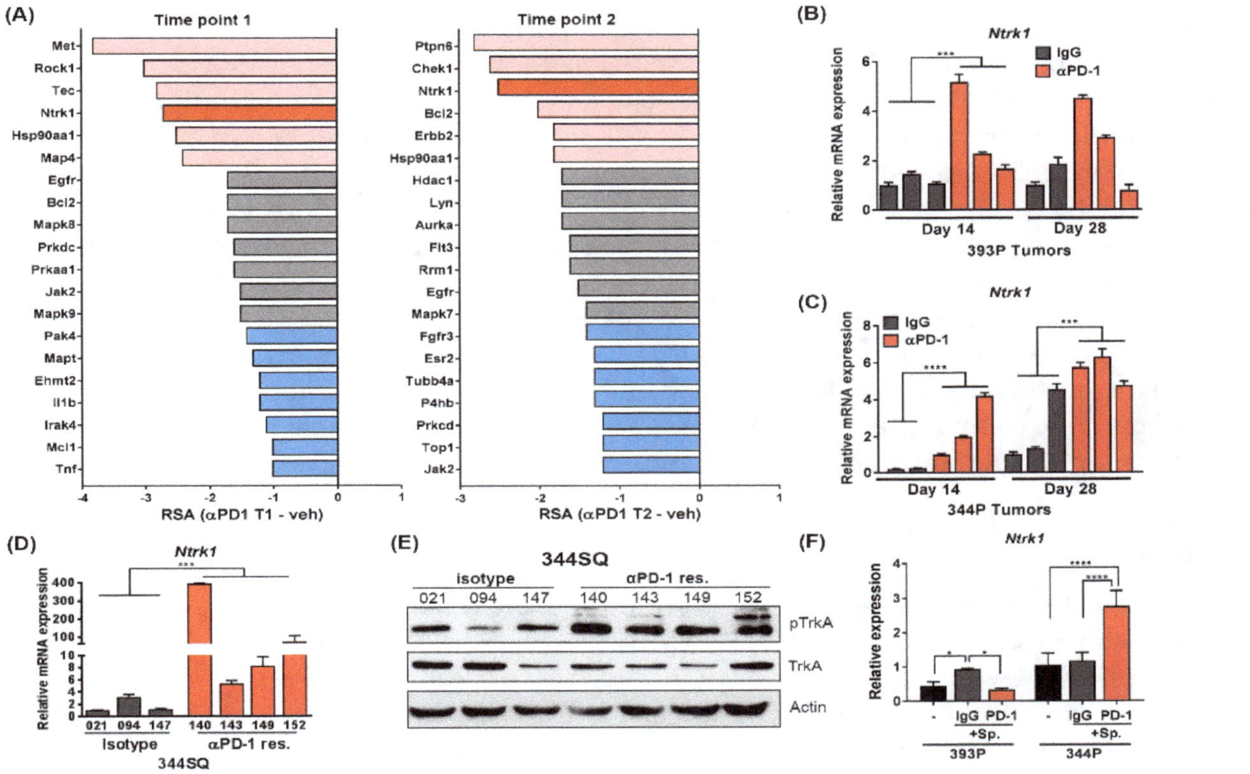

Figure 2. Ntrk1 shRNA drops out significantly from 344P tumors treated with anti-PD-1 and is upregulated in tumor cells treated with anti-PD-1 antibody. (**A**) Results from FDAome shRNA dropout screen in 344P tumors graphed as a differential score. The RSA from the isotype treatment condition for each gene was subtracted from the RSA from the same gene in the anti-PD-1 treatment group. Time point 1 is shown to the left, and time point 2 to the right. The top 10% of hits are depicted and these are divided into three groups, with the most significant shown in red. Ntrk1 is highlighted in bold red in both graphs. (**B**) Real-time PCR (qPCR) data for Ntrk1 expression in 393P tumors treated with anti-PD-1 or isotype control for 14 or 28 days. Expression values are normalized against L32 reference gene, relative to one isotype treated tumor sample. (**C**) Ntrk1 expression was analyzed in 344P tumors as described in panel B. (**D**) 344SQ tumor cells implanted in syngeneic mice were treated with isotype control or anti-PD-1 antibody. Tumors were collected after development of resistance to PD-1 blockade (~week 6), cell lines were derived from the tumors, and Ntrk1 expression analyzed via qPCR. The numbers below bars denote the individual mouse from which the cell line was derived. (**E**) Cell lines described in panel D were probed for phospho-TrkAY674/675 levels by Western blotting. (**F**) 393P and 344P cells were cultured in vitro either alone (-) or in the presence of splenocytes (sp.) at a 5:1 ratio of splenocytes to tumor cells. The treatment of either IgG or PD-1 blocking antibody was added to the co-culture and after 4 days, splenocytes were washed out and tumor cells were collected for RNA. Ntrk1 expression was analyzed using qPCR.

2.3. Transcript Level and Protein Activity of Ntrk1 Are Increased in PD-1 Treated Tumors

Because Ntrk1 dropped out significantly in the FDAome hairpin screen with a PD-1 blocking antibody, we next wanted to determine if the levels of Ntrk1 expression are elevated in tumors treated with immune checkpoint inhibitors. 393P and 344P tumors treated with an IgG control or anti-PD-1 antibody were collected for RNA after 14 or 28 days of treatment. Quantitative real-time PCR (qPCR) revealed that Ntrk1 transcript levels were significantly enhanced in two of the 393P tumors after 14 days of treatment, whereas the 344P tumors showed a more consistent and significant upregulation of Ntrk1 at both time points of treatment (Figure 2B,C). Additionally, another mesenchymal KP murine cell line, 344SQ, was used to derive primary lines from tumors after the development of resistance to PD-1 treatment, which we have previously shown to typically occur between weeks 5 and 7 of treatment [22]. When re-implanted into wildtype mice, these cells showed no response to anti-PD-1 treatment (Supplementary Figure S3). Compared to isotype treated 344SQ tumors, three of four independent 344SQ PD-1 resistant cell lines showed upregulation of Ntrk1 transcript levels, as well as increased phosphorylation of TrkA protein as shown by western blot (Figure 2D,E). Specifically, the PD-1 resistant cells showed increased expression of the fully glycosylated, mature 140 kDa species of phospho-TrkA, suggesting that downstream signaling of TrkA is more active in these cells. Lastly, 393P and 344P cells were cultured alone or co-cultured with total splenocytes in vitro and treated with an IgG or a PD-1 blocking antibody. Ntrk1 was again found to be significantly upregulated in 344P cells co-cultured with splenocytes that were treated with a PD-1 blocking antibody compared to the isotype control (Figure 2F).

Taken together, these data indicate that anti-PD-1 treatment in tumors or in cell lines co-cultured with an immune compartment upregulates Ntrk1 transcription and activation status, suggesting this pathway may be aberrantly activated as a result of an activated T cell response.

2.4. Baseline Expression of Ntrk1 Is Higher in Mesenchymal Murine and Human Lung Cancer Cell Lines and Is Necessary for Invasion and Migration

Previously, our lab generated a panel of KP murine cell lines and profiled them based on their epithelial and mesenchymal status [19,20]. Using these lines, we assayed baseline Ntrk1 expression and found that Ntrk1 levels and phosphorylation correlate with cells in a mesenchymal state (Figure 3A,B), which may explain the differential findings between 393P and 344P from the screen. Similarly, a small panel of human cells delineated by epithelial or mesenchymal status showed the same trend, with Ntrk1 expression correlating with a mesenchymal status. Additionally, cells driven into a mesenchymal state via Zeb1 induction or a more epithelial state with miR-200 induction, as described previously [21,24,25], also confirmed that Ntrk1 expression is higher in cells pushed into a mesenchymal state (Supplementary Figure S4). Because Ntrk1 expression is higher in mesenchymal cells, we generated stable shRNA-mediated knockdowns in the mesenchymal 344P and 344SQ murine lines and assayed the effect of Ntrk1 knockdown on the ability of these cells to migrate and invade a microenvironment. We found that Ntrk1 knockdown significantly reduced the ability of 344SQ cells to migrate and invade using transwell assays (Figure 3C). Additionally, when plated on a 50% Matrigel:50% collagen type I matrix, the ability of multicellular aggregates to invade was also significantly reduced with Ntrk1 depletion (Figure 3D). Conversely, we generated cell lines stably overexpressing the human cDNA of Ntrk1 in the 393P epithelial murine cell line. Compared to vector control cells, the overexpression of Ntrk1 was sufficient to stimulate invasion and migration (Figure 3E,F). We also analyzed whether another member of the same family, Ntrk3, can impact KP cancer cell biology in a similar manner as Ntrk1. We generated cell lines overexpressing the human cDNA of Ntrk3 in the epithelial 393P cells and determined that these also demonstrate increased invasion and migration (Figure S5). These data indicate that both Ntrk1 and Ntrk3 can regulate cell migration and invasion in KP mutant lung cancer cells, and the expression of Ntrk1 correlates with a more aggressive, mesenchymal state.

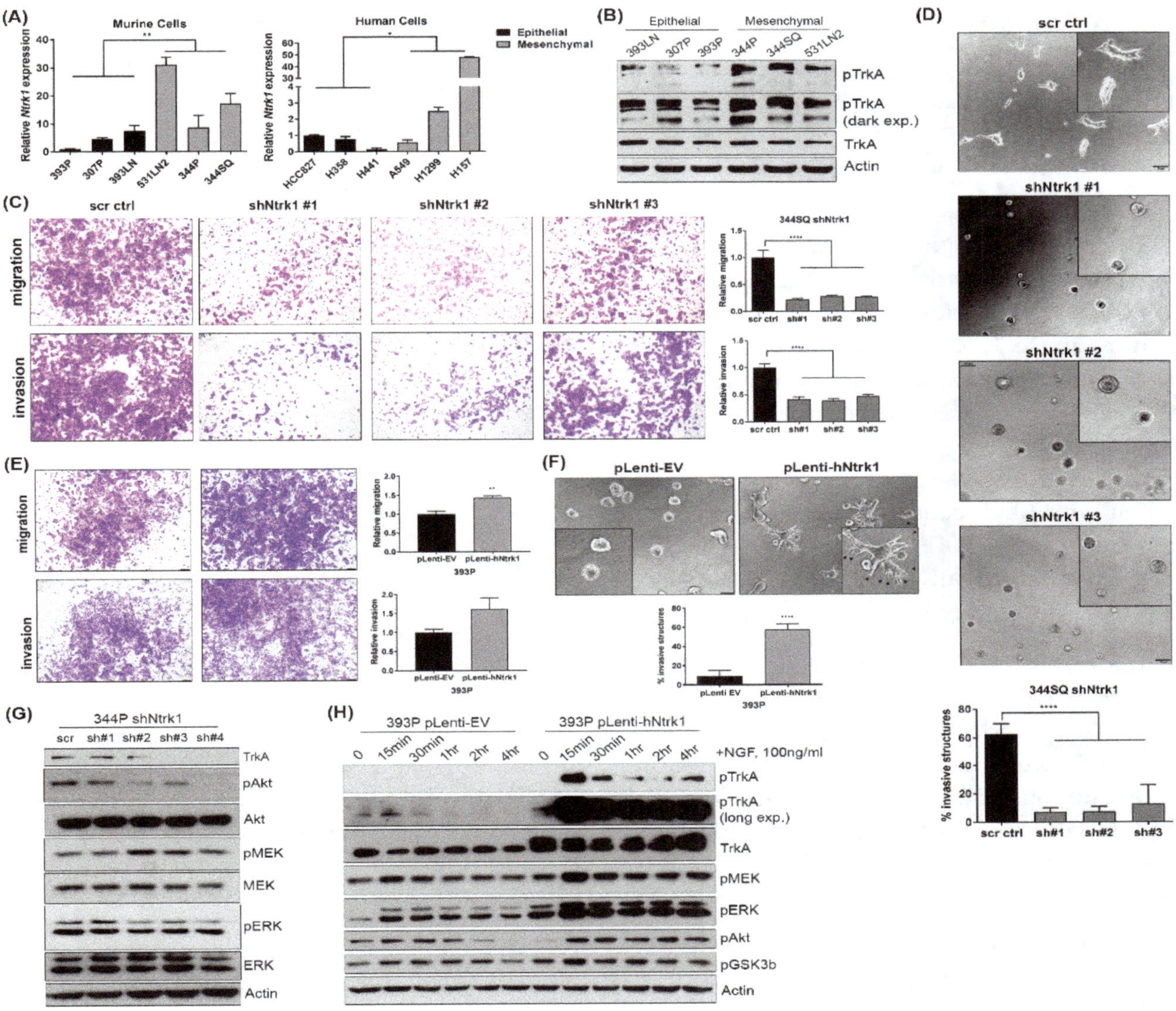

Figure 3. Ntrk1 expression correlates with cells in a mesenchymal state and regulates cell migration, invasion, and AKT and MAPK signaling pathways. (**A**) Real-time qPCR data for Ntrk1 expression in 3 epithelial and 3 mesenchymal murine KP lung cancer cell lines (left) and in 3 epithelial and 3 mesenchymal human lung cancer cell lines (right). (**B**) Western blot showing phospho-TrkA expression in murine KP lung cancer cells as a function of epithelial and mesenchymal status. Actin was used as a loading control. (**C**) Ntrk1 was stably depleted using 3 different shRNA sequences. 344SQ Ntrk1 knockdown cells were plated in triplicate in transwell chambers with Matrigel to measure invasion or without to measure migration. After 16 hours, cells that had migrated or invaded were fixed and stained with crystal violet. Representative images of a single chamber are shown. Quantifications were done using ImageJ and are graphed to the right as a fold change compared to non-targeting scrambled control cells. (**D**) 344SQ shNtrk1 cells were plated on a 50% Matrigel:50% collagen type I matrix. Images were taken after 3 days and the percentage of invasive structures was quantified and graphed below. (**E**) Human cDNA encoding for Ntrk1 was stably introduced into 393P cells. These cells were plated in migration and invasion transwell assays as described in panel C. Representative images are shown and quantifications are graphed to the right. (**F**) 393P Ntrk1 overexpressing cells were plated on a Matrigel and collagen type 1 mixed matrix as described in panel D. Invasive structures were quantified and are shown in the graph below. (**G**) Western blot analysis of 344P Ntrk1 knockdown cells to examine protein expression of TrkA to confirm knockdown and signaling pathways including AKT and MEK/ERK. Actin was used as a loading control. (**H**) 393P empty vector (EV) and Ntrk1 overexpression cells were stimulated with NGF over the course of 4 hours and protein collected for western blot analysis of phospho-TrkA, and AKT and MEK/ERK signaling pathways.

2.5. Ntrk1 Activates AKT and MAPK Signaling in KP Lung Cancer Cell Lines to Regulate Cell Growth

Additional analysis of Ntrk1-modulated cells revealed that Ntrk1 regulates not only invasion and migration but also cell growth. Specifically, knockdown of Ntrk1 results in a significant reduction of cell growth over time, whereas overexpression of Ntrk1—or exogenous addition of nerve growth factor (NGF) to stimulate TrkA signaling—can stimulate cell growth in epithelial 393P cells (Supplementary Figure S6).

To determine if Ntrk1 regulates known downstream signaling pathways involved in cell growth and survival, we performed western analysis of Ntrk1 knockdown cell lines. Compared to scrambled control cells, depletion of Ntrk1 decreased both protein kinase B (PKB/AKT) and extracellular receptor kinase 1/2 (ERK1/2) phosphorylation (Figure 3G). Similarly, we utilized the Ntrk1 and Ntrk3 overexpression cells and stimulated signaling with exogenous NGF or NT-3, respectively. In both Ntrk1 and Ntrk3 overexpression cells, AKT and ERK1/2 were quickly and robustly activated, with long term kinetics compared to the control cell line (Figure 3H and Supplementary Figure S5). We also investigated endogenous signaling cascades regulated by TrkA in KP lung cancer cells. In the 393P and 344P cells stimulated with an NGF ligand, phospho-TrkA was higher at baseline in the mesenchymal 344P cells compared to the 393P cells, as observed in Figure 3B (Supplementary Figure S6). Additionally, AKT and ERK1/2 signaling cascades were activated in both cell lines, though the kinetics and degree of response differed between them (Supplementary Figure S6).

To determine if either AKT or MAPK signaling regulates the cell growth phenotype observed with Ntrk1 overexpression, we utilized either MK2206, an AKT specific inhibitor, or trametinib, a mitogen-activated protein kinase kinase (MAP2K/MEK) specific inhibitor. Utilizing MTT viability assays, we determined that while AKT inhibition does inhibit the viability of Ntrk1 overexpression cells, exogenous stimulation of TrkA signaling via NGF was sufficient to circumvent this repression (Supplementary Figure S6), suggesting that an independent pathway regulates cell growth. By contrast, the addition of trametinib significantly inhibited cell viability, and this was not able to be rescued via exogenous NGF addition.

Taken together, our data indicate that Ntrk1 and Ntrk3 both regulate downstream signaling to AKT and MAPK in KP lung cancer cells, but the regulation of cell growth by Ntrk1 mainly occurs via MAPK signaling cascades.

2.6. Ntrk1 Overexpression Promotes Tumor Growth In Vivo and Augments the Tumor Infiltrating Immune Compartment by Promoting CD8+ T Cell Exhaustion

Because Ntrk1 was originally identified from the FDAome hairpin screen as being necessary for tumor cell survival when under immune-mediated pressure via PD-1 blockade, we wanted to determine if Ntrk1 modulates the immune compartment within tumors. To address this, we implanted the Ntrk1 overexpressing and control cells subcutaneously into 129/sv wildtype mice to assay the effects on the immune microenvironment. The overexpression of Ntrk1 significantly enhanced tumor size in vivo (Figure 4A), corroborating the in vitro growth data. Flow cytometry data collected from four-week tumors revealed that Ntrk1 overexpression correlated with a significant reduction of the total T cell infiltrate within the primary tumor, likely due to the significant reduction in total CD8+ T cells, with no significant effect observed on the CD4+ population (Figure 4B–D). Additionally, we found that Ntrk1 overexpression also impacted the functionality of CD8+ cells, with the Ntrk1-expressing tumors presenting with an almost three-fold increase in the level of PD-1+ CD8+ T cells (Figure 4E,F). These cells were also double positive for Tim3, suggesting this population of CD8+ cells were exhausted. In vitro co-culture assays also confirmed that Ntrk1 overexpression can reduce the proliferative capabilities of immune cells as measured by flow cytometry, whereas depleting Ntrk1 promotes the proliferation of immune cells (Supplementary Figure S7).

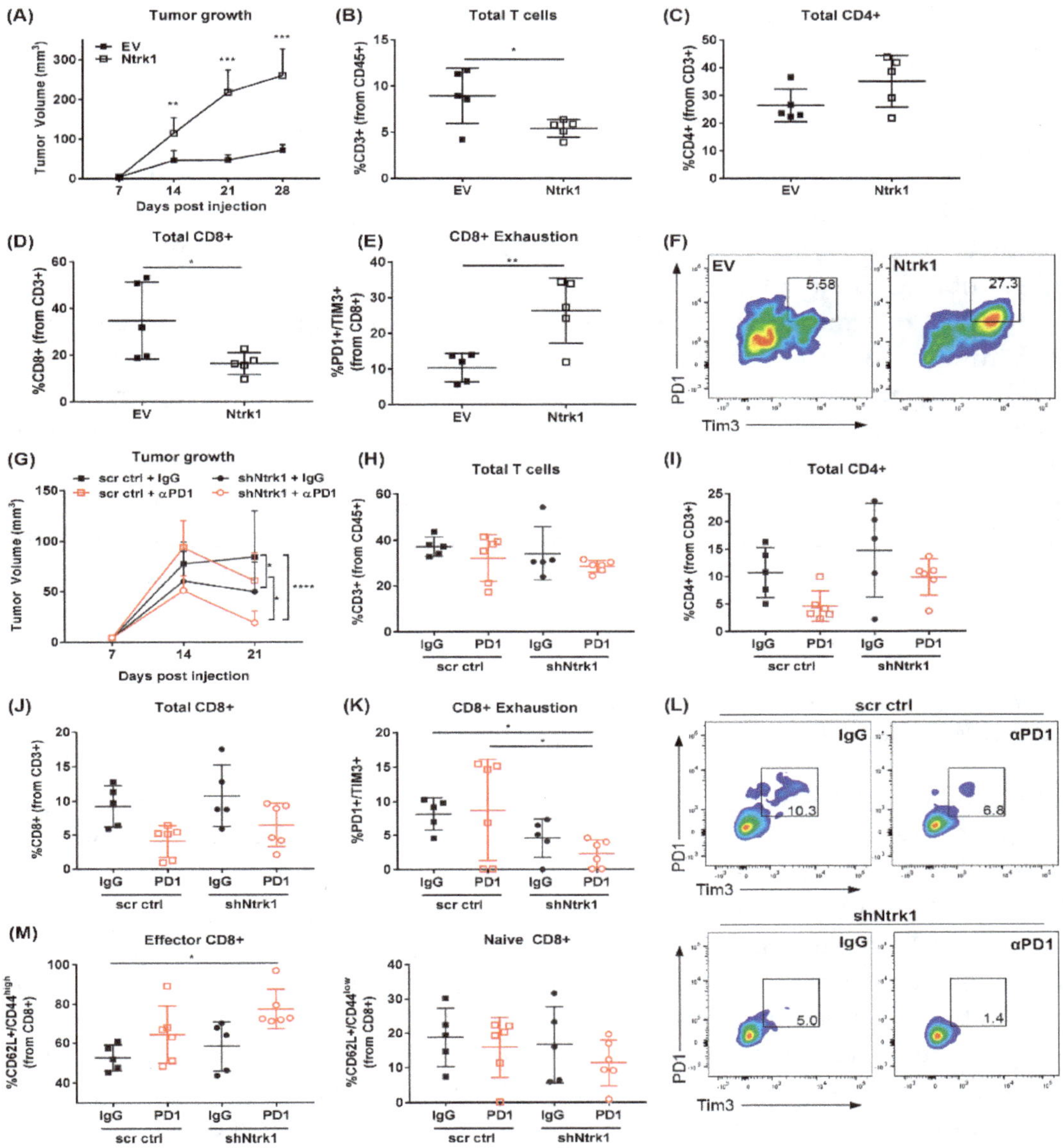

Figure 4. Ntrk1 modulates tumor growth as well as CD8+ T cell exhaustion and activity in vivo. (**A**–**F**) 393P EV and Ntrk1 cells were implanted subcutaneously into 129/sv wildtype mice. After 4 weeks of growth, tumors were collected and processed for flow cytometry analysis of immune cell populations. $n = 5$ mice/cell line. (**A**) Tumor growth was monitored weekly via caliper measurements. (**B**) The percentage of CD3+ T cells in the microenvironment was gated from live CD45+ cells. (**C**) CD4+ T cells were calculated as a percentage of total CD3+. (**D**) CD8+ T cells were calculated as percentage of CD3+ T cells. (**E**) T cell exhaustion was measured as PD-1+/TIM3+ from the CD8+ population. (**F**) A representative dot plot of PD1+/TIM3+ T cells from each condition. (**G**–**M**) 344P cells with stable depletion of Ntrk1 were implanted subcutaneously into 129/sv wildtype mice and compared to a non-targeting control cell line. One week post-implantation, tumors were then treated with either IgG control or PD-1 blocking antibody for 2 weeks, at which point tumors were collected and processed for flow cytometry analysis. (**G**) Tumor growth was monitored weekly via caliper measurements. (**H**) The total CD3+ T cells was quantified from total live CD45+ cells in tumors. (**I**) CD4+ T cells were calculated from total CD3+ cells. (**J**) CD8+ T cells were quantified as a percentage of total CD3+ T cells. (**K**) PD-1+/TIM3+ exhausted T cells were calculated as described in panel E. (**L**) Representative dot plots from each condition showing PD1+/TIM3+ T cells. (**M**) Effector (left graph) and naïve (right graph) CD8+ T cells were calculated as a percentage from total CD8+ T cells. Effector cells were characterized as CD62L+/CD44high and naïve cells as CD62L+/CD44low.

These data suggest that Ntrk1 expression promotes tumor growth at least in part by promoting T cell exhaustion.

2.7. Combination of Ntrk1 Knockdown with PD-1 Blockade Significantly Reduces Tumor Growth and CD8+ T Cell Exhaustion In Vivo

To further explore the function of Ntrk1 in immunosuppression, we subcutaneously implanted 344P Ntrk1 knockdown or scrambled control cells and treated them either with an IgG control or a PD-1 blocking antibody. The depletion of Ntrk1 alone was sufficient to reduce tumor burden, with the addition of anti-PD-1 treatment further repressing tumor growth (Figure 4G). Tumors were analyzed for infiltrating immune subpopulations using flow cytometry, and while knockdown had no impact on total levels of the immune populations (Figure 4H–J), we found a trend towards decreased CD8+ exhaustion with Ntrk1 knockdown alone, and this was further enhanced with the addition of an anti-PD-1 antibody (Figure 4K,L). Additionally, the population of CD62L+/CD44^{high} effector CD8+ T cells was also significantly increased (Figure 4M), so that the proportion of active CD8 to exhausted CD8 was significantly altered with PD-1 blockade in Ntrk1 depleted tumors. Together with the overexpression analyses, the data demonstrate that Ntrk1 modulates immune functionality with a consistent impact on CD8+ activity and exhaustion.

2.8. Ntrk1 Expression Impacts Jak Signaling and Correlates with PD-L1 Levels in Cells Co-Cultured with an Immune Compartment and in Tumor Samples

To determine how Ntrk1 may be modulating tumor growth and the immune microenvironment, we examined Jak/Stat signaling as a function of Ntrk1 expression; this is a known pathway utilized by tumors to promote immunosuppression. By western blot, we found that Ntrk1 knockdown in 344SQ mesenchymal cells did result in decreased phosphorylation of Jak1 and Stat3 as compared to scrambled control cells (Figure 5A). Additionally, stimulation of TrkA signaling via exogenous NGF also increased phospho-Jak1 levels consistently in the 393P cells, whereas phospho-Jak1 levels were high in the 344P cells initially and then fluctuated throughout the time course with NGF stimulation (Figure 5B). One of the well-studied immunosuppressive molecules altered downstream of Jak signaling is Irf1, which in turn triggers the transcription of CD274 or PD-L1. Thus, we assayed whether Ntrk1 can directly impact the expression of PD-L1. In co-culture assays with Ntrk1 knockdown cells, we found that at baseline, Irf1 and PD-L1 expression levels are lower in knockdown versus control cells and this becomes more drastic when knockdown cells are co-cultured with splenocytes (Figure 5C). Conversely, we found a robust and significant increase in Irf1 and PD-L1 expression in Ntrk1 overexpressing cells when cultured with splenocytes (Figure 5D). The upregulation of PD-L1 by Ntrk1 has functional consequences on T cell proliferation. As demonstrated previously, Ntrk1 expression can decrease immune cell proliferation. However, the addition of an anti-PD-L1 antibody to a co-culture of Ntrk1 overexpressing cells with splenocytes can restore immune cell proliferative capabilities (Supplementary Figure S7). Ntrk1 overexpressing cells also demonstrate a robust increase of PD-L1 expression at 5:1 and 20:1 ratios of splenocytes to tumor cells at the protein level (Figure 5E). Importantly, this upregulation of PD-L1 could be partially reversed when cells were treated with LOXO-101, a pan-Trk inhibitor. These findings were consistent in Ntrk1 overexpressing tumors, with increased PD-L1 levels when compared to vector control tumors (Figure 5F). As expected, treatment with Ruxolitinib, a Jak1/2 inhibitor, significantly inhibited the upregulation of both Irf1 and PD-L1 as a consequence of co-culture with the immune compartment in both vector and Ntrk1-overexpressing cells (Supplementary Figure S8), suggesting that Trk signaling is just one upstream molecule that impacts Jak-dependent upregulation of PD-L1.

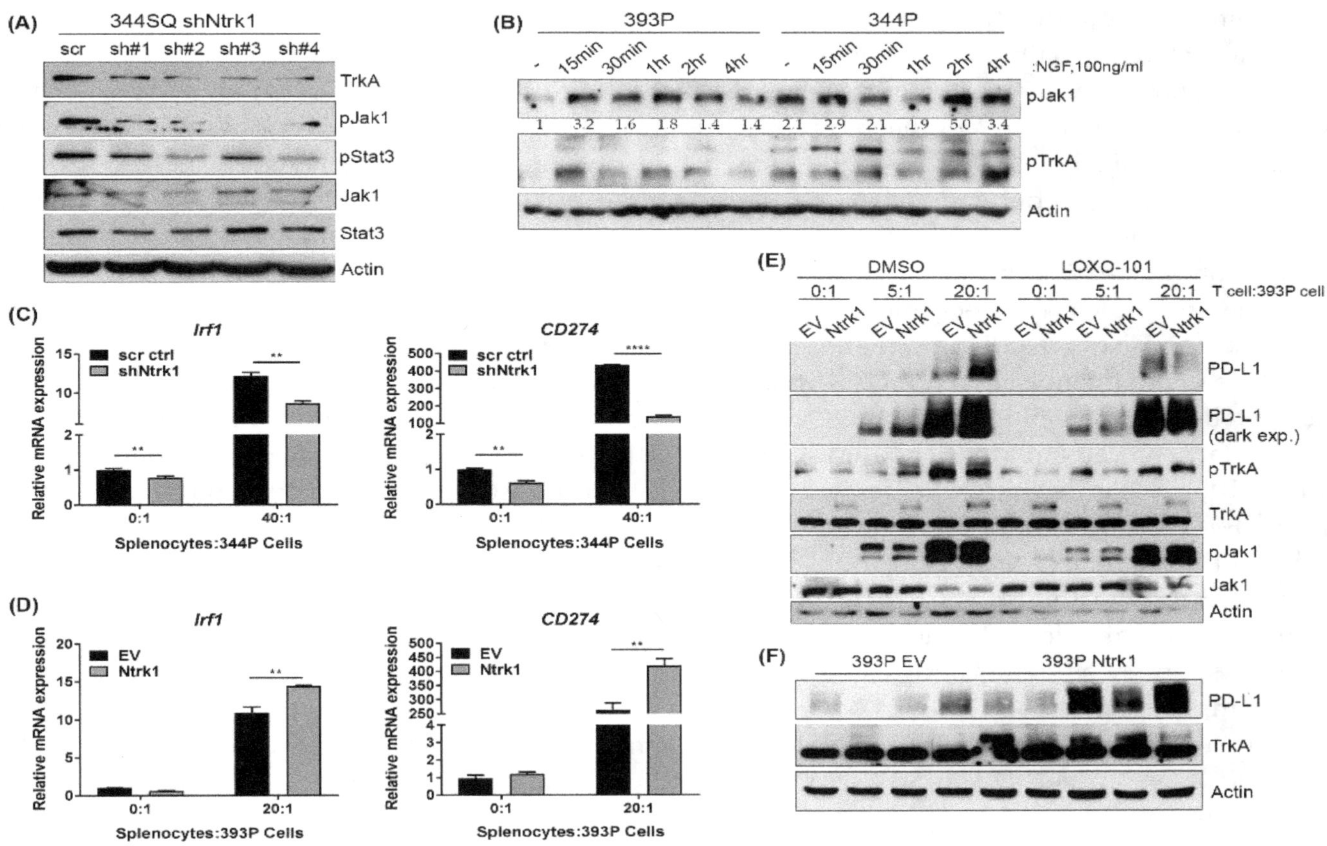

Figure 5. Ntrk1 can regulate JAK/STAT signaling to promote expression of PD-L1. (**A**) Western blot analysis of 344SQ Ntrk1 knockdown cells probing for phospho-Jak1 and phospho-Stat3. Actin was used as a loading control. (**B**) Western blot analysis of 393P and 344P cell lines stimulated with NGF at 100ng/ml over a short time course to assay activation of phospho-Jak1 and phospho-TrkA. Densitometry calculations of phospho-Jak1 intensity relative to actin were normalized to 393P (-) and are shown below the phospho-Jak1 blot. (**C**) Real-time qPCR analysis of CD274 (PD-L1) expression in 344P Ntrk1 knockdown cells when co-cultured with total splenocytes. (**D**) 393P Ntrk1 overexpression cells were co-cultured with total splenocytes and assayed using qPCR for expression of CD274. (**E**) 393P Ntrk1 overexpression cells were cultured alone (0:1) or co-cultured with total splenocytes at 5:1 and 20:1 ratios. Either DMSO control or LOXO-101, a pan Trk-inhibitor, were added to the co-culture at the time of seeding. After 3 days, tumor cells were assayed for protein expression of PD-L1, phospho-TrkA, and phospho-Jak1. (**F**) Western blot analysis of PD-L1 expression in 393P empty vector (EV) control and Ntrk1 overexpression tumors.

Interestingly, although signaling cascades and biological phenotypes such as invasion and migration are similar between Ntrk1 and Ntrk3 expressing cells, the overexpression of Ntrk3 in 393P cells has no impact on PD-L1 expression when in co-culture with splenocytes (Supplementary Figure S7). Thus, the regulation of PD-L1 and other immunosuppressive molecules downstream of Jak/Stat signaling cascades may be a unique function of Ntrk1 in KP mutant lung cancer.

Together, these data demonstrate that Ntrk1 expression can modulate KP lung cancer biology as well as the immune microenvironment via Jak1 signaling to promote the expression of immunosuppressive molecules including PD-L1.

3. Discussion

The data generated from the in vivo FDAome dropout screen provide compelling evidence for the use of in vivo functional genomic screens to identify novel tumor cell genes and/or pathways that promote immunosuppression and thus may contribute to immunotherapy resistance. We and others have demonstrated the utility of these screens, in the context of immunotherapy or in the context of other tumor biology hallmark dependencies (i.e., cellular growth), to provide preliminary evidence for novel drug targets as well as stimulate new research questions. For example, human patient-derived xenografts and genetically engineered mouse models have been utilized to perform loss-of-function screens using a shRNA library targeting known epigenetic regulators in pancreatic cancer to identify novel tumor survival dependencies [26]. This group provided strong evidence for *WDR5* as being essential for pancreatic tumorigenesis and thus targeting it as a potential therapeutic strategy to further explore for pancreatic cancer patients.

Recently, functional genomic screens have moved towards the CRISPR-Cas9 system for gene editing as it has several advantages over shRNA-based screens, including complete gene knockout as well as greater genomic coverage with larger libraries. Two recent screens did so in the context of tumor cell-immune cell interactions. One was completed in vitro with human T cells in co-culture with melanoma cells to identify tumor genes essential for the effector functions of T cells [27]. The other CRISPR-Cas9 screen was performed in vivo with anti-PD-1 treatment in combination with GM-CSF-secreting, irradiated tumor cell vaccine (GVAX) [28]. This screen contained ~2500 genes and identified hits in the IFNγ response and antigen presentation pathways as expected, but also less understood hits such as *PTPN2*. From these two studies alone, the breadth of knowledge and the resources available to develop hypothesis-driven research about tumor cell influence on immune system response was significantly expanded and will continue to provide additional knowledge about these complex processes.

To contribute to these efforts and better understand response and resistance to immune checkpoint inhibitors in a complex system, we performed a clinically relevant FDAome in vivo dropout screen using a Kras/p53 mutant syngeneic mouse model of lung cancer. This model and the GEM model from which the KP mutant cell lines were originally derived [19] closely recapitulate the progression of human lung cancer disease, with development of metastatic lesions throughout the body, as well as heterogeneity of immune infiltrate and response to immunotherapy agents [19–22,29]; thus, the similarity to *KRAS*-driven human lung cancer validates the use of these models to address specific immune-related questions, as well as to perform mechanistic and therapeutic studies. We identified Ntrk1 as a top lead hit as being essential for tumor cell survival in vivo when challenged with an anti-PD-1 antibody and therefore a potential avenue of acquired resistance. Molecular studies revealed that Ntrk1 regulates KP lung cancer cell intrinsic biological processes such as cell signaling to AKT and MAPK to promote cellular growth as well as regulation of in vitro invasive capacity. In vivo analyses demonstrated that Ntrk1 also augments immune infiltrate and functionality. Specifically, Ntrk1 expression can promote CD8+ T cell exhaustion within the tumor microenvironment, suggesting that its expression may contribute to CD8+ T cell dysfunction and thus diminish response to PD-1 inhibition.

We now provide the first evidence that Ntrk1 can regulate the expression of the immunosuppressive molecule PD-L1, likely due to modulation of Jak/Stat signaling cascade. In melanoma, loss-of-function *JAK1/JAK2* mutations were discovered in a minority of patients after relapse on the anti-PD-1 treatment pembrolizumab; therefore, it is a potential avenue of acquired resistance to immune checkpoint blockade [30]. Our data may indicate a distinct mechanism by which this pathway becomes aberrantly hyperactivated in lung cancer cells to promote immunosuppression and resistance to immune checkpoint inhibition. Ntrk1 can promote activation of Jak1 and Stat3, and Ntrk1 depletion reduces this signaling and downstream PD-L1 expression. There is little evidence in the literature connecting Ntrk1 to Jak signaling, so this mechanism needs to be further explored. However, previous work in neuronal cells demonstrated that neurotrophin-dependent stimulation of downstream transcription and neuronal cell elongation can be blocked by depletion of Stat3 [31], suggesting that Stat3 does function downstream of neurotrophin receptors. Additionally, knockout of gp130, a type I cytokine receptor, can diminish NGF-induced neurite extension, thus linking Ntrk1 signaling and cytokine signaling. However, both of these studies were limited to neuronal cells and lacked further mechanistic studies to determine whether Ntrk1 directly interacts with these cytokine response elements. Thus, the mechanism for Ntrk1-dependent activation of Jak/Stat signaling remains to be fully elucidated. Additionally, other immunosuppressive molecules that are upregulated as a result of Ntrk1 overexpression in addition to PD-L1 need to be explored to understand the full impact of Ntrk1 upregulation on various immune subpopulations and their functionality within tumors.

In vivo functional genomics screens to address specific immune-related questions such as undiscovered mechanisms of acquired resistance to the anti-PD-1 antibody will drive the field forward and bolster our understanding of the regulatory pathways driving tumor cell evasion of immune detection and death. The goal of the work described was to identify novel therapeutic combinations to improve patient response to immunotherapy. Our data indicate that Ntrk1 may be one such hit that could be carried forward clinically to improve patient response to a single agent PD-1 blocking antibody. In some solid tumor types such as lung cancer, Ntrk1 genetic rearrangements occur infrequently (~1–3% of lung adenocarcinomas), leading to fusion proteins with constitutive kinase activity. Targeted therapies have recently been FDA approved, with most patients showing durable responses [32–36]. Importantly, our preliminary in vivo screen and supporting data suggest that a significantly broader patient population may benefit from these well-tolerated Trk inhibitors in the context of immune checkpoint blockade.

4. Materials and Methods

4.1. Cell Culture and Reagents

The human lung cancer cell lines used in these studies were H1299, H157, A549, H441, H358, and HCC827. Murine lung cancer cells were created from $Kras^{LA1/+}/p53^{R172H\Delta g/+}$ genetically engineered mice as previously described [19]. All lung cancer cell lines were cultured in Roswell Park Memorial Institute (RPMI) + 10% Fetal Bovine Serum (FBS). A total of 293T cells were cultured in Dulbecco's Modified Eagle's Medium (DMEM) + 10% FBS and were used to generate lentiviral particles for creating stable cell lines. The miR-200ab inducible H1299 cells and Zeb1-inducible 393P cells were generated using the pTRIPz plasmid as previously described by our laboratory [21,24]. Expression of mir-200ab or Zeb1 was induced using 2 μg/mL of doxycycline. Ntrk1 overexpression cells were generated by subcloning human Ntrk1 cDNA from pCMV5 TrkA (Addgene plasmid #15002; http://n2t.net/addgene:15002; RRID:Addgene_15002 [37]) into the pLenti-puro vector backbone using EcoRI and AgeI restriction cut sites. Human Ntrk3 cDNA was cloned into the pLD6E2F vector. The Ntrk1 shRNA sequences that were used in these studies were as follows: sh#1: 5′-TCAAGCGCCAGGACATCATT; sh#2: 5′-GTGGCTGCTGGTATGGTATATCT; sh#3: 5′-TCTATAGCACAGACTATTACC; sh#4: 5′-TTGGAGTCTGCGCTGACTAAT.

NGF and NT-3 ligands were obtained from Sigma (St. Louis, MO, USA) and used at a final concentration of 100 ng/mL. MK2206, LOXO-101, trametinib, and ruxolitinib inhibitors were obtained from SelleckChem (Houston, TX, USA). Anti-PD-L1 (clone 10F.9G2), PD-1 (clone RMP1-14), and isotype control antibodies (Rat IgG2b and IgG2a, respectively) were obtained from BioXCell (West Lebanon, NH, USA).

4.2. Animal Studies

Cancer cells were prepared at a concentration of 1×10^6 cells in 100μl of serum free media. The cells were subcutaneously implanted into the right flanks of male and female syngeneic 129/sv mice of at least three months of age. Tumors were allowed to grow for 3–4 weeks, depending on the study. Where indicated, mice were treated with an anti-PD-1 or isotype control antibody via i.p. injections biweekly (100 μL per dose for a total of 200 μg). After euthanasia, tumors were measured both by calipers and weight and subsequently collected for flow cytometry analyses or sequencing for the FDAome screen (see below). All animal experiments were reviewed and approved by the Institutional Animal Care and Use Committee at the University of Texas MD Anderson Cancer Center (protocol #00001271).

4.3. FDAome Dropout Screen

Murine lung cancer cell lines (393P and 344P) were infected at a multiplicity-of-infection (MOI) of 0.3 with a pooled shRNA lentiviral library targeting 192 genes associated with FDA-approved target therapies (10 independent shRNAs/gene). The FDAome expressing cells were implanted into 129/Sv mice at 1.0×10^6 cells/mouse in triplicate for each condition. Once tumor size reached ~150 mm^3 as measured by calipers, mice were either treated with an isotype control or PD-1 blocking antibody as described above. Tumors were collected after 10 days (time point 1) or 17 days (time point 2) in the 344P model, or after 25 days in the 393P model.

The shRNA-coupled barcodes were detected deploying high-throughput sequencing technology (for detailed procedures and primer sequences see the following reference) [26]. Raw counts for the screen endpoints and a reference population, isolated after transduction, were normalized using the variance stabilizing transformation in R (version 3.3.2) with the DESeq2 in R. A fold change in barcode abundance was estimated by dividing the normalized counts by the reference. Four independent shRNA targeting essential genes (Rpl30, Psma1) or the negative control luciferase (LUC) were cloned with five unique barcodes each and incorporated in the library as positive and negative controls (20 reagents/control, see Table S1). One LUC hairpin showed an apparent off-target effect, whereas one hairpin for Psma1 did not show a robust drop out; however, this result was not reflective of poor screen performance as the trend was consistent across the five barcodes. After excluding those hairpins, the separation of positive and negative controls was evaluated by the robust strictly standardized mean (SSM, Table S1). Fold change distribution was converted to percentiles, and biological replicates were collapsed for RSA analysis. The RSA logP-values and ranks are provided in Table S2.

4.4. Cell Viability and Growth Assays

Cell growth in Ntrk1 knockdown or overexpression cells was measured by plating an equal cell number at day 0 and then counting viable cells (using Trypan blue exclusion) every day over a three-day period. Cell growth in Ntrk3 overexpression cells was measured in 3D cultures. These cells were plated on top of a thick Matrigel layer in 8 well chamber slides as single cells. NT-3 ligand was added at the time of cell seeding. Growth was monitored over six days and media refreshed every other day. Images from day 6 were used to measure 3D structure diameter using ImageJ software (version 1.5h). Two independent chambers were quantified for each condition.

Cell viability in the presence of either dimethyl sulfoxide (DMSO,) MK2206 (1 μM), or trametinib (1 μM) was measured using a 3-(4,5-Dimethylthiazol-2-yl)-2,5-Diphenyltetrazolium Bromide (MTT) reagent (Sigma, St. Louis, MO, USA). Cells were plated in a 96 well plate and the drug was added at the time of seeding at the indicated concentrations. After 72 h, an MTT reagent (1.5 mg/mL) was added to each well, incubated for one hour, then supernatant aspirated and precipitate solubilized in DMSO. Absorbance values were read using an Epoch plate reader at 570 nm and 630 nm (background), and background absorbance values were subtracted from 570 nm values.

4.5. Invasion and Migration Assays

Cells were plated in an equal number in 8 μm Transwell inserts (BD Biosciences) placed in 24 well plates as described previously [19]. Cells were incubated overnight for 16 h and then stained with a crystal violet solution. Chambers were then imaged by brightfield microscopy on an Olympus IX73 (Olympus, Center Valley, PA, USA), and ImageJ software was used to count cells that had migrated/invaded through the insert pores.

3D cultures were completed as previously described [19]. Briefly, either 100% Matrigel or a Matrigel/collagen type I mixture (50:50) were used to coat 8 well chamber slides. Collagen was used at a final concentration of 1.5–2.0 mg/mL. Single tumor cells were plated on top of the matrix (1500 cells/chamber) in media containing 2% Matrigel. Cells then grew over a period of 3–5 days and invasive structures were manually counted as a percentage of total structures in each well. 30–50 structures were counted per well, and each condition was plated in triplicate.

4.6. Co-Culture Assays

Spleens were extracted from 129/Sv mice bearing either 393P or 344P tumors. These were then mechanically processed and filtered to obtain single cells. Red blood cells were lysed using red blood cell (RBC) Lysis buffer (BioLegend, San Diego, CA, USA). Splenocytes were frozen in 90% FBS/10% DSMO. After thaw, viable splenocytes were counted using Trypan blue exclusion and incubated with a far red proliferation dye (Life Technologies, Carlsbad, CA, USA). After 30 min at 37 °C, the dye was washed out with complete media, and stained splenocytes were plated at various ratios with matched tumor cells (i.e., splenocytes from 393P tumors were plated with 393P tumor cells in co-culture) in media supplemented with 5 μg/mL of anti-CD-3 and anti-CD28 (Thermo). Where indicated, an anti-PD-L1 antibody was added at the time of seeding at a concentration of 20 μg/mL. The percentage of far red positive splenocytes was then measured by flow cytometry using a FACSCanto II machine (BD Biosciences, San Jose, CA, USA).

4.7. Flow Cytometry Analysis for Immune Subpopulations

Tumors were processed for flow cytometry into single cells using mechanical and enzymatic digestion (enzyme mixture—collagenase, DNAse, and hyaluronidase). Red blood cells were lysed as described above and viable tumor cells counted. The following antibodies were used to stain immune cell populations: Ghost violet 510 Live/Dead, Pacific Blue CD45, PE-594 CD3, PE/Cy7 CD8, APC/Cy7 CD4, BV605 PD-1, APC Tim3, FITC CD62L, BV711 CD44 (BioLegend).

Samples were run on an LSR Fortessa machine. Single color compensation controls were performed using compensation beads (Thermo Fisher Scientific, Waltham, MA, USA) to correct for overlap in signal among antibodies. Spleen samples were used to set a gating strategy for CD3+/CD4+ and CD3+/CD8+ T cells. FlowJo software (version 10) was used to perform all downstream analyses on subpopulations.

4.8. Western Blot Analysis

Cells were harvested and lysed in radioimmunoprecipitation assay buffer (RIPA) lysis buffer supplemented with phenylmethylsulfonyl fluoride (PMSF), a protease inhibitor (Cell Signaling), and phosphatase inhibitors (Sigma). Lysates were separated by SDS-PAGE (BioRad, Hercules, CA, USA), transferred to nitrocellulose or polyvinylidene fluoride (PVDF) (BioRad) membranes, and probed with the following primary antibodies: phospho-TrkA(Y674/675), phospho-TrkA(Y785), TrkA, phospho-MEK, MEK, phospho-ERK, ERK, phospho-AKT, AKT, phospho-GSK3b, phospho-Jak1, Jak1, phospho-Stat3, Stat3 (Cell Signaling, Danvers, MA, USA), phospho-TrkC, total TrkC (Thermo Fisher), PD-L1 (Abcam, Cambridge, MA, USA), and actin (ProteinTech, Rosemont, IL, USA).

4.9. RNA Extraction and Real-Time qPCR

RNA was extracted from cells in vitro using a TRIzol reagent (Thermo Fisher). Tumor cell RNA was extracted using the mirVana RNA extraction kit (Life Technologies). Briefly, tumors were collected and snap frozen, then processed in 300 μL of lysis buffer using homogenization. RNA was then extracted as directed by the kit protocol.

All RNA samples were quantified, and reverse transcription was performed with 2 μg of RNA using qSCRIPT cDNA SuperMix (Quantabio, Beverly, MA, USA). Real-time PCR was performed using primer sets specific for each gene (obtained from Origene, Rockland, MD, USA) and the SYBR® Green PCR Master Mix (Life Technologies). L32 (60S ribosomal gene) was used to normalize expression across samples.

4.10. Statistical Analyses

All analyses were performed using GraphPad Prism software (version 7.01). Unpaired Student's *t* tests were used in comparison of two conditions, and one-way ANOVA was used for comparisons of three or more conditions. Tukey's test was used to correct for multiple comparisons. All analyses were 2-tailed and *p*-values < 0.05 were regarded as significant.

5. Conclusions

Functional genomics screening in vivo generates novel scientific questions in the context of a complex ecosystem within a whole animal. The FDAome in vivo dropout screen revealed Ntrk1 as a novel regulatory molecule of both KP tumor cell intrinsic biology and extrinsic immune microenvironment factors. Our data indicate that Ntrk1 regulates KP tumor cell invasion, migration, as well as signaling downstream to survival and growth pathways. Additionally, Ntrk1 augments the immune profile within tumors, pushing them towards a dysfunctional, exhausted state. Together, these data suggest that targeted Trk inhibitors may have utility in combination therapy strategies with immune checkpoint inhibitors to improve lung cancer patient response and survival.

Supplementary Materials:
Figure S1: 344P and 393P response to anti-PD-1 treatment in vivo, Figure S2: Ntrk1 shRNA does not demonstrate significant dropout from 393P tumors treated with anti-PD-1 antibody, Figure S3: Cell lines derived from anti-PD-1 resistant tumors maintain resistance when re-challenged with anti-PD-1 antibody in vivo, Figure S4: Ntrk1 expression correlates with the mesenchymal status of cells, Figure S5: Overexpression of Ntrk3 increases cell migration, invasion, 3D growth, and signaling via MAPK and AKT pathways, Figure S6: Ntrk1 promotes cellular growth through MAPK signaling, Figure S7: T cell proliferative capacity is inhibited as a function of Ntrk1 expression through PD-L1 activity, Figure S8: Treatment with a Jak1/2 inhibitor blocks upregulation of Irf1 and PD-L1 in splenocyte co-culture, Table S1: Positive and negative controls for FDAome dropout screen, Table S2: RSA values and rank scores for the FDAome shRNA dropout screen with a PD-1 blocking antibody.

Author Contributions: Conceptualization, J.M.K. and D.L.G.; Data curation, J.M.K., B.L.R., L.G., D.D., R.M. and M.D.P.; Formal analysis, J.M.K., M.D.P., J.K., A.C., C.B. and T.H.; Funding acquisition, D.L.G.; Methodology, J.M.K., B.L.R. and D.L.G.; Resources, J.K., A.C., T.H. and D.L.G.; Supervision, D.L.G.; Visualization, J.J.F.; Writing—original draft, J.M.K.; Writing—review & editing, J.M.K., B.L.R., J.J.F., L.G., D.D., C.B. and D.L.G.

References

1. National Cancer Institute. SEER Stat Fact Sheets: Lung and Bronchus. Available online: http://seer.cancer.gov/statfacts/html/lungb.html (accessed on 9 June 2016).
2. American Cancer Society. Cancer Facts & Figures 2015. Available online: http://www.cancer.org/research/cancerfactsstatistics/cancerfactsfigures2015/ (accessed on 9 June 2016).
3. Davis, R.J.; Van Waes, C.; Allen, C.T. Overcoming barriers to effective immunotherapy: MDSCs, TAMs, and Tregs as mediators of the immunosuppressive microenvironment in head and neck cancer. *Oral Oncol.* **2016**, *58*, 59–70. [CrossRef] [PubMed]
4. Wu, A.A.; Drake, V.; Huang, H.-S.; Chiu, S.; Zheng, L. Reprogramming the tumor microenvironment: Tumor-induced immunosuppressive factors paralyze T cells. *OncoImmunology* **2015**, *4*, e1016700. [CrossRef] [PubMed]
5. Spranger, S. Mechanisms of tumor escape in the context of the T-cell-inflamed and the non-T-cell-inflamed tumor microenvironment. *Int. Immunol.* **2016**, *28*, 383–391. [CrossRef] [PubMed]
6. Pardoll, D.M. The blockade of immune checkpoints in cancer immunotherapy. *Nat. Rev.* **2012**, *12*, 252–264. [CrossRef] [PubMed]
7. Keir, M.E.; Butte, M.J.; Freeman, G.J.; Sharpe, A.H. PD-1 and Its Ligands in Tolerance and Immunity. *Annu. Rev. Immunol.* **2008**, *26*, 677–704. [CrossRef] [PubMed]

8. Borghaei, H.; Paz-Ares, L.; Horn, L.; Spigel, D.R.; Steins, M.; Ready, N.E.; Chow, L.Q.; Vokes, E.E.; Felip, E.; Holgado, E.; et al. Nivolumab versus Docetaxel in Advanced Nonsquamous Non-Small-Cell Lung Cancer. *N. Engl. J. Med.* **2015**, *373*, 1627–1639. [CrossRef] [PubMed]
9. Brahmer, J.R.; Tykodi, S.S.; Chow, L.Q.; Hwu, W.-J.; Topalian, S.L.; Hwu, P.; Drake, C.G.; Camacho, L.H.; Kauh, J.; Odunsi, K.; et al. Safety and Activity of Anti-PD-L1 Antibody in Patients with Advanced Cancer. *N. Engl. J. Med.* **2012**, *366*, 2455–2465. [CrossRef]
10. Topalian, S.L.; Hodi, F.S.; Brahmer, J.R.; Gettinger, S.N.; Smith, D.C.; McDermott, D.F.; Powderly, J.D.; Carvajal, R.D.; Sosman, J.A.; Atkins, M.B.; et al. Safety, Activity, and Immune Correlates of Anti-PD-1 Antibody in Cancer. *N. Engl. J. Med.* **2012**, *366*, 2443–2454. [CrossRef]
11. Hugo, W.; Zaretsky, J.M.; Sun, L.; Song, C.; Moreno, B.H.; Hu-Lieskovan, S.; Berent-Maoz, B.; Pang, J.; Chmielowski, B.; Cherry, G.; et al. Genomic and Transcriptomic Features of Response to Anti-PD-1 Therapy in Metastatic Melanoma. *Cell* **2016**, *165*, 35–44. [CrossRef]
12. Koyama, S.; Akbay, E.A.; Li, Y.Y.; Herter-Sprie, G.S.; Buczkowski, K.A.; Richards, W.G.; Gandhi, L.; Redig, A.J.; Rodig, S.J.; Asahina, H.; et al. Adaptive resistance to therapeutic PD-1 blockade is associated with upregulation of alternative immune checkpoints. *Nat. Commun.* **2016**, *7*, 10501. [CrossRef]
13. Page, D.B.; Postow, M.A.; Callahan, M.K.; Allison, J.P.; Wolchok, J.D. Immune Modulation in Cancer with Antibodies. *Annu. Rev. Med.* **2014**, *65*, 185–202. [CrossRef] [PubMed]
14. Romero, D. PD-1 says goodbye, TIM-3 says hello. *Nat. Rev. Clin. Oncol.* **2016**, *13*, 203. [CrossRef] [PubMed]
15. Tumeh, P.C.; Harview, C.L.; Yearley, J.H.; Shintaku, I.P.; Taylor, E.J.M.; Robert, L.; Chmielowski, B.; Spasić, M.; Henry, G.; Ciobanu, V.; et al. PD-1 blockade induces responses by inhibiting adaptive immune resistance. *Nature* **2014**, *515*, 568–571. [CrossRef] [PubMed]
16. Eberhard, D.A.; Johnson, B.E.; Amler, L.C.; Goddard, A.D.; Heldens, S.L.; Herbst, R.S.; Ince, W.L.; Jänne, P.A.; Januario, T.; Klein, P.; et al. Mutations in the Epidermal Growth Factor Receptor and in KRAS Are Predictive and Prognostic Indicators in Patients with Non-Small-Cell Lung Cancer Treated With Chemotherapy Alone and in Combination With Erlotinib. *J. Clin. Oncol.* **2005**, *23*, 5900–5909. [CrossRef]
17. Skoulidis, F.; Byers, L.A.; Diao, L.; Papadimitrakopoulou, V.A.; Tong, P.; Izzo, J.; Behrens, C.; Kadara, H.; Parra, E.R.; Canales, J.R.; et al. Co-occurring genomic alterations define major subsets of KRAS—Mutant lung adenocarcinoma with distinct biology, immune profiles, and therapeutic vulnerabilities. *Cancer Discov.* **2015**, *5*, 860–877. [CrossRef]
18. Skoulidis, F.; Goldberg, M.E.; Greenawalt, D.M.; Hellmann, M.D.; Awad, M.M.; Gainor, J.F.; Schrock, A.B.; Hartmaier, R.J.; Trabucco, S.E.; Gay, L.; et al. STK11/LKB1 Mutations and PD-1 Inhibitor Resistance in KRAS-Mutant Lung Adenocarcinoma. *Cancer Discov.* **2018**, *8*, 822–835. [CrossRef] [PubMed]
19. Gibbons, D.L.; Lin, W.; Creighton, C.J.; Rizvi, Z.H.; Gregory, P.A.; Goodall, G.J.; Thilaganathan, N.; Du, L.; Zhang, Y.; Pertsemlidis, A.; et al. Contextual extracellular cues promote tumor cell EMT and metastasis by regulating miR-200 family expression. *Genome Res.* **2009**, *23*, 2140–2151. [CrossRef]
20. Gibbons, D.L.; Lin, W.; Creighton, C.J.; Zheng, S.; Berel, D.; Yang, Y.; Raso, M.G.; Liu, D.D.; Wistuba, I.I.; Lozano, G.; et al. Expression Signatures of Metastatic Capacity in a Genetic Mouse Model of Lung Adenocarcinoma. *PLoS ONE* **2009**, *4*, e5401. [CrossRef]
21. Chen, L.; Gibbons, D.L.; Goswami, S.; Cortez, M.A.; Ahn, Y.-H.; Byers, L.A.; Zhang, X.; Yi, X.; Dwyer, D.; Lin, W.; et al. Metastasis is regulated via microRNA-200/ZEB1 axis control of tumor cell PD-L1 expression and intratumoral immunosuppression. *Nat. Commun.* **2014**, *5*, 5241. [CrossRef]
22. Chen, L.; Diao, L.; Yang, Y.; Yi, X.; Rodriguez, B.L.; Li, Y.; Villalobos, P.A.; Cascone, T.; Liu, X.; Tan, L.; et al. CD38-Mediated Immunosuppression as a Mechanism of Tumor Cell Escape from PD-1/PD-L1 Blockade. *Cancer Discov.* **2018**, *8*, 1156–1175. [CrossRef]
23. Peng, D.H.; Kundu, S.T.; Fradette, J.J.; Diao, L.; Tong, P.; Byers, L.A.; Wang, J.; Canales, J.R.; Villalobos, P.A.; Mino, B.; et al. ZEB1 suppression sensitizes KRAS mutant cancers to MEK inhibition by an IL17RD-dependent mechanism. *Sci. Transl. Med.* **2019**, *11*, eaaq1238. [CrossRef] [PubMed]
24. Ungewiss, C.; Rizvi, Z.H.; Roybal, J.D.; Peng, D.H.; Gold, K.A.; Shin, D.-H.; Creighton, C.J.; Gibbons, D.L. The microRNA-200/Zeb1 axis regulates ECM-dependent β1-integrin/FAK signaling, cancer cell invasion and metastasis through CRKL. *Sci. Rep.* **2016**, *6*, 18652. [CrossRef] [PubMed]
25. Peng, D.H.; Ungewiss, C.; Tong, P.; Byers, L.A.; Wang, J.; Canales, J.R.; Villalobos, P.A.; Uraoka, N.; Mino, B.; Behrens, C.; et al. ZEB1 Induces LOXL2-Mediated Collagen Stabilization and Deposition in the Extracellular Matrix to Drive Lung Cancer Invasion and Metastasis. *Oncogene* **2016**, *36*, 1925–1938. [CrossRef] [PubMed]

26. Carugo, A.; Genovese, G.; Seth, S.; Nezi, L.; Rose, J.L.; Bossi, D.; Cicalese, A.; Shah, P.K.; Viale, A.; Pettazzoni, P.F.; et al. In Vivo Functional Platform Targeting Patient-Derived Xenografts Identifies WDR5-Myc Association as a Critical Determinant of Pancreatic Cancer. *Cell Rep.* **2016**, *16*, 133–147. [CrossRef] [PubMed]
27. Patel, S.J.; Sanjana, N.E.; Kishton, R.J.; Eidizadeh, A.; Vodnala, S.K.; Cam, M.; Gartner, J.J.; Jia, L.; Steinberg, S.M.; Yamamoto, T.N.; et al. Identification of essential genes for cancer immunotherapy. *Nature* **2017**, *548*, 537–542. [CrossRef] [PubMed]
28. Manguso, R.T.; Pope, H.W.; Zimmer, M.D.; Brown, F.D.; Yates, K.B.; Miller, B.C.; Collins, N.B.; Bi, K.; LaFleur, M.W.; Juneja, V.R.; et al. In vivo CRISPR screening identifies Ptpn2 as a cancer immunotherapy target. *Nature* **2017**, *547*, 413–418. [CrossRef] [PubMed]
29. Winslow, M.M.; Dayton, T.L.; Verhaak, R.G.W.; Kim-Kiselak, C.; Snyder, E.L.; Feldser, D.M.; Hubbard, D.D.; DuPage, M.J.; Whittaker, C.A.; Hoersch, S.; et al. Suppression of Lung Adenocarcinoma Progression by Nkx2-1. *Nature* **2011**, *473*, 101–104. [CrossRef] [PubMed]
30. Zaretsky, J.M.; García-Diaz, Á.; Shin, D.S.; Escuin-Ordinas, H.; Hugo, W.; Hu-Lieskovan, S.; Torrejon, D.Y.; Abril-Rodriguez, G.; Sandoval, S.; Barthly, L.; et al. Mutations Associated with Acquired Resistance to PD-1 Blockade in Melanoma. *N. Engl. J. Med.* **2016**, *375*, 819–829. [CrossRef] [PubMed]
31. Ng, Y.P.; Cheung, Z.H.; Ip, N.Y. STAT3 as a Downstream Mediator of Trk Signaling and Functions. *J. Boil. Chem.* **2006**, *281*, 15636–15644. [CrossRef]
32. Amatu, A.; Sartore-Bianchi, A.; Siena, S. NTRK gene fusions as novel targets of cancer therapy across multiple tumour types. *ESMO Open* **2016**, *1*, e000023. [CrossRef]
33. Farago, A.F.; Le, L.P.; Zheng, Z.; Muzikansky, A.; Drilon, A.; Patel, M.; Bauer, T.M.; Liu, S.V.; Ou, S.-H.I.; Jackman, D.; et al. Durable Clinical Response to Entrectinib in NTRK1-Rearranged Non-Small Cell Lung Cancer. *J. Thorac. Oncol.* **2015**, *10*, 1670–1674. [CrossRef] [PubMed]
34. Okimoto, R.A.; Bivona, T.G. Tracking down response and resistance to TRK inhibitors. *Cancer Discov.* **2016**, *6*, 14–16. [CrossRef] [PubMed]
35. Vaishnavi, A.; Capelletti, M.; Le, A.T.; Kako, S.; Butaney, M.; Ercan, D.; Mahale, S.; Davies, K.D.; Aisner, D.L.; Pilling, A.B.; et al. Oncogenic and drug sensitive NTRK1 rearrangements in lung cancer. *Nat. Med.* **2013**, *19*, 1469–1472. [CrossRef] [PubMed]
36. TRK Inhibitor Shows Early Promise. *Cancer Discov.* **2015**, *6*. [CrossRef]
37. Yano, H.; Cong, F.; Birge, R.B.; Goff, S.P.; Chao, M.V. Association of the Abl tyrosine kinase with the Trk nerve growth factor receptor. *J. Neurosci. Res.* **2000**, *59*, 356–364. [CrossRef]

Permissions

All chapters in this book were first published by MDPI; hereby published with permission under the Creative Commons Attribution License or equivalent. Every chapter published in this book has been scrutinized by our experts. Their significance has been extensively debated. The topics covered herein carry significant findings which will fuel the growth of the discipline. They may even be implemented as practical applications or may be referred to as a beginning point for another development.

The contributors of this book come from diverse backgrounds, making this book a truly international effort. This book will bring forth new frontiers with its revolutionizing research information and detailed analysis of the nascent developments around the world.

We would like to thank all the contributing authors for lending their expertise to make the book truly unique. They have played a crucial role in the development of this book. Without their invaluable contributions this book wouldn't have been possible. They have made vital efforts to compile up to date information on the varied aspects of this subject to make this book a valuable addition to the collection of many professionals and students.

This book was conceptualized with the vision of imparting up-to-date information and advanced data in this field. To ensure the same, a matchless editorial board was set up. Every individual on the board went through rigorous rounds of assessment to prove their worth. After which they invested a large part of their time researching and compiling the most relevant data for our readers.

The editorial board has been involved in producing this book since its inception. They have spent rigorous hours researching and exploring the diverse topics which have resulted in the successful publishing of this book. They have passed on their knowledge of decades through this book. To expedite this challenging task, the publisher supported the team at every step. A small team of assistant editors was also appointed to further simplify the editing procedure and attain best results for the readers.

Apart from the editorial board, the designing team has also invested a significant amount of their time in understanding the subject and creating the most relevant covers. They scrutinized every image to scout for the most suitable representation of the subject and create an appropriate cover for the book.

The publishing team has been an ardent support to the editorial, designing and production team. Their endless efforts to recruit the best for this project, has resulted in the accomplishment of this book. They are a veteran in the field of academics and their pool of knowledge is as vast as their experience in printing. Their expertise and guidance has proved useful at every step. Their uncompromising quality standards have made this book an exceptional effort. Their encouragement from time to time has been an inspiration for everyone.

The publisher and the editorial board hope that this book will prove to be a valuable piece of knowledge for researchers, students, practitioners and scholars across the globe.

List of Contributors

Rabia Boulahssass and Olivier Guerin
Geriatric Coordination Unit for Geriatric Oncology (UCOG) PACA Est CHU de Nice, 06000 Nice, France
FHU OncoAge, 06000 Nice, France
University Côte d'Azur, 06000 Nice, France

Sebastien Gonfrier and Noémie Champigny
Geriatric Coordination Unit for Geriatric Oncology (UCOG) PACA Est CHU de Nice, 06000 Nice, France

Véronique Hofman
Laboratory of Clinical and Experimental Pathology, CHU Nice, FHU OncoAge, University Côte d'Azur, 06100 Nice, France
Team 4, IRCAN, FHU OncoAge, University Côte d'Azur, CNRS, INSERM, 06107 Nice CEDEX 02, France
Hospital-Integrated Biobank (BB-0033-00025), CHU Nice, FHU OncoAge, University Côte d'Azur, 06100 Nice, France

Elodie Long-Mira and Sandra Lassalle
Laboratory of Clinical and Experimental Pathology, Hospital-Integrated Biobank (BB-0033-00025), Nice Hospital University, FHU OncoAge, Université Côte d'Azur, Nice 06000, France
Team 4, Institute for Research on Cancer and Aging, Nice (IRCAN), INSERM U1081/UMR CNRS 7284, FHU OncoAge, Université Côte d'Azur, Nice 06107, France

Paul Hofman and Marius Ilié
Inserm U1081, CNRS UMR7284, Institut de Recherche sur le Cancer et le Vieillissement (IRCAN), FHU OncoAge, Université Côte d'Azur, 06107 Nice, France
Laboratory of Clinical and Experimental Pathology, CHU Nice, FHU OncoAge, University Côte d'Azur, 06100 Nice, France
Hospital-Integrated Biobank (BB-0033-00025), CHU Nice, FHU OncoAge, University Côte d'Azur, 06100 Nice, France
Laboratory of Clinical and Experimental Pathology, Hospital-Integrated Biobank (BB-0033-00025), Nice Hospital University, FHU OncoAge, Université Côte d'Azur, Nice 06000, France
Team 4, Institute for Research on Cancer and Aging, Nice (IRCAN), INSERM U1081/UMR CNRS 7284, FHU OncoAge, Université Côte d'Azur, Nice 06107, France

Eric François
Department of Medical Oncology, Lacassagne Center, 06000 Nice, France

Emma Guilbaud and Laurent Yvan-Charvet
Institut National de la Santé et de la Recherche Médicale (Inserm) U1065, Université Côte d'Azur, Centre Méditerranéen de Médecine Moléculaire (C3M), Atip-Avenir, Fédération Hospitalo-Universitaire (FHU) Oncoage, 06204 Nice, France

Emmanuel L. Gautier
Institut National de la Santé et de la Recherche Médicale (Inserm) UMR_S 1166, Sorbonnes Universités, Hôpital de la Pitié Salpêtrière, 75013 Paris, France

Jonathan Benzaquen and Charles Marquette
Department of Pulmonary Medicine and Oncology, Université Côte d'Azur, CHU de Nice, FHU OncoAge, 06100 Nice, France
Institute of Research on Cancer and Ageing (IRCAN), Université Côte d'Azur, FHU OncoAge, CNRS, INSERM, 06107 Nice, France

Jacques Boutros
Department of Pulmonary Medicine and Oncology, Université Côte d'Azur, CHU de Nice, FHU OncoAge, 06100 Nice, France

Hervé Delingette
Asclepios Project Team, Sophia Antipolis-Mediterranee Research Centre, Université Côte d'Azur, FHU OncoAge, Inria, 06902 Sophia Antipolis, France

Barbara Pardini
Department of Experimental Therapeutics, The University of Texas MD Anderson Cancer Center, Houston, 1515 Holcombe Boulevard, Unit 422, Houston, TX 77030, USA
Department of Medical Sciences, University of Turin, Turin 10126, Italy
Italian Institute for Genomic Medicine (IIGM), Turin 10126, Italy

George A. Calin
Department of Experimental Therapeutics, The University of Texas MD Anderson Cancer Center, Houston, 1515 Holcombe Boulevard, Unit 422, Houston, TX 77030, USA
Center for RNA Interference and Non-Coding RNAs, The University of Texas MD Anderson Cancer Center, Houston, TX 77030, USA
Department of Leukemia, The University of Texas MD Anderson Cancer Center, Houston, TX 77030, USA

Elisabeth Smolle
Division of Pulmonology, Department of Internal Medicine, Medical University Graz, 8036 Graz, Austria

Martin Pichler
Department of Experimental Therapeutics, Division of Medicine, The UT MD Anderson Cancer Center, Houston, TX 77030, USA

Rama Soundararajan, Ignacio I. Wistuba, Fei Yang and Sendurai A. Mani
Department of Translational Molecular Pathology, The University of Texas MD Anderson Cancer Center, Houston, TX 77030, USA

Lauren A. Byers and Emily B. Roarty
Department of Thoracic/Head-Neck Medical Oncology, The University of Texas MD Anderson Cancer Center, Houston, TX 77030, USA

Stacy Moulder, Debasish Tripathy and Bora Lim
Department of Breast Medical Oncology, The University of Texas MD Anderson Cancer Center, Houston, TX 77030, USA

Xiang Zhang and Jeffrey M. Rosen
Department of Molecular and Cellular Biology, Baylor College of Medicine, Houston, TX 77030, USA

Navin Varadarajan
Department of Chemical and Biomolecular Engineering, University of Houston, Houston, TX 77204, USA

Chantale Bernatchez
Departments of Melanoma Medical Oncology–Research and Translational Molecular Pathology, The University of Texas MD Anderson Cancer Center, Houston, TX 77030, USA

Jeffrey T. Chang
Department of Integrative Biology and Pharmacology, The University of Texas Health Sciences Center, Houston, TX 77030, USA

Alejandro Contreras
Department of Pathology (Anatomical), The University of Texas MD Anderson Cancer Center, Houston, TX 77030, USA

Jing Wang
Department of Bioinformatics and Computational Biology, The University of Texas MD Anderson Cancer Center, Houston, TX 77030, USA

Michelle Barton
Department of Epigenetics and Molecular Carcinogenesis, The University of Texas MD Anderson Cancer Center, Houston, TX 77030, USA

Simon Heeke
Laboratory of Clinical and Experimental Pathology, CHU Nice, FHU OncoAge, University Côte d'Azur, 06100 Nice, France
Team 4, IRCAN, FHU OncoAge, University Côte d'Azur, CNRS, INSERM, 06107 Nice CEDEX 02, France

Charles-Hugo Marquette
Team 4, IRCAN, FHU OncoAge, University Côte d'Azur, CNRS, INSERM, 06107 Nice CEDEX 02, France
Department of Pneumology and Oncology, CHU Nice, FHU OncoAge, University Côte d'Azur, 06100 Nice, France

Yutong Sun
Department of Molecular and Cellular Oncology, the University of Texas MD Anderson Cancer Center, Houston, TX 77030, USA

Li Ma
Department of Experimental Radiation Oncology, the University of Texas MD Anderson Cancer Center, Houston, TX 77030, USA

Robert J. Cardnell and Lauren Averett Byers
Department of Thoracic/Head and Neck Medical Oncology, The University of Texas MD Anderson Cancer Center, Houston, TX 77030, USA

Anna Maria Rachiglio, Francesca Fenizia, Matilde Lambiase, Cristin Roma, Antonella De Luca and Nicola Normanno
Cell Biology and Biotherapy Unit, Istituto Nazionale Tumori-IRCCS-Fondazione G. Pascale, 80131 Naples, Italy

Maria Carmela Piccirillo and Francesco Perrone
Clinical Trials Unit, Istituto Nazionale Tumori-IRCCS-Fondazione G. Pascale, 80131 Naples, Italy

Domenico Galetta and Elisabetta Sara Montagna
Medical Oncology, National Cancer Research Center "Giovanni Paolo II", 70126 Bari, Italy

Lucio Crinò
Istituto Scientifico per lo Studio e la Cura dei Tumori (IRST), 47014 Meldola (FC), Italy

Bruno Vincenzi
Medical Oncology, Campus Bio-Medico University of Rome, 00128 Rome, Italy

Emiddio Barletta
Medical Oncology, "G. Rummo" Hospital, 82100 Benevento, Italy

Carmine Pinto
Medical Oncology, AUSL-IRCCS di Reggio Emilia, 42123 Reggio Emilia, Italy

Francesco Ferraù
Medical Oncology, "S. Vincenzo" Hospital, 98039 Taormina (ME), Italy

Agnese Montanino and Alessandro Morabito
Medical Oncology, Thoraco-Pulmonary Department, Istituto Nazionale Tumori-IRCCS-Fondazione G. Pascale, 80131 Naples, Italy

Vienna Ludovini
Department of Medical Oncology, Santa Maria della Misericordia Hospital, 06129 Perugia, Italy

Gaetano Rocco
Thoracic Surgery, Thoraco-Pulmonary Department, Istituto Nazionale Tumori-IRCCS-Fondazione G. Pascale, 80131 Naples, Italy

Gerardo Botti
Surgical Pathology Unit, Istituto Nazionale Tumori-IRCCS-Fondazione G. Pascale, 80131 Naples, Italy

Cécile Badoual and Hélène Roussel
Department of Pathology, Hôpital Européen Georges Pompidou, APHP, Paris 75015, France
INSERM U970, Université Paris Descartes Sorbonne Paris-Cité, Paris 75015, France

Fiona Henderson
Department EMEA, Indica Labs, 2469 Corrales Rd Bldg. A-3 Corrales, NM 87048, USA

Léa Berland and Marame Hamila
Laboratory of Clinical and Experimental Pathology, Hospital-Integrated Biobank (BB-0033-00025), Nice Hospital University, FHU OncoAge, Université Côte d'Azur, Nice 06000, France

Eric Tartour
INSERM U970, Université Paris Descartes Sorbonne Paris-Cité, Paris 75015, France
Department of Immunology, Hôpital Européen Georges Pompidou, Paris 75015, France

Edwin Roger Parra, Alejandro Francisco-Cruz and Ignacio Ivan Wistuba
Department of Translational Molecular Pathology, The University of Texas MD Anderson Cancer Center, 2130 West Holcombe Blvd, Houston, TX 77030, USA

Hsiao-Ling Chen and Hsiu-Mei Chang
Department of Pharmacy, Kaohsiung Municipal Ta-Tung Hospital, Kaohsiung 80145, Taiwan

Yu-Kang Tu
Institute of Epidemiology and Preventive Medicine, National Taiwan University, Taipei 100225, Taiwan
Department of Medical Research, National Taiwan University Hospital, Taipei 100225, Taiwan

Tai-Huang Lee
Department of Internal Medicine Kaohsiung Municipal Ta-Tung Hospital, Kaohsiung Medical University, Kaohsiung 88145, Taiwan

Kuan-Li Wu, Yu-Chen Tsai and Mei-Hsuan Lee
Division of Pulmonary and Critical Care Medicine, Department of Internal Medicine, Kaohsiung Medical University Hospital, Kaohsiung Medical University, Kaohsiung 88708, Taiwan

Chih-Jen Yang
Division of Pulmonary and Critical Care Medicine, Department of Internal Medicine, Kaohsiung Medical University Hospital, Kaohsiung Medical University, Kaohsiung 88708, Taiwan
Department of General Medicine, Kaohsiung Medical University Hospital, Kaohsiung Medical University, Kaohsiung 88708, Taiwan
Faculty of Medicine, College of Medicine, Kaohsiung Medical University, Kaohsiung 88708, Taiwan
Respiratory Therapy, College of Medicine, Kaohsiung Medical University, Kaohsiung 88708, Taiwan

Jen-Yu Hung
Department of Internal Medicine Kaohsiung Municipal Ta-Tung Hospital, Kaohsiung Medical University, Kaohsiung 88145, Taiwan
Division of Pulmonary and Critical Care Medicine, Department of Internal Medicine, Kaohsiung Medical University Hospital, Kaohsiung Medical University, Kaohsiung 88708, Taiwan
Faculty of Medicine, College of Medicine, Kaohsiung Medical University, Kaohsiung 88708, Taiwan

Inn-Wen Chong
Department of General Medicine, Kaohsiung Medical University Hospital, Kaohsiung Medical University, Kaohsiung 88708, Taiwan
Faculty of Medicine, College of Medicine, Kaohsiung Medical University, Kaohsiung 88708, Taiwan
Respiratory Therapy, College of Medicine, Kaohsiung Medical University, Kaohsiung 88708, Taiwan
Department of Biological Science & Technology, National Chiao Tung University, Hsinchu 300, Taiwan

Nicholas Ayache
Epione Team, Inria, FHU OncoAge, Université Côte d'Azur, 06902 Sophia Antipolis, France

Pascal Barbry, Philippe Blancou, Frédéric Checler, Nicolas Glaichenhaus and Bernard Mari
CNRS UMR7275, Institut de Pharmacologie Cellulaire et Moléculaire, FHU OncoAge, Université Côte d'Azur, 06560 Valbonne, France

Michel Barlaud
i3S Sophia Antipolis, FHU OncoAge, Université Côte d'Azur, 06560 Sophia Antipolis, France

Audrey Bel and Taycir Skhiri
Centre d'Innovation et d'Usages en Santé (CIUS), FHU OncoAge, Université Côte d'Azur, 06000 Nice, France

Sylvie Chevillard
Laboratoire de Cancérologie Expérimentale, Institut François Jacob, CEA Direction de la Recherche Fondamentale, FHU OncoAge, Université Côte d'Azur, 92265 Fontenay-aux-Roses, France

Gael Cristofari, Eric Gilson and Véronique Paquis-Flucklinger
Inserm U1081, CNRS UMR7284, Institut de Recherche sur le Cancer et le Vieillissement (IRCAN), FHU OncoAge, Université Côte d'Azur, 06107 Nice, France

Mathilde Demory
Ville de Nice, Mairie de Nice, FHU OncoAge, Université Côte d'Azur, 06364 Nice, France

Vincent Esnault
Nephrology Department, CHU Nice, FHU OncoAge, Université Côte d'Azur, 06001 Nice, France

Claire Falandry
Geriatric Unit, Centre Hospitalier Lyon Sud, Hospices Civils de Lyon, FHU OncoAge, Université Claude Bernard Lyon 1, 69310 Pierre-Benite, France
Laboratoire CarMeN, Inserm U1060, INRA U139, INSA Lyon, Ecole de Médecine Charles Mérieux, Université Claude Bernard Lyon 1, 69921 Oullins, France

Olivier Guérin and Frédéric Prate
Geriatric Coordination Unit for Geriatric Oncology (UCOG) PACA Est, CHU Nice, FHU OncoAge, Université Côte d'Azur, 06000 Nice, France

Joel Guigay
Oncology Department, Centre Antoine Lacassagne, FHU OncoAge, Université Côté d'Azur, 06189 Nice, France

Charles-Hugo Marquette
Department of Pulmonary Medicine and Oncology, CHU Nice, FHU OncoAge, Université Côte d'Azur, 06000 Nice, France

Pierre Saintigny
Département de Médecine, INSERM 1052, CNRS 5286, Centre de recherche en cancérologie de Lyon, Centre Léon Bérard, FHU OncoAge, Université Claude Bernard Lyon 1, 69008 Lyon, France

Barbara Seitz-Polsky
CNRS UMR7275, Institut de Pharmacologie Cellulaire et Moléculaire, FHU OncoAge, Université Côte d'Azur, 06560 Valbonne, France
Laboratory of Immunology, CHU Nice, FHU OncoAge, Université Côte d'Azur, 06200 Nice, France

Ellen Van Obberghen-Schilling
CNRS, Inserm, iBV, Centre Antoine Lacassagne, FHU OncoAge, Université Côte d'Azur, 06108 Nice, France

Emmanuel Van Obberghen
CNRS, LP2M, FHU OncoAge, Université Côte d'Azur, 06107 Nice, France

Jessica M. Konen, B. Leticia Rodriguez, Jared J. Fradette and Laura Gibson
Department of Thoracic/Head & Neck Medical Oncology, University of Texas MD Anderson Cancer Center, 1515 Holcombe Blvd, Houston, TX 77030, USA

Denali Davis
Department of Chemistry, Indiana University of Pennsylvania, 1011 South Drive, Indiana, PA 15705, USA

Rosalba Minelli
Department of Genomic Medicine, University of Texas MD Anderson Cancer Center, 1515 Holcombe Blvd, Houston, TX 77030, USA

Michael D. Peoples, Jeffrey Kovacs and Christopher Bristow
Center for Co-Clinical Trials, University of Texas MD Anderson Cancer Center, 1515 Holcombe Blvd, Houston, TX 77030, USA

Alessandro Carugo and Timothy Heffernan
Institute for Applied Cancer Science, University of Texas MD Anderson Cancer Center, 1515 Holcombe Blvd, Houston, TX 77030, USA

Don L. Gibbons
Department of Thoracic/Head & Neck Medical Oncology, University of Texas MD Anderson Cancer Center, 1515 Holcombe Blvd, Houston, TX 77030, USA
Department of Molecular and Cellular Oncology, University of Texas MD Anderson Cancer Center, 1515 Holcombe Blvd, Houston, TX 77030, USA

Index

www.ingramcontent.com/pod-product-compliance
Lightning Source LLC
LaVergne TN
LVHW081028210926
848485LV00004B/977